ULTRASOUND
SECRETS

ULTRASOUND SECRETS

Vikram Dogra, MD
Associate Professor of Radiology
Case Western Reserve University School of Medicine
Director, Division of Ultrasound
Associate Program Director, Radiology Residency
Director, Cross-sectional Imaging Fellowship Program
University Hospitals of Cleveland
Cleveland, Ohio

Deborah J. Rubens, MD
Professor of Radiology and Surgery
Associate Chair of Special Imaging
Associate Director, Center for Biomedical Ultrasound
Department of Radiology
University of Rochester Medical Center
Rochester, New York

HANLEY & BELFUS
An Affiliate of Elsevier

HANLEY & BELFUS
An Affiliate of Elsevier

The Curtis Center
Independence Square West
Philadelphia, Pennsylvania 19106

Note to the reader: Although the techniques, ideas, and information in this book have been carefully reviewed for correctness, neither the authors nor the publisher can accept any legal responsibility for any errors or omissions that may be made. Neither the authors nor the publisher makes any guarantee, expressed or implied, with respect to the material contained herein.

Library of Congress Control Number: 2003113800

ULTRASOUND SECRETS   ISBN 1-56053-594-6

Printed in the United States of America

Last digit is the print number: 9 8 7 6 5 4 3 2 1

CONTENTS

CONTENTS

CONTRIBUTORS

Osbert Adjei, M.D.
Instructor, Department of Radiology, University of Rochester Medical Center, Rochester, New York

Marat Bakman, M.D.
Department of Radiology, University of Rochester Medical Center, Rochester, New York

Christopher Bang, D.O.
Department of Radiology, University of Rochester Medical Center; Strong Memorial Hospital, Rochester, New York

Sheila C. Berlin, M.D.
Assistant Professor, Division of Pediatric Radiology, Department of Radiology, Case Western Reserve University School of Medicine; University Hospitals of Cleveland, Cleveland, Ohio

Shweta Bhatt, DMRD, DMRE
Research Fellow, Department of Radiology, Case Western Reserve University School of Medicine; University Hospitals of Cleveland, Cleveland, Ohio

Shannon C. Campbell, M.D.
Department of Radiology, University of Rochester Medical Center, Strong Memorial Hospital, Rochester, New York

Nancy L. Carson, M.B.A., RDMS, R.V.T.
Supervisor of Radiology Ultrasound, Department of Radiology, University of Rochester Medical Center, Rochester, New York

Vernon D. Cook, M.D.
Associate Professor, Department of Obstetrics and Gynecology, University of Louisville School of Medicine, Louisville, Kentucky

Jodie C. Crowley, B.S., RDMS
Clinical Instructor (Adjunct Faculty), Diagnostic Medical Sonography, Department of Medical Sciences, Rochester Institute of Technology; Strong Memorial Hospital, University of Rochester Medical Center, Rochester, New York

Jeanne A. Cullinan, M.D.
Associate Professor, Department of Radiology, University of Rochester Medical Center; Strong Memorial Hospital, Rochester, New York

Cheri X. Deng, Ph.D.
Assistant Professor, Department of Biomedical Engineering, Case Western Reserve University, Cleveland, Ohio

Vikram Dogra, M.D.
Associate Professor, Department of Radiology, Case Western Reserve University School of Medicine; Director, Division of Ultrasound; Associate Program Director, Radiology Residency; Director, Cross-sectional Imaging Fellowship Program, University Hospitals of Cleveland, Cleveland, Ohio

David A. Dombroski, M.D.
Assistant Professor, Department of Radiology, University of Rochester Medical Center; Strong Memorial Hospital, Rochester, New York

Patrick J. Fultz, M.D.
Associate Professor, Department of Radiology, University of Rochester Medical Center, Rochester, New York

Hamad Ghazle, M.S., RDMS
Director and Associate Professor, Department of Medical Sciences, Diagnostic Medical Sonography Program, Rochester Institute of Technology; University of Rochester Medical Center; Strong Memorial Hospital, Rochester, New York

Mark A. Hall, B.S., RDMS
Assistant Lead Sonographer, Division of Ultrasound, Department of Radiology, University of Rochester Medical Center, Rochester, New York

Amy R. Harrow, M.D.
Department of Radiology, University of Rochester Medical Center, Rochester, New York

Nancy E. Judge, M.D.
Associate Professor, Department of Reproductive Biology, Case Western Reserve University School of Medicine; Maternal-Fetal Medicine Specialist, MacDonald Women's Hospital, Cleveland, Ohio

William T. Kuo, M.D.
Department of Radiology, University of Rochester Medical Center, Rochester, New York

Noam Lazebnik, M.D.
Associate Professor of Obstetrics and Gynecology and Genetics, Department of Obstetrics and Gynecology, Case Western Reserve University School of Medicine; Staff Physician, University Hospitals of Cleveland, Cleveland, Ohio

Roee S. Lazebnik, Ph.D.
Department of Biomedical Engineering, Case Western Reserve University School of Medicine, Cleveland, Ohio

Ryan K. Lee, M.D.
Department of Radiology, University of Rochester Medical Center, Rochester, New York

Tara Maria McElroy, M.D.
Department of Obstetrics and Gynecology, Case Western Reserve University School of Medicine; MacDonald Women's Hospital, Cleveland, Ohio

Melissa T. Myers, M.D.
Assistant Professor, Division of Pediatric Radiology, Department of Radiology, Case Western Reserve University School of Medicine; Rainbow Babies and Children's Hospital, Cleveland, Ohio

Dean A. Nakamoto, M.D.
Assistant Professor, Department of Radiology, Case Western Reserve University School of Medicine; Section Head, Abdominal Imaging, University Hospitals of Cleveland, Cleveland, Ohio

Mayumi Oka, M.D.
Neuroradiology Division, Department of Radiology and Radiological Science, Johns Hopkins Hospital, Baltimore, Maryland

Raj Mohan Paspulati, M.D.
Assistant Professor, Department of Radiology, Case Western Reserve University School of Medicine; University Hospitals of Cleveland, Cleveland, Ohio

Deborah J. Rubens, M.D.
Professor of Radiology and Surgery; Associate Chair of Special Imaging; Associate Director, Center for Biomedical Ultrasound, Department of Radiology, University of Rochester Medical Center, Rochester, New York

David M. Schmanke, RDMS, R.T.
Division of Ultrasound, Department of Radiology, University of North Carolina Hospital at Chapel Hill, Chapel Hill, North Carolina

Dinesh M. Shah, M.D.
Professor, Department of Obstetrics, Gynecology, and Women's Health, University of Louisville School of Medicine; University of Louisville Hospital, Louisville, Kentucky

John Strang, M.D.
Associate Professor, Department of Radiology, University of Rochester Medical Center; Strong Memorial Hospital, Rochester, New York

Labib Syed, M.D.
Department of Radiology, University of Rochester Medical Center, Rochester, New York

Stephen W. Tamarkin, M.D.
Assistant Professor, Department of Radiology, Case Western Reserve University School of Medicine; Chief of Body Imaging, MetroHealth Medical Center, Cleveland, Ohio

Pauravi Shah Vasavada, M.D.
Assistant Professor, Department of Radiology, Case Western Reserve University School of Medicine; Rainbow Babies and Children's Hospital, Cleveland, Ohio

Susan L. Voci, M.D.
Assistant Professor and Director of Ultrasound, Department of Radiology, University of Rochester Medical Center, Rochester, New York

Pranav Krishnakant Vyas, M.D.
Assistant Professor, Department of Radiology, Case Western Reserve University School of Medicine; Rainbow Babies and Children's Hospital, University Hospitals of Cleveland, Cleveland, Ohio

Andrea Zynda-Weiss, M.D.
Department of Radiology, University of Rochester Medical Center; Strong Memorial Hospital, Rochester, New York

FOREWORD

The rapid advances to and refinement of modern imaging systems have provided a wide array of diagnostic tools to the practicing radiologist. Ultrasound has enjoyed considerable enhancements as a result of improved materials, electronics, and computer processing, similar to CT and MRI. Over the years, computer algorithms and technical refinements in materials have pushed the resolution and quality of these systems to levels never imagined.

State-of-the-art ultrasound remains one of the essential imaging tools in today's highly competitive and demanding health care landscape. In some areas, such as flow and multidimensional real-time imaging, ultrasound is superior to all other modalities. In other situations, it is truly complementary, providing unique information that CT and MRI do not.

Although numerous ultrasound books are on the market, this one is quite special. The authors contributing to this book are exceptional in their academic knowledge and professional experiences. The authors provide essential information about ultrasound, including information on diagnosis, theory, and practical insights into germane technical details. The question-and-answer format is an effective approach. By raising awareness of the problem at the onset, the information provided in the answer is better assimilated.

Because I know many of the authors personally, I am confident of the success of this work and its value to its readers. I am very proud of all the contributors to this fine book.

John R. Haaga, M.D.
Chairman and Professor
Department of Radiology
Case Western Reserve University
  School of Medicine
University Hospitals of Cleveland
Cleveland, Ohio

PREFACE

This book is inspired by our medical students, residents, fellows, and sonographers. Their questions and desire for knowledge motivate and inspire us all to keep learning. In organizing this book, we have included detailed, disease-oriented questions as well as practical how-to issues that are not often found in books or journals but are nonetheless encountered daily in the practice of sonography. Our intention is that the topics presented will improve the reader's understanding of ultrasound and the ever-increasing role it plays in patient care. We welcome readers' comments and questions as we explore the future secrets that ultrasound holds for us.

We would like to thank Marianne Chaloupek, Adrienne Jones, and Holly Stiner for their secretarial assistance in the preparation of the manuscript. We would also like to thank Joseph Molter and Margaret Kowaluk for their assistance in preparing the images for the book. In addition, our sincere thanks go to Cecelia Bayruns at Elsevier for her assistance in coordinating the production of the book.

Vikram Dogra, M.D.
Deborah J. Rubens, M.D.

COLOR PLATES

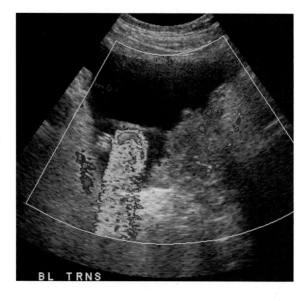

FIGURE 1. Twinkle artifact (*see also* Chapter 3, Figure 1B, page 14).

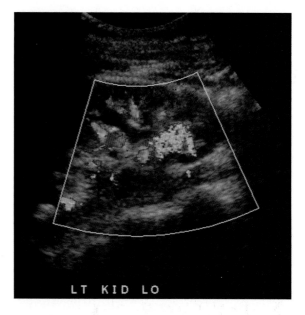

FIGURE 2. Twinkle artifact identifying renal calculi (*see also* Chapter 3, Figure 2B, page 15).

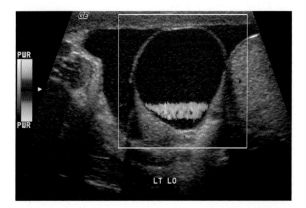

FIGURE 3. Pseudoflow (*see also* Chapter 3, Figure 4A, page 16).

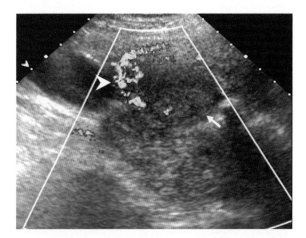

FIGURE 4. Ovarian torsion (*see also* Chapter 13, Figure 1B, page 106).

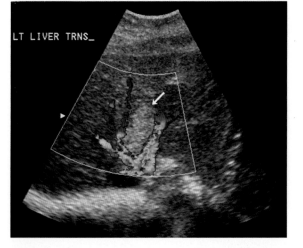

FIGURE 5. Liver hemangioma (*see also* Chapter 16, Figure 7B, page 143).

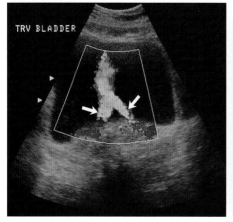

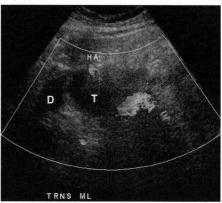

FIGURE 6. Bladder jets (*see also* Chapter 18, Figure 6, page 172).

FIGURE 7. Pancreatic tumor (*see also* Chapter 20, Figure 8B, page 189).

FIGURE 8. Pancreatic tumor (*see also* Chapter 20, Figure 8D, page 190).

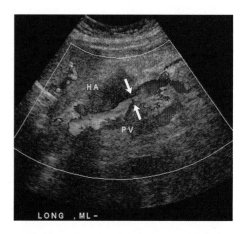

FIGURE 9. Portal vein thrombosis (*see also* Chapter 25, Figure 4, page 227).

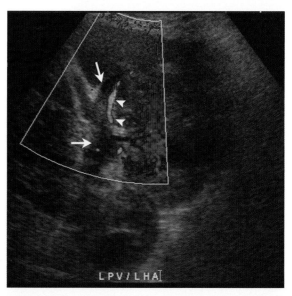

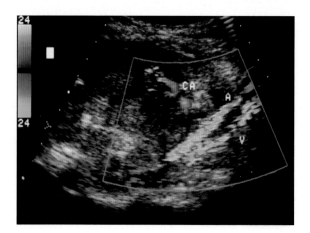

FIGURE 10. Pancreas transplant with venous thrombosis (*see also* Chapter 26, Figure 16A, page 249).

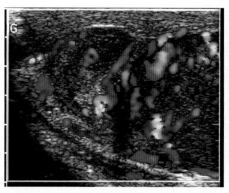

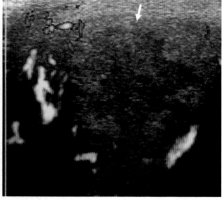

FIGURE 11. Epididymo-orchitis (*see also* Chapter 27, Figure 2, page 252).

FIGURE 12. Testicular torsion (*see also* Chapter 27, Figure 3, page 254).

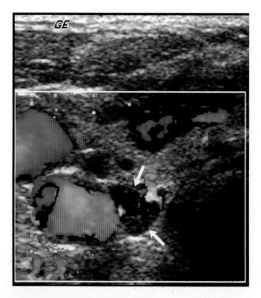

FIGURE 13. Parathyroid adenoma (*see also* Chapter 28, Figure 7B, page 267).

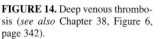

FIGURE 14. Deep venous thrombosis (*see also* Chapter 38, Figure 6, page 342).

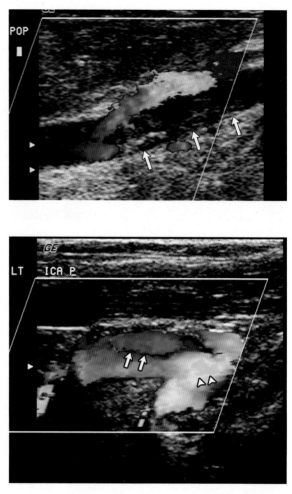

FIGURE 15. Flow reversal (*see also* Chapter 39, Figure 6, page 356).

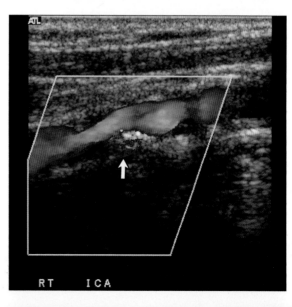

FIGURE 16. Carotid plaque (*see also* Chapter 39, Figure 9C, page 362).

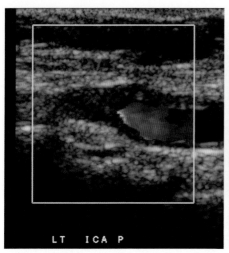

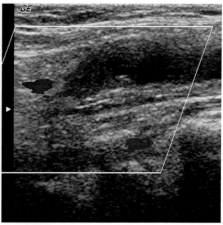

FIGURE 17. Internal carotid artery occlusion (*see also* Chapter 39, Figure 11A, page 363).

FIGURE 18. String sign (*see also* Chapter 39, Figure 12A, page 364).

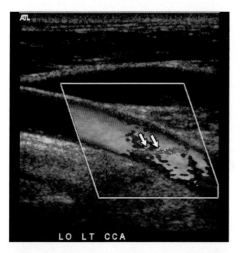

FIGURE 19. Carotid dissection (*see also* Chapter 39, Figure 13B, page 366).

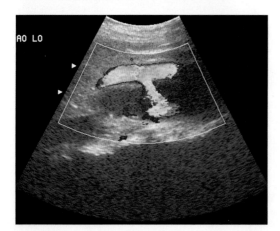

FIGURE 20. Aortic dissection (*see also* Chapter 40, Figure 3B, page 374).

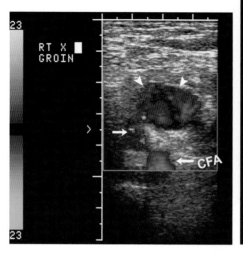

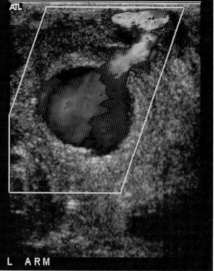

FIGURE 21. Pseudoaneurysm (*see also* Chapter 42, Figure 1A, page 379).

FIGURE 22. Pseudoaneurysm (*see also* Chapter 42, Figure 2A, page 380).

FIGURE 23. Arteriovenous fistula in renal transplant. High-velocity venous flow (blue) appears when all other vessels are arterial (red) and directed into the kidney (*see also* Chapter 42, Figure 3A, page 383).

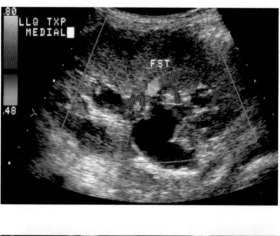

FIGURE 24. Arteriovenous fistula (*see also* Chapter 42, Figure 3C, page 384).

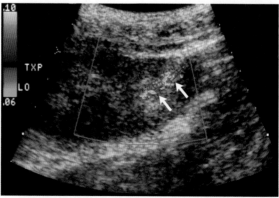

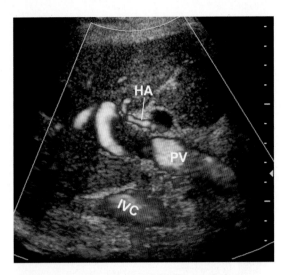

FIGURE 25. Portal vein clot (*see also* Chapter 46, Figure 6, page 408).

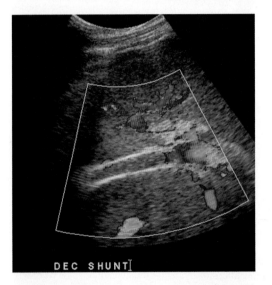

FIGURE 26. Occluded transjugular intrahepatic portosystemic shunt (*see also* Chapter 46, Figure 14, page 414).

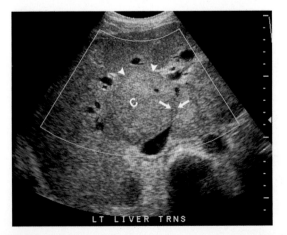

FIGURE 27. Budd-Chiari syndrome (*see also* Chapter 46, Figure 18A, page 418).

I. Ultrasound Physics

1. BASIC ULTRASOUND TECHNOLOGY

John Strang, M.D.

1. What is an ultrasound wave?

An ultrasound wave is a sound wave over specific frequencies. A sound wave is a compression/rarefaction wave; molecules are compressed or spread apart in the direction that the wave travels. The range of human audible sound is 20–20,000 Hz. The range of grayscale ultrasound is 2–15 MHz; Doppler frequencies are slightly lower.

2. What are the units of frequency, wavelength, and speed of sound?

- Frequency (F) = cycles/sec (Hertz)
- Megahertz (MHz) = millions of cycles/second
- Wavelength (λ) = distance per complete wave
- Speed of sound = distance/time. Speed of sound is different for different materials in the body. For biologic soft tissues, the speed of sound varies between 1480 and 1580 m/sec. Speed is much faster in bone: 4080 m/sec; in air much slower: 330 m/sec.

3. What is the relationship between frequency and wavelength?

Frequency $\times$ wavelength = speed of sound. For a given speed of sound, they are reciprocal. Increasing the frequency decreases the wavelength, and vice versa.

4. What is the relationship of frequency to sound absorption?

Higher frequencies are absorbed more rapidly than lower frequencies. Low frequencies have better penetration.

5. What is the relationship of frequency to spatial resolution?

Higher frequencies have shorter wavelengths. Shorter wavelengths can distinguish between reflectors that are closer together. Therefore, higher frequencies have better spatial resolution but limited penetration.

6. How can deeper tissues be seen better?

Good contact is important. The operator should use a low enough frequency to penetrate the area of interest and consider using harmonic imaging to reduce superficial noise.

7. How can more superficial tissues be seen better?

Again, good contact between the skin, gel, and probe is needed. Penetration is not an issue, so the operator can use a higher frequency and get the benefit of better spatial resolution. A stand-off pad may be used when the object is too superficial for the focal zone of the transducer.

8. What does tissue do to ultrasound waves?

Tissue absorbs (turns to heat), refracts (bends, like a lens bends a light wave), scatters, and reflects sound. Reflection can be diffuse (like a projection screen) or specular (like a mirror).

9. Why can't ultrasound go through air?

Sound does, of course, but ultrasound is poorly transmitted between water and air. This is called *impedance mismatching*. Almost all the sound is reflected at an air–water interface. This works in both directions. For example, the sound of a propeller that churns up water is very loud to listeners in a submarine but is muffled to a listener on the boat.

10. Why can't ultrasound go through bone?

It does, but again, there is an impedance mismatch between the bone and the soft tissue, causing most of the sound to be reflected at the interface.

11. What is a specular reflector?

A specular reflector is like a mirror: the sound wave is reflected at whatever angle it strikes the reflector. The echo is very bright if the sound wave strikes perpendicular to the reflector.

12. What is a diffuse reflector?

A diffuse reflector is like a motion picture screen; that is, the sound is reflected in all directions (so it does not matter where one sits). The angle of incidence is of lesser importance. Most tissues in the body are diffuse reflectors.

13. What is absorption?

Absorption is the amount of energy of an ultrasound wave that is lost per amount of tissue it passes through. This is a proportional process (like compound interest or exponential decay); a percent is lost through a given depth. The rate of loss is also inversely proportional to the frequency: the higher the frequency, the faster the loss. Decibels measure the energy of sound on a logarithmic scale, so a loss of approximately 3 dB means that the sound energy is half as strong. The rate of absorption depends on the tissue type, but is approximately 0.5–1 dB/cm/MHz. For a 5-Mhz wave, then, the sound energy loses 2.5–5 dB/cm, or half its energy every centimeter.

14. How does ultrasound work (in a nutshell)?

The ultrasound transducer receives a short electrical pulse and generates a corresponding pressure wave pulse. This pulse is only several cycles long. The pulsed wave propagates down through the tissue, away from the transducer. The tissue absorbs, scatters, reflects and refracts the wavefront. The reflected waves head back to the transducer. (The tissue also absorbs, scatters, reflects, and refracts the returning sound wave.) The transducer switches to receive mode and, as it receives pressure waves, converts them into electrical pulses. After a fixed period of time, the transducer stops receiving and transmits the next pressure wave.

15. Does each pressure wave make an image?

No. Each pressure wave makes one vertical line of an image. Each image is composed of many vertical lines. These vertical lines can be arranged as parallel lines or as a fan (as with a sector transducer).

16. What is a transducer?

A transducer converts one form of energy to another. Ultrasound transducers convert electricity and pressure waves. Currently this is done with a piezoelectric crystal (*piezo* means "pressure"). In the future, this may be done directly.

17. What is a phased-array transducer?

This probe has an array of crystals that can be energized in a series. Some phased-arrays transducers can be steered electronically, triggering a wave that enters the tissue at an angle.

18. How does ultrasound determine the depth that the echo came from?
Depth is determined by measuring the length of time from pulse formation at the transducer until it returns to the transducer. It is assumed that the wave traveled at the average speed of sound in tissue (1540 m/sec), and that it had to travel the distance twice, so depth $= 1/2 \times T \times 1540$ (m/sec).

19. What does the brightness of the echo mean?
The brightness corresponds to the strength of the reflected wave. Tissue reflects sound to varying degrees and is echogenic; simple fluid reflects little sound and is hypoechoic or anechoic.

20. What is the acoustic power?
Acoustic power is how powerfully an echo is transmitted. In general, a stronger echo gives a better image, but the strength is limited by the Food and Drug Administration (FDA) due to concerns about biologic heating and tissue effects.

21. What is the temporal resolution (frame rate) of ultrasound? What does it depend on?
The temporal resolution is the speed at which the images are refreshed. This depends on:
- The number of vertical lines in an image (each line is painted separately, so more lines means lower temporal resolution)
- How long each vertical line takes to create, which is a function of depth of field. Deeper imaging takes longer for the sound to penetrate and return.
- The combination of grayscale, color, and spectral Doppler, because each is done with separate waves.

Typical frame rates are between 10 and 30 Hz. In general, cardiac imaging requires the fastest frame rates to visualize the moving valves.

22. If the human eye sees flicker at frame rates less than ~25 Hz and ultrasound frame rates can be as low as 10 cycles/sec, why don't humans see the ultrasound image flickering?
The screen is refreshed at normal monitor rates so the screen does not appear to flicker, but the image that is displayed on the screen is only refreshed at the frame rate. Low frame rates have a noticeable lag and can look jerky.

23. What is the dynamic range?
The dynamic range refers to how the image is displayed. The ultrasound transducers can detect a tremendous range of sound energies, up to 120 dB, but the human visual system can only detect a small range of differences. The dynamic range adjusts the display. A wide dynamic range (60 dB) displays a wide range of reflected intensities as shades of gray, but as a result the shades are not very different. A narrow range displays fewer of the intensities as shades of gray, with a greater difference between those intensities. Dynamic range is analogous to window width on computed tomography (CT).

24. What is time gain compensation (TGC) depth-related compensation?
Sound is largely absorbed by human tissue. Therefore, the strength of the echo returning from 10 cm deep (which has passed through 20 cm of tissue) is many times weaker than the strength of the echo returning from 2 cm deep. TGC allows the operator to amplify (increase the gain of) the displayed echoes from deeper tissue. (It is called *time gain compensation* because depth is determined by time elapsed since the echo was created.) Because different tissues in different people absorb and scatter sound to different degrees, TGC cannot be programmed automatically.

25. What is A-mode ultrasound?
A-mode is for amplitude. This is the simplest form of ultrasound; it is only one voxel wide, as if from a pencil beam. The display is depth versus echogenicity, but this has been replaced by B-mode.

26. What is B-mode ultrasound?

B-mode is brightness mode. It is what is usually thought of as ultrasound. It is a two-dimensional image, with the brightness of each pixel in the image corresponding to the strength of the echo. It is made up of a number of A-mode images displayed next to each other.

27. What is M-mode ultrasound?

After A and B comes M. M is for motion. It is a two-dimensional image, with the dimensions being depth and time. This is A-mode mapped against time, giving very high temporal resolution, and is used for motion of heart valves (a task that has strong echogenic interfaces and needs high temporal resolution because it is so fast.)

28. What is the focal zone? Fresnel zone? Frauenhofer zone?

The ultrasound wavefront is complex and interacts with itself. In the near field (Fresnel zone), the pressure amplitude varies. In the far field (Frauenhofer zone), the beam diverges and the energy reduces. Between them, at the narrowest part of the beam, is the focal zone, which gives the best spatial resolution. In practice, one can focus the transducer to a selected depth (or depths) and this improves the image at that depth. The price of multiple focal zones is a low frame rate.

29. What is Doppler?

The frequencies of sound emitted from objects moving toward another object are increased and are decreased when the object moves away. It does not matter whether that sound is generated by the object (e.g., a train whistle) or is generated by something else and reflected by the moving object (ultrasound). The faster an object is moving, the greater the frequency shift.

30. What is duplex?

Duplex ultrasound is the use of two display modes simultaneously, usually grayscale two-dimensional ultrasound plus either spectral Doppler or color Doppler ultrasound.

31. What is spectral Doppler ultrasound and how is it used?

Spectral Doppler measures the velocity of moving blood within a small region (the sample gate). This velocity spectrum is then displayed in a rolling graph of velocity versus time. A grayscale image is usually acquired as well, with the site of Doppler acquisition displayed against the grayscale image. Duplex ultrasound, with its dual display of grayscale and spectral Doppler imaging, was a huge advance over continuous wave spectral Doppler (flow probes), which would detect but not localize flow.

Tip: The size of the sample gate can be varied; a larger gate is more sensitive to finding flow but also subject to increased partial volume effects (a greater chance of detecting flow not truly in the sample volume). The marker of direction of flow within the sample gate is visually adjusted by the sonographer for subsequent angle correction to determine velocity.

32. How does ultrasound determine velocity?

Velocity is determined by measuring the Doppler frequency shift and applying angle correction. Doppler shift occurs when the sound wave source (in biology, the red blood cells) are moving toward or away from the transducer. When they are moving toward the transducer, they shorten the wavelength and increase the frequency (the high pitch when a train approaches). When they are moving away, the wavelength is lengthened and the frequency (pitch) decreases. Only the component of motion toward or away from the transducer is measured. If the echo source is moving at an oblique angle relative to the transducer, angle correction mathematically corrects for this obliquity.

33. What is the equation for frequency shift for an object moving directly toward the transducer?

$$\Delta F = 2F_{transmitted} \times (v/c) \quad (v = \text{velocity of the object}, c = \text{speed of sound})$$
$$or \; \Delta F = 2 \, v/\lambda \quad (\lambda = \text{wavelength})$$

34. What is the relationship of frequency shift to velocity? What is a conceptual way to re-member the frequency shift equation?

Velocity is proportional to frequency shift. Ultrasound engineers often think in terms of fre-quency shift; physicians often think in terms of velocity.

Imagine the object is moving toward the transducer and reflects extra waves. The number of extra waves reflected in 1 second depends on how many waves would "fit" in the distance it moves in that 1 second (i.e., v/λ). The factor of 2 comes about because the object is reflecting and there are two sets of waves in that distance: the waves being transmitted and the waves be-ing reflected.

35. In clinical practice, is it necessary to derive or calculate the frequency shift equation?

No. Use it to quiz your mentors before they quiz you.

36. What is the Doppler equation?

$V = \cos \theta \times$ frequency shift (wavelength)

37. What is the cos θ term (or what is angle correction)?

Blood is usually not moving directly at or away from the transducer. Because Doppler mea-sures only that component of motion that is directly at or away from the transducer, the Doppler shift that is measured underestimates the true velocity. Angle correction calculates the true ve-locity based on the measured velocity (acquired by the machine) and the angle of flow (deter-mined by the sonographer). It is a purely mathematical adjustment; it does not change what was measured, but only changes the display.

The key point is that the observed frequency shift only comes from movement that is directly toward or away from the transducer. Movement parallel to the transducer face does not cause a frequency shift. The cos θ adjusts for this. Movement directly toward the transducer ($\theta = 0°$) sees the full frequency shift. Movement at $\theta = 45°$ sees 70% of the shift, at $\theta = 60°$ sees 50% shift, and at $\theta = 90°$ (parallel to the transducer face) sees no shift.

38. Is the Doppler shift equation also of purely academic interest?

No. It has two practical consequences, the first being angle adjustment. The ultrasound ma-chine does not calculate the angle that the blood is traveling. The sonographer determines the an-gle by aligning a line parallel to the direction of blood flow. This introduces human imprecision and occasionally gross human error into the accuracy of the measured velocity.

The second is the nature of the cos θ term. For angles near 0° the angle changes little; for an-gles greater than 60° (mostly parallel flow), the cos θ changes rapidly and human imprecision is magnified.

39. Why should an angle of < 60° be used?

First, the more the blood is moving toward or away from the transducer, the stronger the Doppler signal relative to noise. Second, angle correction becomes sensitive to small errors at an-gles at which the flow is nearly parallel to the transducer. The more the flow is coming at or away from the transducer, the better.

40. What is Doppler aliasing?

The sonographer determines the sensitivity range for frequency shifts. The larger this range, the lower the sensitivity to small frequency shifts. The smaller this range, the greater the sensi-tivity to small shifts (slow velocities). A small range is not always used because higher velocities exceed the range of the small scale and alias (appearing to be multiples of small shifts).

41. What differentiates aliasing from reversed flow?

Most spectral scales have a filter that considers small spectral shifts noise and not true shifts. These are displayed as black on color scales. Therefore, if the velocity goes from positive to negative with a black zone in between, the result is not aliasing, whereas if velocity goes from maximum positive to maximum negative, the result is not physiologic and is aliasing.

42. What is color Doppler ultrasound, and how does it work?

Color Doppler uses Doppler ultrasound to measure a velocity at every voxel within a region. This creates a "velocity map" that is then displayed in color, with each color assigned to a range of velocities. Color Doppler is useful for quickly determining flow versus no flow (with appropriate filters), for finding vessels to interrogate for quantitative velocities with spectral Doppler, and for finding high-velocity jets (e.g., in the carotid artery) to interrogate for quantitative velocities.

Tip: The color map is not angle adjusted, so the velocity map is actually a map of the velocity directly toward or away from the transducer. Therefore, it is not the true maximum velocity. Color Doppler is displayed against a background grayscale image to maintain anatomic landmarks. Color Doppler is slow to acquire, and the speed of acquisition depends on the size of the Doppler interrogated region. Thus, a smaller color region will have a faster frame rate. A noise floor filter is set so that low velocities (which are probably random noise) are not displayed. For displaying slow velocities, however, the noise floor must be lowered.

43. What is power Doppler imaging?

Power Doppler imaging is Doppler imaging without directionality. This makes the Doppler information stronger (answering whether the reflector is moving or not) but with loss of direction and quantitative velocity information.

44. What is spectral broadening?

Spectral broadening occurs when there is a broad range of Doppler frequencies (velocities), such as after stenoses, which cause turbulence and a range of velocities.

45. Are there any bioeffects of ultrasound?

Ultrasound deposits energy as heat. At high powers, ultrasound can cause cavitation.

46. Is Doppler ultrasound safe for pregnancy?

Spectral Doppler deposits more energy (heat) at a point than real-time two-dimensional imaging. Two-dimensional imaging continually sweeps across a field. Spectral Doppler concentrates on a smaller area. Doppler also uses lower frequencies and longer and more frequent pulse trains, which increases energy deposition. Color Doppler, although not concentrating on one point, also produces higher energy depositions. However, there are no studies proving fetal biohzard, and prudent use (minimizing energy transmit gain and imaging time) within ALARA (as low as reasonably achievable) guidelines is standard practice.

47. What is HIFU?

HIFU is high-intensity focused ultrasound, which focuses high acoustic energy at a target. HIFU may prove to be a percutaneous treatment for tumors or a way to coagulate blood.

48. What is harmonic imaging?

Harmonic imaging is transmitting at one frequency, but receiving at a harmonic of the transmit (fundamental) frequency. A harmonic is a multiple of the transmit frequency; that is, 4 MHz is the first harmonic of 2 MHz. The harmonics are created by the nature of the reflecting tissue and how it resonates.

49. What is the advantage of harmonic imaging?

The signal-to-noise ratio of the returned echo is often higher at harmonic frequencies. Subcutaneous fat tends to create a lot of noise at the primary (the transmitted) frequency, which is eliminated with harmonic imaging. Again, ultrasound contrast agents give strong harmonic signals and higher signal-to-noise ratios.

50. What are ultrasound contrast agents, and how do they work?

Ultrasound contrast agents are microbubbles or particles. They are injected intravenously (sometimes after shaking up the agent to create the bubbles). These bubbles vibrate and reflect sound strongly. They are small enough to pass through the lungs.

Ultrasound contrast agents vibrate when struck by sound and often have strong harmonic resonances, vibrating at two or more times the frequency of the stimulating echo train. The ultrasound contrast bubbles are particularly echogenic relative to the surrounding tissue when the echo is transmitted at one frequency but received at a harmonic frequency.

51. What is pulse inversion?

Pulse inversion imaging takes advantage of another property of microbubbles, which are non-linear reflectors, meaning that they respond differently to the positive and negative pressures that compose an ultrasound wave. (A positive wave compresses the bubble; the negative wave lets it expand. A bubble can expand more than it can be compressed.) Pulse inversion sends a pair of waves, with one being the negative or opposite of the other. Linear reflectors (most tissue) reflect them equally, and the result mathematically cancels. Microbubbles do not reflect them equally and thus stand out against the canceled background.

52. What is three-dimensional ultrasound and how does it work?

Direct three-dimensional ultrasound has a two-dimensional array of crystal elements in the transducer. The third dimension is based on the time of the returning echo, just as standard two-dimensional ultrasound uses a one-dimensional transducer and time of returning echo to generate the second dimension.

Computed three-dimensional ultrasound uses a one-dimensional array to make two-dimensional images, which are then swept perpendicular to the array (mechanically or freehand) to acquire the third dimension. This is similar to three-dimensional CT, which is composed of a stack of two-dimensional images.

53. How does extended field-of-view work?

Extended field-of-view uses a one-dimensional array. The ultrasound probe is moved parallel to the array to digitally create a wide two-dimensional image.

54. How can better ultrasound images be obtained?

- Don't be overwhelmed by the number of controls. A sonographer can demonstrate the appropriate knobs.
- Pick an appropriate probe (high frequencies for close penetration, low frequencies for deep penetration)
- Obtain good contact through a good window.
- Don't move the probe too fast.
- Practice, practice, practice.

BIBLIOGRAPHY

1. Burns PN: Contrast agents and bubble behavior. Presented at the First Annual Symposium on Ultrasound Contrast for Radiological Diagnosis, Toronto, 1998.
2. Burns PN: Contrast agents for ultrasound imaging and Doppler. In Rumack CM, Wilson SR, Charboneau JW (eds): Diagnostic Ultrasound, vol 1, 2nd ed. St. Louis, Mosby, 1998, pp 57–83.
3. Fowlkes JB, Holland CK: Biologic effects and safety. In Rumack CM, Wilson SR, Charboneau JW (eds): Diagnostic Ultrasound, vol 1, 2nd ed. St. Louis, Mosby, 1998, pp 35–55.
4. Merritt CRB: Physics of ultrasound. In Rumack CM, Wilson SR, Charboneau JW (eds): Diagnostic Ultrasound, vol 1, 2nd ed. St. Louis, Mosby, 1998, pp 10–33.

2. GRAYSCALE ULTRASOUND ARTIFACTS

Ryan K. Lee, M.D.

1. What is reverberation artifact (RA)?

Reverberation occurs when sound echoes internally in tissue. This can happen multiple times, resulting in additional echoes, which are interpreted as being deeper within the tissues than the original reflector. Reverberation artifacts are recognized by repeating horizontally positioned linear echoes that are equally spaced on the image with decreasing intensity. Harmonic imaging decreases this artifact. For example, in the liver, reverberation can sometimes obscure a cyst or even a mass (Fig. 1).

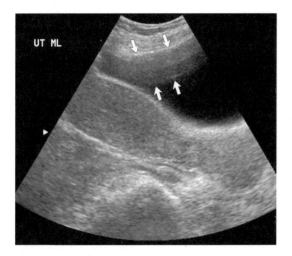

FIGURE 1. Reverberation (*arrows*) fills in anterior bladder.

2. What is ring down artifact?

Ring down artifacts are a type of reverberation artifact. They are most commonly seen with gas bubbles. When sound waves interact with the gas bubbles, they excite the fluid trapped between the bubbles causing the fluid to resonate. This causes multiple artifactual echoes to be displayed as originating deep to the gas bubbles. This artifact can be useful to help detect free intraperitoneal gas (Fig. 2).

3. What is comet tail artifact?

A comet tail artifact is another type of reverberation. When sound waves enter a cholesterol crystal, they reflect internally before returning to the transducer. Each additional internal reverberation produces an artifactual echo that appears deeper than the original echo. As sound is attenuated with each reflection, each deeper artifactual echo is smaller in size, creating a V-shape artifact, hence its description as a comet tail. The comet tail is most often used to describe cholesterol crystals in the gallbladder, either from adenomyomatosis or polyps. This artifact is also seen with surgical clips or other metals (Fig. 3).

4. What is mirror image artifact?

Mirror image artifacts occur because of strong reflectors. Sound is reflected from an obliquely oriented specular reflector (the mirror), then echoes off a secondary reflector, and is reflected back to the transducer to the obliquely oriented strong reflector. Because the computer does not process this internal reflection, it determines the position of an echo based on the prin-

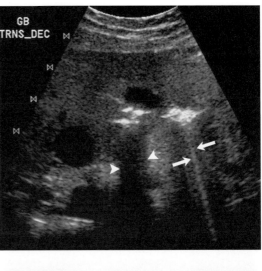

FIGURE 2. Gas can produce sharp shadows (*arrowheads*) when the sound is reflected or can ring down (*arrows*) when the sound reverberates in the gas bubbles.

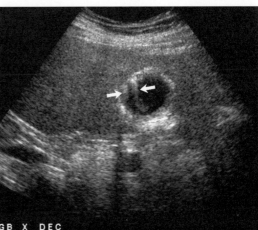

FIGURE 3. Comet tail artifacts (*arrows*) of parallel narrowing echoes arise from reverberation in cholesterol crystals in the gallbladder wall.

ciple that the amount of time a sound wave takes to return is proportional to distance. The result is a mirror image artifact created deep to the strong reflector. The diaphragm is a strong reflector that often causes this artifact. For example, a liver lesion often is reflected by the diaphragm to simulate a lung lesion (Fig. 4).

5. What is acoustic shadowing?
Acoustic shadowing occurs when sound waves encounter a substance that can almost completely attenuate or reflect the beam. Because of this attenuation, there is little to no sound energy to penetrate behind the highly attenuating substance.

This artifact is useful in finding all types of calcifications, such as renal calculi and gallstones (Fig. 5). It can also be a hindrance, such as when rib shadows obscure deeper structures. Acoustic shadowing can also arise from a large impedance mismatch between two tissues, such as gas and soft tissue (see Figure 2). This results in an absence of echoes behind the interface and is often seen when bowel gas prevents the visualization of deeper tissues.

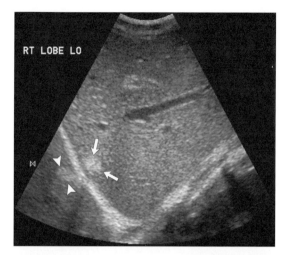

FIGURE 4. Mirror image artifact. A hepatic hemangioma (*arrows*) is reflected by the diaphragm and is mirrored behind it, creating a second pseudolesion (*arrowheads*). In reality, the lung occupies this space.

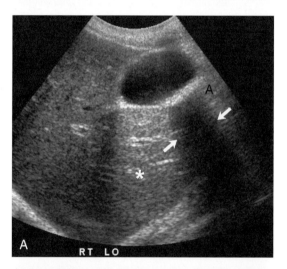

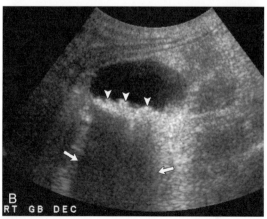

FIGURE 5. *A,* Gallbladder stones are recognized by the sharp acoustic shadows they cast (*arrows*). The discrete stones are not seen in this supine position. The shadow is the key to the abnormality. Also note enhanced through transmission (*asterisk*) behind the gallbladder. *B,* By turning the patient on his side (decubitus), the multiple discrete echogenic stones (*arrowheads*) are seen, accounting for the shadow (*arrows*).

6. What is a refraction artifact?

Sound passing between two types of tissue that have different speeds of sound is refracted. Lens-shaped objects act as acoustic lenses. (This is how an optical lens works; the speed of light is different in glass than in air.) This causes a misregistration artifact because the computer assumes that the echo originated along a straight path. The result is an object that is displayed in the wrong location. This refraction artifact also produces shadowing at the edges of structures (Fig. 6). This sometimes results in duplication of an object. This most commonly occurs at the junction of the rectus muscles and abdominal wall fat where deeper abdominal structures can appear duplicated (also known as a *ghost artifact*). Refraction can be a problem during biopsy because the needle is straight. (This is like spearfishing from the water's surface; the fish is not where it appears to be.) Scanning from different angles usually solves this problem.

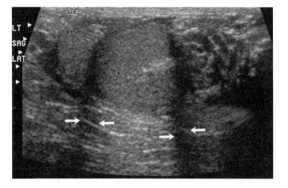

FIGURE 6. Arrows denote the hypoechoic shadows that result from refraction of the beam, so less sound is available to image the tissue in this region.

7. What is *enhanced through transmission*?

Enhanced through transmission occurs behind tissues that absorb or reflect little sound, such as cysts or very homogenous solids (lymphoma). Therefore, objects on the far side of the cyst receive an unattenuated beam. Because of the time gain compensation, deeper echoes are amplified more than superficial echoes. Thus the tissue deep to a cyst appears enhanced (Fig. 7 and see Figure 5A).

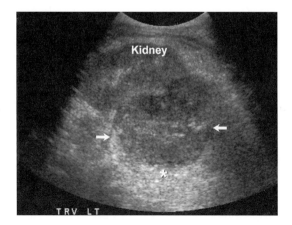

FIGURE 7. Renal abscess (*arrows*) with enhanced through transmission (*asterisk*).

8. What are side lobes?

Most of the ultrasound energy emanates from the central portion of the beam. About 1% of the ultrasound energy, however, radiates outward from the periphery, and these portions of the beam are known as the side lobes. These waves (the side lobes) are normally too weak to generate any significant echoes, but can occasionally cause artifact when they encounter strong reflectors. These artifacts arise because the computer interprets these echoes as arising from the central beam. An example of this artifact is the false impression of echoegenic bile in the gallbladder (pseudosludge) (Fig. 8).

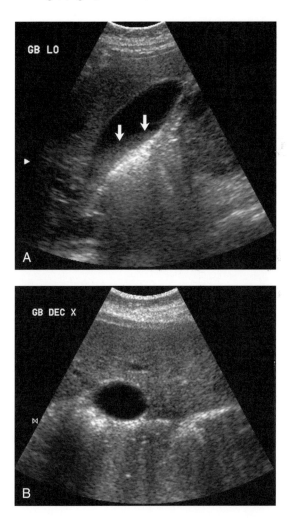

A

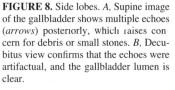

FIGURE 8. Side lobes. *A,* Supine image of the gallbladder shows multiple echoes (*arrows*) posteriorly, which raises concern for debris or small stones. *B,* Decubitus view confirms that the echoes were artifactual, and the gallbladder lumen is clear.

B

9. What is the speed of sound artifact?

The speed of sound artifact occurs when the sound beam passes through a material with a significantly different speed of sound than the assumed normal speed of 1540 m/sec. If the material renders the beam slower, the echoes that pass through are delayed and objects appear deeper than they really are (Fig. 9).

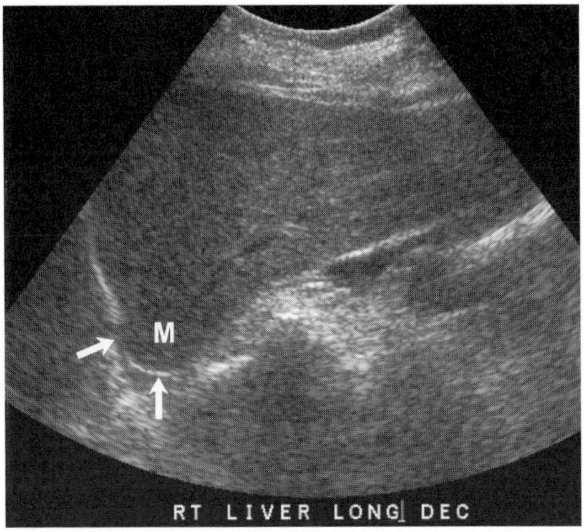

FIGURE 9. Sound artifact. The diaphragm (*arrows*) is artifactually disrupted by a nearly isoechoic mass (*M*) anterior to it. The beam travels slower through the mass, so the echoes from the diaphragm take longer to return to the transducer than those behind a normal liver. Thus, a discrepant diaphragm is shown.

BIBLIOGRAPHY

1. Keogh MB, Cooperberg PL: Is it real or is it an artifact? Ultrasound Q 17:201–210, 2001.
2. Siegal MJ: Pediatric Sonography, 2nd ed. New York, Raven Press, 1995, pp 13–27.
3. Thurston W, Wilson SR: The urinary tract. In Rumack CM, Wilson SR, Charboneau JW (eds): Diagnostic Ultrasound, 2nd ed. St. Louis, Mosby, 1998, pp 329–397.

3. DOPPLER ULTRASOUND ARTIFACTS

Shannon C. Campbell, M.D.

1. What artifacts are unique to Doppler ultrasonography?

The artifacts unique to Doppler ultrasonography include twinkle artifact, pseudoflow artifact, flash artifact, edge artifact, aliasing, artifactual spectral broadening, and artifactual absence of flow.

2. What is twinkle artifact?

Twinkle artifact occurs behind a strongly reflecting interface, such as urinary tract stones or parenchymal calcification, and appears as a quickly fluctuating mixture of Doppler signals with an associated characteristic spectrum with a noisy appearance. The appearance of the twinkling artifact is highly dependent on machine settings and is likely generated by a narrow-band, intrinsic machine noise called *phase* (or clock) *jitter* (Figs. 1 and 2).

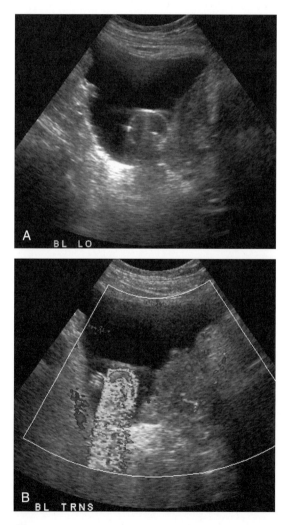

FIGURE 1. Foley catheter. Grayscale (*A*) image shows normal image while color Doppler (*B*) shows intensive mosaic multicolored pixels emanating from the anterior margin of the Foley balloon (see also Color Plates, Figure 1). This is clearly an artifact, dubbed a "twinkle" artifact.

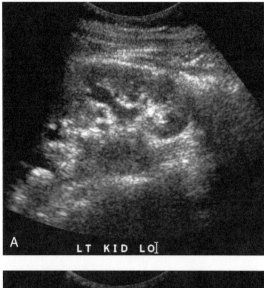

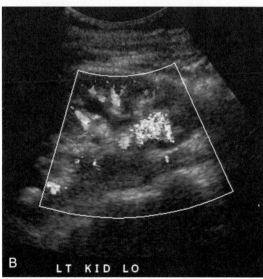

FIGURE 2. Twinkle artifact identifies renal calculi. Grayscale (*A*) image shows a faint echogenic focus in the lower pole and one in the upper pole, which are difficult to separate from the sinus. No shadows are seen. Color Doppler image (*B*) shows intense "twinkle" multicolored pixels behind the stones and normal color display in the renal vessels (see also Color Plates, Figure 2). Without the twinkle, the stones are difficult to diagnose.

3. What causes pseudoflow artifact?

Pseudoflow represents true flow of a substance other than blood, such as ascites or amniotic fluid. Bladder jets are pseudoflow. *Pseudoflow* is a historic misnomer; *pseudoblood* is more accurate (Figs. 3–5). This artifact can be useful for detecting fluid motion or ballottement in complex fluid collections such as hematomas or abscesses, which may mimic solid tissue.

4. What is flash artifact?

Flash artifact is the sudden burst of color signal that encompasses the frame. It can be caused by motion of the transducer or the patient's breathing. The beating heart can cause flash artifact in the adjacent liver (Fig. 6).

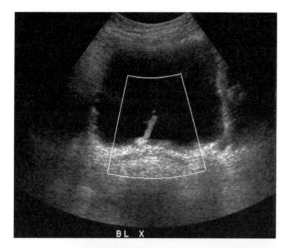

FIGURE 3. Bladder jet. Transverse image though the bladder base shows a normal right bladder jet.

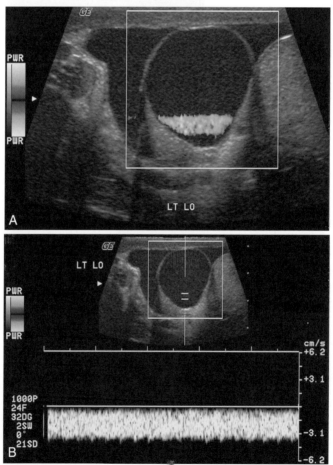

FIGURE 4. Pseudoflow. *A,* Longitudinal view of superior testis and epididymus with cyst. An intense band of color Doppler fills a portion of the cyst. *B,* Spectral Doppler shows monotonous unidirectional flow, indicating motion of fluid or debris within the cyst. (See also Color Plates, Figure 3.)

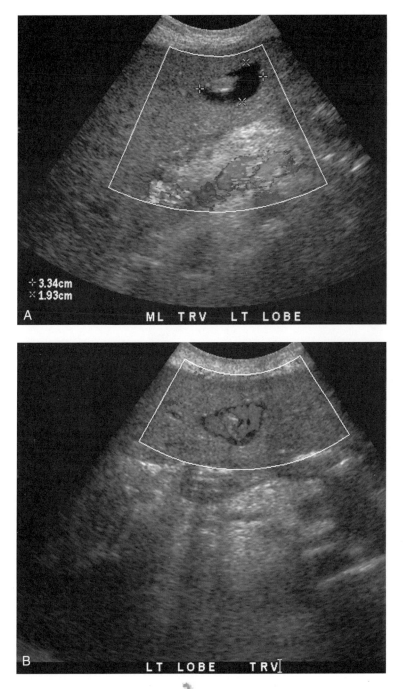

FIGURE 5. Pseudoflow in ascites. Transverse grayscale image (*A*) through the falciform ligament shows anechoic fluid surrounding it. Fluid fills with color (*B*) on color Doppler image.

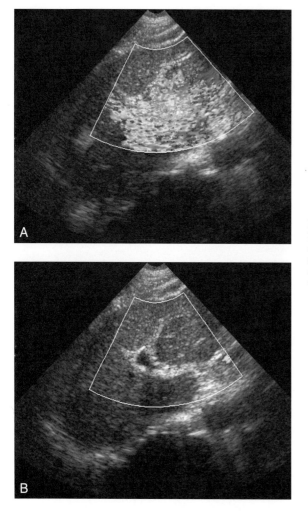

FIGURE 6. Flash artifact. *A,* Color Doppler images show a multicolored cloud of pixels that fill the color box after respiratory motion. *B,* A second or 2 later, the image shows only true vascular flow.

5. What is color bleed?

Color bleed is the extension of color beyond the region of flow and beyond the vessel walls. Color bleed can be minimized by decreasing the color gain.

6. What is edge artifact?

Edge artifact occurs at the interface of strong reflectors and appears as color along the rim of calcified structures such as gallstones or cortical bone (Fig. 7).

7. What is aliasing?

Aliasing arises from an incorrect measurement of the signal frequency resulting from an insufficient sampling rate. It manifests as a mix of color signals in the area of measurement ambiguity. On spectral display this appears as a "wrap around" of the areas of high frequencies to below the baseline. Aliasing occurs when the Doppler shift frequency exceeds half the pulse repetition frequency (PRF) (Fig. 8).

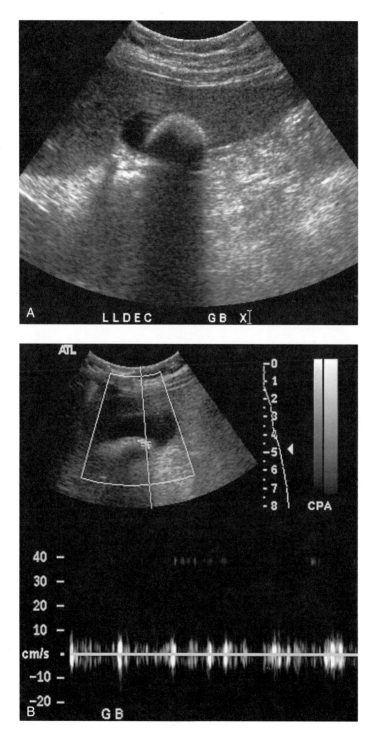

FIGURE 7. Gallstone with edge artifact. *A*, Grayscale image of a large gallstone. *B*, Power Doppler image simulating flow at the stone surface. Spectral tracing (*B*) shows only noise and no flow. This was present on color Doppler as well as power Doppler imaging.

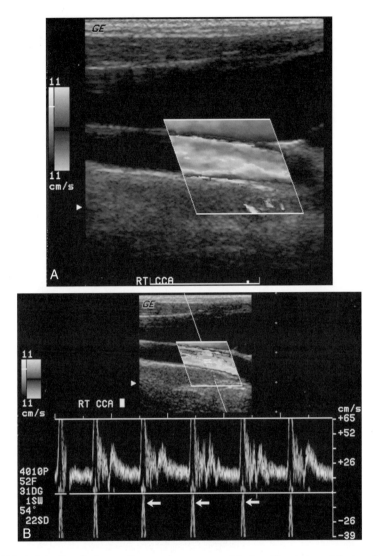

FIGURE 8. *A,* Color Doppler image of a normal common carotid artery. Flow is toward the transducer and should be displayed as red. However, the higher velocity flow centrally (yellow to blue) exceeds the positive color Doppler scale toward the transducer and wraps around to the negative side. Thus, it is displayed as if it is flowing away from the transducer as does the adjacent jugular vein. *B,* Spectral Doppler tracing in a normal common carotid artery. The velocity scale is too low; the normal systolic velocity peak exceeds the scale above the baseline and wraps around to display below the baseline (*arrows*).

8. How can aliasing be eliminated?

Aliasing can be eliminated primarily by increasing the PRF or decreasing the Doppler shift frequency (by using a lower frequency transducer).

9. What is meant by artifactual spectral broadening? What causes this artifact?

In spectral broadening, a large range of flow velocities are present on spectral waveform at a given point in the cardiac cycle, typifying high-grade stenosis. Artifactual spectral broadening has an identical appearance and may be caused by placement of the sample volume near the vessel wall, an inappropriately large sample volume, or excessively large system gain.

10. What is the mirror image artifact?

This artifact is the same in Doppler as in grayscale. A strong specular reflector reflects the Doppler signal to and from the object, increasing the time to return to the transducer. In Doppler, this is most common from the pleural surface, mirroring either subclavian artery or vein. The spectral Doppler mirrors as well as the color Doppler signal (Fig. 9).

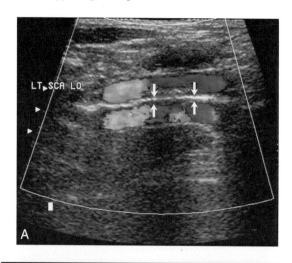

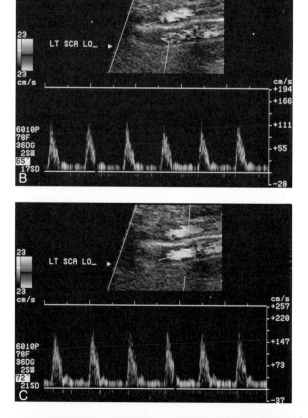

FIGURE 9. Mirror image. Color Doppler image of the normal subclavian artery shows a duplicated identical vessel below the pleural surface (*arrows*). Spectral Doppler of the true vessel (*B*) is identical to that of the mirror image (*C*).

11. What are the sources of artifactual absence or decrease of Doppler flow signal?

Doppler signal may be lost in many ways. It may be lost by use of a probe of too high frequency, resulting in tissue attenuation and decreased penetration. High settings of wall filters, which are used to help eliminate low-frequency noise, can also eliminate the signals from low-velocity blood flow. Doppler angles > 60° result in inaccurate velocity measurements, and a Doppler angle of 90° results in no flow.

12. What steps can be taken to detect slow or decreased flow when one of these sources is present?

Selection of an appropriate frequency probe (lower frequency for deeper vessels, higher frequency for superficial vessels) is important for signal detection. Wall filters should be set at the lowest level possible while preserving low-frequency noise reduction. Doppler angles should be < 60°.

13. What are the pitfalls of misinterpreting Doppler artifacts?

Pseudoflow may be interpreted as a real vascular phenomenon causing, for example, misdiagnosis of collateral vessels in a patient with ascites when the ascites may not be related to liver disease. Flash artifact can cause confusion about the vascularity of an otherwise anechoic structure, such as a simple renal cyst. Artifactual spectral broadening may lead to diagnosis of a high-grade stenosis in a vessel when in fact the vessel is normal. Slow flow may be diagnosed as thrombosis when Doppler angle is inappropriate or wall filters are high. When the low-frequency signal is eliminated by wall filters, the resistive indices calculated are inaccurate.

14. How can Doppler artifacts be useful?

The presence of twinkle artifact can help identify stones. The presence of bladder jets is helpful in evaluating patients for urinary tract obstruction.

BIBLIOGRAPHY

1. Keogh, CF, Cooperberg PL: Is it real or is it an artifact? Ultrasound Q 17:201–210, 2001.
2. Lee JY, Kim SH, Cho JY, Han D: Color and power Doppler twinkling artifacts from urinary stones: Clinical observations and phantom studies. Am J Roentgen 176:1441–1445, 2001.
3. Mitchell DG: Color Doppler imaging: Principles, limitations, and artifacts. Radiology 177:1–10, 1990.
4. Pozniak MA, Zagzebski JA, Scanlan KA: Spectral and color Doppler artifacts. Radiographics 12:35–44, 1992.
5. Rahmouni A, Bargoin R, Herment A, et al: Color Doppler twinkling artifact in hyperechoic regions. Radiology 199:269–271, 1996.
6. Rumack CM, Wilson SR, Charboneau JW: Diagnostic Ultrasound, 2nd ed. St. Louis, Mosby, 1998, pp 29–32.
7. Taylor KJ, Holland S: Doppler US. Part I. Basic principles, instrumentation, and pitfalls. Radiology 174:297–307, 1990.

4. CONTRAST AGENTS FOR ULTRASOUND IMAGING

Cheri X. Deng, Ph.D.

BASICS OF ULTRASOUND CONTRAST AGENTS

1. What are ultrasound contrast agents (UCAs)?

UCAs are small particles in fluid suspension designed to enhance ultrasound image contrast. These particles have a diameter of 1–5 μm and are either gas filled or contain gases and are suspended in fluid. When injected into the bloodstream, they can increase the backscattered ultrasound signals and result in better image contrast.

2. Why use UCAs?

UCAs improve ultrasound imaging capability by increasing imaging sensitivity for slow flow in deep and small vessels, which is important in early disease detection, diagnosis, and monitoring. Figure 1 shows ultrasound images of the heart after contrast agent injection.

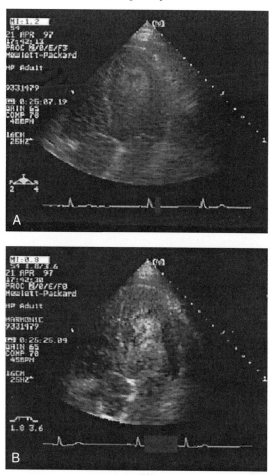

FIGURE 1. Apical four-chamber view of a human heart after an IV administration of Levovist. *A*, Fundamental imaging (i.e., transmitting and receiving at 3 MHz). *B*, Second harmonic B-mode imaging (i.e., transmitting at 1.8 MHz and receiving at 3.6 MHz). (From Frinking PJA, Bouakaz A, Kirkhorn J, et al: Ultrasound contrast imaging: Current and new potential methods. Ultrasound Med Biol 26:965–975, 2000, with permission.)

3. How do UCAs enhance image contrast?

UCAs are capable of producing much stronger backscatter than regular blood or tissue due to the substantial differences in compressibility and density between the filling gas inside the bubbles and the surrounding blood.

4. What are the clinical applications of UCAs?

UCAs are used in a wide range of applications, including the identification of cardiac structures, determination of perfusion area such as the detection of myocardial perfusion and infarction, and quantification of cardiac output. There are many reports of contrast-assisted imaging for liver lesion characterization, breast tumor detection, and prostate cancer detection. Application of UCAs also represents one potential approach for tumor angiogenesis by providing enhanced capability to measure tumor flow and vascular volume. Ultrasound contrast imaging makes it possible to characterize structural and functional features of tumor vascularity from an earlier stage.

5. What are the basic properties of UCAs?

UCAs are usually stabilized by a thin shell made of biocompatible material such as human serum albumin in order to keep the gas inside from dissolving into blood. They are small enough to pass through the pulmonary circulation. UCAs can substantially increase the backscattered ultrasound signal or ultrasound image contrast in B-mode or Doppler imaging.

6. What are the common UCAs and their status?

There are, in general, five types of agents in ultrasound imaging with different physical properties: free gas bubbles, capsulated gas bubbles, colloidal suspensions, emulsions, and aqueous solutions. The most successful agents are those stabilized microbubble agents that can pass through the lung capillary circulation and that are stable enough to reach the left heart after an IV injection. All current UCAs are able to reach the left ventricle cavity of the heart and are based on free-gas bubbles or are stabilized by encapsulation to avoid rapid disappearance.

More than 10 UCAs are currently under investigation and being tested in clinical trials. However, only three transpulmonary agents are commercially available: Levovist (Schering AG, Berlin, Germany, approved in Europe), Albunex, and Optison (Mallinckrodt, St. Louis, USA). Only Albunex and Optison are cleared by the Food and Drug Administration (FDA) in the United States for cardiac applications.

7. What are the basic physical phenomena involved with UCAs?

The most important phenomenon involved in UCA interactions is the scattering phenomenon. Scattering of ultrasound occurs when an ultrasound field is traveling through a medium that contains localized inhomogeneities such as small particles or bubbles. Because of the large difference between the acoustic impedances of the gas inside the bubbles and the surrounding liquid, UCAs are efficacious scatterers of ultrasound, capable of producing much stronger backscatter than regular blood or normal tissue. Such bubbles react to external ultrasound pressure field with volume pulsations, absorbing and radiating ultrasound energy, thus generating a scattered field and reducing the transmitted field. Scattering is especially pronounced at the resonant frequency of a contrast agent: for an air-filled bubble in water, this frequency (in megahertz) is approximately equal to $3/R$, where R is the bubble radius in micrometers. For example, the resonant frequency for a 1-μm bubble is 3 MHz, which is close to the frequency range used in diagnostic ultrasound.

8. What are the nonlinear phenomena associated with UCAs?

Depending on the magnitude of the incident ultrasound field, the pulsation is linear or nonlinear with respect to the applied pressure. When the applied pressure amplitude is sufficiently large (e. g., > 100 kPa), contrast agent bubbles respond nonlinearly. Nonlinear interaction phenomena include harmonic and subharmonic generation. Acoustic emission has also been observed. The spectrum of the scattered ultrasound signal contains higher harmonics of the incident or fundamental frequency in addition to the original incident frequency. A highly nonlinear system, contrast agent bubbles can even generate subharmonic backscatter at a frequency equal to half of the incident frequency.

9. How can UCAs be destroyed by ultrasound?

When the incident pressure is large enough, contrast agent bubbles can be destroyed or disrupted by the ultrasound field. The disruption of contrast agent particles is caused by the rapid collapsing of bubble or the degeneration of the shell either in a rapid or gradual fashion. Disruption can generate stimulated acoustic emission (SAE) or broad-spectrum emission, which can produce strong, transient backscatter enhancement.

10. What are the physical principles of interaction of UCAs with ultrasound?

The dynamic interaction of ultrasound with small gas bubbles involves the following two factors: (1) the extreme acoustic impedance difference between the enclosed gas and the host liquid and (2) the resonant behavior as a result of stiffness and inertia. The stiffness arises from the compressibility of the enclosed volume of gas, and the inertia arises from the surrounding mass that oscillates with the bubble driven by the incident ultrasound.

When an ultrasound field impinges on a bubble in a liquid, the bubble expands and contracts in response to the pressure variation, and the sound field is scattered because of the acoustic impedance mismatch. If the relative changes in volume are small, linear theory applies; otherwise, nonlinear phenomena must be considered.

11. Why is it important to characterize UCAs?

Because the scattered ultrasound field depends on the characteristics of the scattering contrast agent bubbles, it carries information regarding the scatterers. Thus, the measured scattered ultrasound can be used to extract important parameters describing the contrast agent and the medium. Innovative measurement techniques are being developed to obtain such information from the interrogated medium. The most basic measurement technique is the measurement of the backscatter from a contrast agent medium.

12. How are UCAs characterized?

A pulse-echo system is usually used, and radiofrequency (RF) backscattered signals are digitized for analysis. Frequency domain methods are used to study the spectrum of the backscattered signals. Quantitative backscatter measurement techniques can be implemented to study both linear scattering and nonlinear performance of contrast agents. Attenuation and sound speed in contrast agent suspensions can also be measured from the backscatter signals. Effects of other factors (e.g., concentration of contrast agent bubbles on the backscattered power) have also been studied.

CLINICAL APPLICATIONS OF ULTRASOUND CONTRAST AGENTS

13. What is the basic clinical contrast-assisted imaging method?

Numerous studies have demonstrated the benefit of backscatter enhancement achieved by introduction of contrast agents in ultrasound examinations. These studies showed that clinical application of UCAs improves fundamental B-mode image clarity and increases Doppler signal amplitude. By increasing the effective reflectivity of the blood, UCAs enable better delineation of tumor boundaries, better detection of endocardial borders (for assessment of wall motion abnormities), and better detection of blood flow in small, deep vessels.

14. What are the nonlinear imaging modalities or techniques?

Because of the strong nonlinear phenomena that UCAs exhibit in an ultrasound field, nonlinear imaging techniques have been developed to exploit the nonlinear properties of contrast agents. Techniques such as harmonic, subharmonic, and pulse-inversion B-mode imaging exploit the nonlinear characteristics of contrast agent bubbles and require the relatively stable presence of contrast agent populations for optimal performance.

15. What is harmonic imaging?

Second harmonic B-mode imaging is a method in which the ultrasound system generates images from backscattered signals at the harmonic frequency of the transmitted fundamental frequency. Because contrast agent bubbles exhibit stronger nonlinearity than surrounding tissue, these harmonic signals arise primarily from the agent in the blood. Thus, B-mode images generated from harmonic echo signals preferentially display vascular volumes and blood-perfused tissues.

16. Describe subharmonic imaging.

Subharmonic imaging has been proposed to generate images based on B-mode presentations derived from the backscattered subharmonic signals of the transmitted frequency signal. Because subharmonic signal generation is minimal in tissue, subharmonic imaging has the potential to supply better differentiation of blood and tissue, yet the development of transducers and imaging strategy is essential for successful application of subharmonic imaging.

17. What is pulse-inversion imaging?

Another imaging technique exploiting the nonlinear properties of contrast agent is pulse-inversion imaging, in which a sequence of two phase-inverted pulses is transmitted into tissue and the sum of the two responses is processed for imaging. For a linear medium, the sum of the two responses is zero because the second response is the inverted replica of the first response. The sum of the two responses for a nonlinear medium is not zero because of waveform deformation through nonlinear propagation. The sum depends on the nonlinearity of the medium and can include all the even harmonic components (not just the second harmonic signal) in the backscattered echo; this helps achieve better imaging resolution than harmonic imaging and harmonic power Doppler imaging (Fig. 2).

18. What is power Doppler imaging?

The power Doppler imaging technique displays the power signal amplitude of Doppler signals to indicate flow existence rather than flow direction, as in the conventional Doppler techniques. Because most Doppler techniques are multipulse techniques, they are susceptible to tissue motion. In some cases, tissue motion can generate Doppler signals that often are comparable with or overshadow the contrast agent signals. Just as in harmonic B-mode imaging, harmonic power Doppler imaging displays the power of the second harmonic Doppler signals, which are primarily returned from contrast agents to differentiate flow and tissue.

19. What other contrast agent–specific imaging modes are implemented in clinical scanners?

Recent developments of clinical contrast imaging include power pulse inversion (PPI), power modulation (Philips Medical System, Bothell, WA), and an agent detection imaging mode (Acuson Corporation, Mountain View, CA). PPI combines pulse inversion harmonics with power Doppler techniques to further increase sensitivity to contrast agents. This new technology uses additional pulses to virtually eliminate the tissue signal from the contrast signal. Contrast agents are displayed in color while tissue is displayed in high-resolution grayscale. This new technology allows the display of minute amounts of contrast while simultaneously displaying a high-resolution two-dimensional image, all in real time, to allow the physician to clearly distinguish blood containing contrast from surrounding tissue.

Power modulation is based on a multipulse technique in which the acoustic amplitude of the transmitted pulse is changed. Two transmission amplitudes are used: full and half amplitude. This transmission amplitude change induces changes in the response of the contrast agent. Received echoes from the half-amplitude–transmitted pulse are adjusted in amplitude and subsequently subtracted from the full-amplitude echoes. This procedure removes most of the linear responses at the fundamental frequency, and the remaining echoes contain mainly nonlinear signals from the microbubbles. Power modulation is also used with a low-frequency wide band transducer. The low-frequency transducer increases the depth of field and transmits the ultrasound energy more uniformly throughout the image. The combination of power modulation and wide band transducer

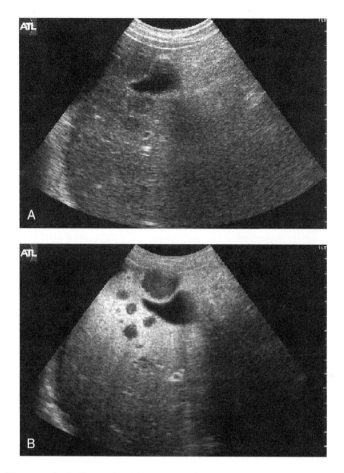

FIGURE 2. Metastases in the liver using (*A*) conventional ultrasound (US) and (*B*) pulse-inversion ultrasound with US contrast. In this example, where the metastases are visible in the conventional image, the contrast between sound tissue and metastases is clearly increased. (From Skoldbye B, Pedersen MH, Struckmann J, et al: Improved detection and biopsy of solid liver lesions using pulse-inversion ultrasound scanning and contrast agent infusion. Ultrasound Med Biol 28:439–444, 2002, with permission.)

allows ultraharmonic imaging, which results in a better elimination of tissue artifacts and therefore increased contrast-to-tissue ratio.

The agent detection imaging mode (Cadence Contrast Agent Imaging) offered by Acuson (Acuson Corporation, Mountain View, CA) provides progressive contrast agent imaging through power contrast imaging, color harmonic imaging, and low mechanical index optimization.

20. What are transient imaging techniques?

Microbubble contrast agents can be destroyed by ultrasound. Transient imaging techniques (e.g., flash echo imaging or triggered imaging) and release-burst imaging employ transient enhanced scattering from ultrasonic contrast agents for optimal imaging capability of contrast agents.

Release-burst imaging is a novel contrast imaging approach that optimally employs the transient characteristic of UCAs. It is based on a combination of multiple high-frequency, broadband detection pulses and a separate release burst. The detection pulses are used to survey the target before and after transient enhanced scattering, which is forced by the release burst. The presence of the contrast agent is detected by correlating or subtracting the before and after burst signals.

Because the time interval between the two detection pulses is minimal (approximately 200–400 μs, depending on, for example, the scan depth and size of the region), the subtraction of the RF data can be performed in real time and is less susceptible to acquisition instabilities.

21. How are UCAs used for blood flow measurement?

UCAs have been used in blood flow measurements to assist conventional flow measurement methods such as Doppler techniques, and flow measurement techniques have been developed using contrast agents. UCAs are contained entirely within the vascular space, travel at the same velocities as the blood flow, and can be relatively stable over a period of time that is suitable for ultrasonic examination. In addition to increasing Doppler signal amplitudes for flow measurement, contrast agents are useful in other methods for flow rate and perfusion measurements, such as in indicator-dilution blood flow analysis. More recently, destruction flow estimation methods have been reported.

Following the indicator-dilution principle, time-video intensity (indicator dilution) curves from media with contrast agents are used to estimate flow rates. Destruction methods exploit ultrasound manipulation of contrast agent bubbles including destruction and radiation force displacement. Such time-domain techniques measure backscatter before and after an induced change in the flowing contrast agent population. The time curve of backscatter is then used to estimate local flow rate and perfusion.

22. How are UCAs used for functional imaging and perfusion estimation?

Tracking the passage of a bolus of contrast agent bubbles through a region of interest gives functional information on its circulation. The clinical applications can be divided into those that interrogate the entire organ and those that study only one region, such as a tumor. Tracking is done by characterizing the transit time of inflow and outflow or by monitoring the "reperfusion," which estimates perfusion from the time for a region of tissue to be repurfused with contrast agents after a destruction of contrast agent takes place.

RECENT DEVELPOMENTS AND FUTURE DIRECTIONS

23. Summarize the recent developments in ultrasonic contrast-assisted imaging.

Significant advances in the field of UCAs can be expected in terms of innovative signal processing concepts, advanced UCA materials, UCAs targeted to adhere to specific tissue sites and used for targeted imaging, and disrupted UCAs used to release therapeutic compounds.

Contrast-assisted ultrasonic imaging is expanding beyond image contrast enhancement and assessment of microvascular perfusion. To overcome the fact that UCAs often cannot specifically differentiate abnormal from normal tissues except by revealing altered blood flow patterns, site-specific UCAs are being developed to potentially provide specific information regarding healthy and pathologic tissues by improving the capability to delineate and localize various tissue pathologies or cell surface markers. Applications of these agents include diagnosis, therapy, biopsy, and resection. Site-specific UCAs have been used for imaging of targeted tissue, including use as markers for imaging of inflammation, thrombus, and angiogenesis, and as an adjunct device for enhanced drug delivery and gene therapy.

24. What are targeted contrast agents and why are they useful?

Site-targeted contrast agents have modified shell materials with attached ligands (antibodies, peptides) and plasmid DNA for targeting. These agents are sometimes designed to remain undetected until they have selectively bound to specific entities, such as thrombus, based on the use of a fibrin-specific antibody. Some agents have also been developed to target inflammation.

These new site-targeted agents do not behave as flow tracers; instead, they are retained within diseased tissue. This specificity is helpful in diagnosis of specific disease and offers potential for targeted delivery of therapeutic compounds.

25. What are the potentials of therapeutic use of UCAs?

UCAs can be used as drug carriers to achieve localized ultrasound-mediated drug release at the desired site when the drug-carried particles are disrupted by ultrasound pulse. When the contrast agent bubbles are destroyed by ultrasound triggering, cavitation activities are generated and enhance transport of genetic material into the cells across the cell membrane, potentially to be used for gene transfection and drug delivery into cells.

BIBLIOGRAPHY

1. Deng CX, Lizzi FL: A review of physical phenomena associated with ultrasonic contrast agents and illustrative clinical applications. Ultrasound Med Biol 28:277–286, 2002.
2. Ferrara KW, Merritt CRB, Burns PN, et al: Evaluation of tumor angiogenesis with US: Imaging, Doppler and contrast agents. Acad Radiol 7:824–839, 2000.
3. Frinking PJA, Bouakaz A, Kirkhorn J, et al: Ultrasound contrast imaging: Current and new potential methods. Ultrasound Med Biol 26:965–975, 2000.
4. Goldberg BB, Liu JB, Forsberg F: Ultrasound contrast agents: A review. Ultrasound Med Biol 20:319–333, 1994.
5. Lanza GM, Wallace K, Scott MJ, et al: A novel site-targeted ultrasonic contrast agent with broad biomedical applications. Circulation 94:3334–3340, 1996.
6. Linder JR, Song J, Christiansen J, et al: Ultrasound assessment of inflammation and renal tissue injury with microbubbles targeted top-selectin. Circulation 104:2107–2112, 2001.
7. Ophir J, Parker KJ: Contrast agents in diagnostic ultrasound. Ultrasound Med Biol 15:319–333, 1989.
8. Porter TR, Xie F: Transient myocardial contrast after initial exposure to diagnostic ultrasound pressures with minute doses of intravenously injected microbubbles. Demonstration and potential mechanisms. Circulation 92:2391–2395, 1995.
9. Unger EC, McCreey TP, Sweitzer R: Ultrasound enhances gene expression of liposomal transfection. Radiology 32:723–727, 1997.
10. Wei K, Jayaweera AR, Firoozan S, et al: Quantification of myocardial blood flow with ultrasound-induced destruction of microbubbles administered as a constant venous infusion. Circulation 95:473–483, 1998.

II. Obstetrics

5. NUCHAL TRANSLUCENCY AND GENETIC SCREENING

Noam Lazebnik, M.D., and Roee S. Lazebnik, Ph.D.

1. What is a genetic sonogram?

A genetic sonogram is a targeted screening ultrasound study to detect the presence of fetal structural anomalies and sonographic fetal anomalies. Sonographic markers are also noted; although they are not necessarily anomalies, they confer higher risk for fetal chromosome abnormality.

2. Describe the rationale for a genetic screening.

All pregnancies have a baseline risk of 3–4% for major congenital anomalies. The etiology for these birth defects includes chromosomal disorders, single gene disorders, multifactorial disorders, and teratogenic or environmental effects. The most common chromosomal abnormality in liveborn babies is Down syndrome (trisomy 21), followed by trisomies 18 and 13. The risk for these abnormalities and sex chromosome abnormalities (47,XXX; 47,XXY; 47,XYY) increases with advancing maternal age. Structural chromosomal abnormalities, such as translocations, deletions, and Turner's syndrome (45,X), are not related to maternal age.

Most newborns with a chromosomal abnormality, including Down syndrome, are born to women younger than 35 years, because most babies are born to younger women. Trisomies 18 and 13, and to a lesser degree trisomy 21, are associated with ultrasonographically recognizable abnormalities. Thus, sonographic examination of the fetus for recognizable abnormal markers is a logical choice.

3. Is there a time frame for genetic sonogram?

The genetic sonogram can be performed at the end of the first trimester at 10–14 weeks' gestation or during the second trimester at 16–20 weeks' gestation.

4. How do the first and second trimester genetic sonograms differ?

The first trimester sonogram can confirm gestational age by measuring the crown rump length (CRL) and is used to quantify the nuchal translucency width. Because of the early gestational age, comprehensive study of the fetal organs cannot be done.

In a second trimester genetic sonogram, the entire fetal anatomy as well as a limited number of abnormal fetal ultrasonic markers can be studied.

FIRST TRIMESTER GENETIC SONOGRAM

5. What are the nuchal translucency and nuchal fold?

Nuchal translucency (NT) is a term used to describe a sonolucent area in the nuchal region (back of the neck) of the fetus and is typically observed during the first trimester between 11 weeks, 0 days, of gestation, and 13 weeks, 6 days of gestation.

The nuchal fold (NF) is the soft tissue in the posterior neck area. It is measured in the sub-occipital-bregmatic plane at the level of the cerebellum. The nuchal fold is studied in the second trimester between 15 and 20 weeks.

6. Describe the purpose of a first trimester genetic sonogram.

A first trimester genetic sonogram is used to look for signs of aneuploidy (a chromosome number that is not an exact multiple of the haploid number n = 23) or triploidy. Although the NT is by far the most helpful marker, the detection of other anomalies during the first trimester are reported among fetuses with aneuploidy, including anterior abdominal wall defects, encephalo-cele, and limb and heart deformities. Growth parameters, although significantly reduced among fetuses with trisomies 13 and 18 and triploidy, were not significantly reduced among fetuses with trisomy 21 or 45,X, or with sex chromosome trisomies.

7. Describe the clinical rationale for an NT study.

Numerous studies have confirmed the association between a thickened fetal nuchal membrane and fetal aneuploidy. It is established that this is the most sonographically reliable marker of aneuploidy in the first trimester.

8. When is an NT study performed?

To obtain precise and reliable risk assessment using nuchal translucency, it is critical that the measurement occur between 11 weeks, 0 days, and 13 weeks, 6 days. Measurements must consider the CRL of the fetus for accurate gestational age. Measurements outside this time window are not reliable to determine individual specific risk.

9. Describe the method used to study NT width.

Fetal NT is defined as a sagittal measurement between the muscles of the cervical spine and the inner layer of the echogenic skin. Because the measured distance is small, it is of utmost importance to establish a highly specific and reproducible method to measure the translucency width. The image must be magnified to distinguish the fetal skin from the amnion. Care needs to be taken not to confuse this finding with an unfused amnion, encephalocele, nuchal cord, or amniotic sheath. This measurement should be feasible to perform transabdominally in > 90% of fetuses. However, to ensure precise measurements, one might occasionally need to perform this measurement transvaginally (Fig 1).

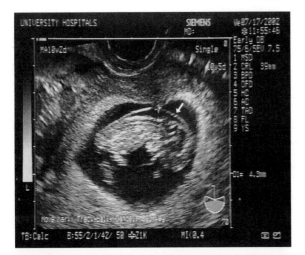

FIGURE 1. Abnormally thickened nuchal translucency in a first trimester fetus with Down syndrome (*arrow*).

10. How should one interpret the NT width study result?

A threshold of 3 mm was used in many studies for an abnormal NT. Currently, the more accepted method bases the cutoff on a progressive rise, using the 95th percentile as the threshold for an abnormal measurement. This results in a more sensitive and specific indicator for the detection of abnormal fetuses. The nuchal thickness normally increases with increasing CRL and medians have been established for each gestational age. Using these medians, the risk for trisomies can be calculated by multiplying the background risk based on maternal age and gestational age by a likelihood ratio, which depends on the degree of deviation in NT thickness from the normal median for that CRL.

11. Could a first trimester nuchal translucency study be used in twins gestation?

Researchers showed that in a twins pregnancy, the first trimester use of individual fetal NT thickness allowed the calculation of specific risk for each fetus. It was also concluded that this physical marker can specifically identify a fetus at increased risk.

12. Is there additional benefit for an NT study in twins gestation?

An NT screening was shown to be useful in monochorionic twin pregnancies to predict the subsequent development of severe twin-to-twin transfusion syndrome (TTS). It has been suggested that the underlying hemodynamic changes associated with TTS may manifest as increased fetal NT thickness between 10 and 14 weeks' gestation.

13. What is the detection rate of fetuses with abnormal chromosomes through a first trimester genetic sonogram?

When measured according to well-defined guidelines, increased NT identifies about 80% of fetuses with chromosomal abnormalities, with a false-positive rate of 5%.

14. Could the detection rate for Down syndrome during the first trimester study be further improved?

Two maternal serum markers were found effective in screening for fetal Down syndrome during the first trimester: (1) maternal serum free-beta human chorionic gonadotropin (hCG) (about twice normal) and (2) maternal serum pregnancy-associated plasma protein (PAPP-A) (about 0.4 times normal). These markers can be combined to achieve a detection rate for fetal Down syndrome of approximately 62%, with a false-positive rate of 5%. When risk figures generated by maternal age and these markers are combined with the first trimester NT measurement, the detection efficiency for fetal Down syndrome increases to 87%, with a false-positive rate of 5%.

15. Does ethnic origin affect the accuracy of a first trimester study for chromosomal abnormalities?

In a first trimester study of white women, Afro-Caribbean women, and Asian women, the median maternal serum marker (MoMs) for free-beta hCG and PAPP-A were 21% and 57% higher, respectively, after weight correction in Afro-Caribbean women and 4% and 17% higher, respectively, in Asian women, than in white women. It is estimated that correcting for maternal weight and ethnicity would increase the detection rate by a modest 1.4%. However, the effect on an individual's risk could be a twofold increase in the patient specific risk for trisomy 21.

16. Could a first trimester screening identify specific risk figures for cases with chromosome abnormalities other than Down syndrome?

By combining NT studies with maternal serum free-beta hCG and PAPP-A, researchers can develop specific risk figures for cases with fetal triploidy (type I and II), trisomies 18 and 13, and cases of fetal sex chromosome abnormalities (45,X, 47,XXX, 47,XXY, and 47,XYY).

17. What is the natural history of fetuses with increased NT?

A potential disadvantage of screening during the first trimester of pregnancy is that earlier screening preferentially identifies those chromosomally abnormal pregnancies that are destined to miscarry or because the patient might elect to discontinue the pregnancy. Thus, natural history data are limited. The outcome of fetuses with increased NT thickness and trisomy 21, whose parents chose to continue with the pregnancy, has been reported in the literature. During the second trimester, the NT resolved in the majority of cases and evolved into nuchal edema in a small number of cases. Therefore, resolution of translucency with advancing gestation is not indicative of a normal karyotype. In the same study, all pregnancies resulted in live births, suggesting that increased NT does not necessarily identify those trisomic fetuses that are destined to die in utero.

18. If a fetus with increased NT is shown to have normal chromosomes, should one suspect other fetal abnormalities?

Studies show that fetuses with thickened NT can have normal chromosomes. The Cornelia de Lange, Noonan, Smith-Lemli-Opitz, Joubert, Apert, Fryns, and Roberts syndromes were reported among such cases. In addition, achondrogenesis, ectrodactyly-ectodermal dysplasia, and multiple pterygium syndromes were also reported. In addition, fetuses with abnormally thickened NT and normal chromosomes were shown to be at increased risk for major cardiac anomalies, diaphragmatic hernia, anterior wall defects, and fetal akinesia/dyskinesia syndrome.

19. Is a thickened NF invariably associated with poor fetal outcome?

Studies have concluded that, for the majority of pregnancies in which fetuses with mild nuchal thickening and normal chromosomes were followed up through early life, the outcome was favorable. However, because some of these patients had nonlethal anomalies that were undetectedable in the early stage of pregnancy, they should all be followed up with a detailed obstetric sonogram, including detailed cardiac evaluation at 18 to 22 weeks' gestation. If all examinations are normal, most such children are expected to be normal at birth. However, further long-term follow-up is advised.

SECOND TRIMESTER GENETIC SONOGRAM

20. What options are available for women at risk for fetal chromosome abnormality who choose not to undergo invasive diagnostic testing?

Maternal serum multiple marker screening and genetic sonogram are alternatives for more invasive prenatal diagnostic testing.

21. Describe the maternal multiple marker screen.

The most widely available screening option is the maternal serum multiple marker assay. The test measures four analytes in the maternal blood that are produced by the fetus or placenta. These analytes are alpha-fetoprotein (AFP), hCG, unconjugated estriol (uE3), and inhibin. To obtain accurate risk figures, one must consider fetal number, gestational age, maternal age, weight, and ethnicity. In addition, one needs to include the maternal glycemic status. By measuring all four analytes in conjunction with the above listed maternal data, one can generate individual risk figures for fetal chromosome abnormalities and birth defects. The test is performed between 15 and 22 weeks of pregnancy. This screening blood test is inexpensive, readily available, and practically risk free, and it has a reasonably good detection rate. The disadvantages of this test are (1) the varied detection rates for trisomy 21 in women of different maternal age, (2) the low sensitivity for the detection of chromosomal abnormality other than trisomies 21 and 18, and (3) the increased false-positive rates associated with advancing maternal age.

22. Describe the rationale and clinical utility of a second trimester genetic sonogram.

The use of prenatal ultrasound was proven efficacious for the prenatal diagnosis of chromosomal abnormalities. The first sonographic sign of Down syndrome, the thickened NF, was first described in 1985. Since then, other sonographically identifiable markers have been described as associated with Down syndrome. The genetic sonogram, involving a detailed search for sonographic signs of aneuploidy, can be used to both identify fetuses at high risk for aneuploidy and, when normal, decrease the risk for aneuploidy in a pregnancy in which no sonographic markers are identified. Combining the genetic sonogram with maternal serum screening may be the best method for assessing the aneuploidy risk for women who desire such assessment in the second trimester. Trisomy 18, trisomy 13, and triploidy are typically associated with sonographically identified abnormalities and have a high prenatal detection rate. The use of the described sonographic signs in low-risk women requires further investigation. However, patients at increased risk for aneuploidy because of advanced maternal age or abnormal serum screening can benefit from a genetic sonogram screening for sonographic signs of aneuploidy to adjust their baseline risk of an affected fetus.

23. Describe the ultrasonographic method used to study the NF width.
   In the second trimester, nuchal thickening is measured in the suboccipital-bregmatic planes (including cavum septi pellucidi, cerebral peduncles, cerebellar hemispheres, and cisterna magna) from the back of the skull to the outer skin edge. This should measure less than 6 mm. Care should be taken to avoid imaging an oblique plane, because this can falsely increase the amount of skin thickening (Fig 2).

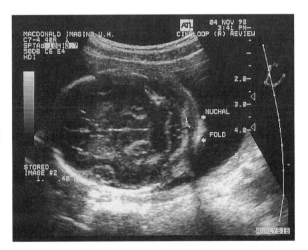

FIGURE 2. Nuchal thickening measurement in the suboccipital-bregmatic planes from the back of the skull to the outer skin edge (*within calipers*).

24. Are all fetal chromosome abnormalities associated with an abnormal sonogram?
   The majority of fetuses with triploidy and trisomies 18 and 13 display major anomalies and thus are recognized ultrasonically. On the other hand, only 25–33% of fetuses with Down syndrome demonstrate major malformations. Therefore, one must look for other ultrasonically detected markers to increase the detection rate for Down syndrome. Furthermore, major fetal malformations such as heart, brain, facial, skeletal, genitourinary, and gastrointestinal defects are known to be strongly associated with severe chromosome abnormality and therefore necessitate fetal chromosome study.

25. Which sonographic markers of the second trimester were reported to be associated with fetal trisomy 21?
   The most commonly used markers are short femur, short humerus, renal pyelectasis, increased NF thickening, echogenic bowel, iliac angle, and echogenic intracardiac focus. Additional sonographic markers such as short ears, hypoplasia of the middle phalanx, hypoplasia of the fifth digit, a shorter frontal lobe, choroid plexus cysts, and separation of the great toe (sandal gap foot) were also reported to confer a higher risk for fetal aneuploidy. However, these are more subtle features and are neither sensitive nor specific.

26. What is the Down syndrome sonographic index and how is it used with the second trimester genetic sonogram?

Starting in 1992, Benacerraf and colleagues developed a sonographic scoring index for the detection of chromosomal abnormalities, Down syndrome in particular. They showed that an NF ≥ 6 mm, major structural defects, short humerus, short femur, and pyelectasis could be quantitatively scored. Two points were given for a thickened NF or a major anomaly, and one point was given for each of three other findings: short femur, short humerus, and pyelectasis. A score ≥ 2 enabled the researchers to detect 81% of fetuses with Down syndrome, with a 4.4% false-positive rate.

27. Which sonographic markers are of highest yield for the detection of fetuses with Down syndrome?

It has been suggested that by using only three ultrasound markers (combination of NF thickening, pyelectasis, and short humerus), the false-positive rate is decreased from 13.4% to 6.7%, without any compromise in the sensitivity (87%). Thickened NF was shown to have the highest yield in detection.

BIBLIOGRAPHY

1. Benacerraf BR: The second-trimester fetuses with Down syndrome: Detection using sonographic features. Ultrasound Obstet Gynecol 7:147–155, 1996.
2. Benacerraf BR, Neuberg D, Bromley B, Frigoletto FD Jr: Sonographic scoring index for prenatal detection of chromosomal abnormalities. J Ultrasound Med 11:449–458, 1992.
3. Cha'ban FK, Van Splunder P, Los FJ, et al: Fetal outcome in nuchal translucency with emphasis on normal fetal karyotype. Prenat Diagn 16:537–541, 1996.
4. Hook EB, Cross PK, Schreinemahers DM: Chromosome abnormality rates at amniocentesis and in liveborn infants. JAMA 249:2034–2038, 1983.
5. Nyberg DA, Luthy DA, Resta RG, et al: Age-adjusted ultrasound risk assessment for fetal Down's syndrome during the second trimester: Description of the method and analysis of 142 cases. Ultrasound Obstet Gynecol 12:8–14, 1998.
6. Sebire NJ, Souka A, Skentou H, et al: Early prediction of severe twin-to-twin transfusion syndrome. Hum Reprod 15:2008–2010, 2000.
7. Shipp TD, Benacerraf BR: Second-trimester genetic sonography in patients with advanced maternal age and normal triple screen. Obstet Gynecol 99:993–995, 2002.
8. Souka AP, Snijders RJ, Novakov A, et al: Defects and syndromes in chromosomally normal fetuses with increased nuchal translucency thickness at 10–14 weeks of gestation. Ultrasound Obstet Gynecol 11:391–400, 1998.
9. Spencer K: Age related detection and false positive rates when screening for Down's syndrome in the first trimester using fetal nuchal translucency and maternal serum free beta hCG and PAPP-A. Br J Obstet Gynaecol 108:1043–1046, 2001.
10. Yagel S, Anteby EY, Rosen L, et al: Assessment of first-trimester nuchal translucency by daily reference intervals. Ultrasound Obstet Gynecol 11:262–265, 1998.

6. FIRST TRIMESTER SONOGRAPHY

Nancy E. Judge, M.D.

1. What scanning approach should be used for the pelvic and fetal structures in first trimester pregnancy studies?

Both transvaginal and transabdominal views will provide complementary information; usually, the transvaginal technique provides superior resolution of intrauterine structures, permitting early identification of sacs, cardiac activity, and optimum embryonic anatomic details. The transabdominal approach allows an overview of the uterine relationship to adjacent pelvic and abdominal structures and may permit visualization of large masses that extend beyond the field of the vaginal probe. Whichever scanning technique is chosen, both sagittal and transverse views, with measurements of the length and height on the sagittal plane and the width on the transverse view, should be obtained for the cervix, uterus, ovaries, and gestational and yolk sacs. Longitudinal measurement of the embryonic pole or crown-rump length can be added as gestation advances (Fig. 1).

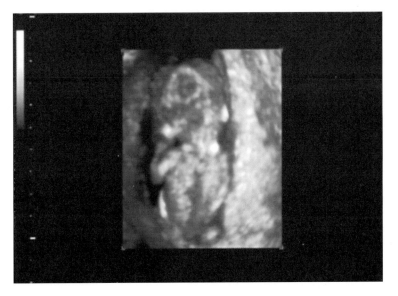

FIGURE 1. Three-dimensional longitudinal image of 13-week embryo.

2. Where should calipers be placed for gestational sac and yolk sac measurement?

The gestational sac should be measured from inner margin to inner margin and should *not* include the echogenic rim, which may vary significantly in width (Fig. 2). The gestational sac and yolk sac diameters should be averaged across three dimensions. In practice, yolk sac diameters are usually uniform and clinically less critical. A single data entry may be appropriate. A gestational sac is expected to be visible once the serum human chorionic gonadotropin (hCG) values exceed 1000–1200 IU.

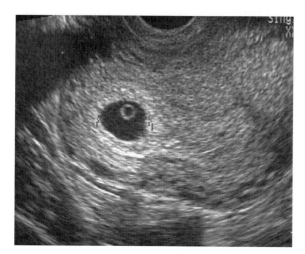

FIGURE 2. Incorrect caliper placement.

3. What is the method error for measurement of the embryonic pole?

The embryonic pole should be measured along its longest axis, with documentation of cardiac activity (if present). The method error is plus or minus 3 days at this stage (Fig. 3). The embryonic measurement is considered more accurate than the gestational sac for dating purposes.

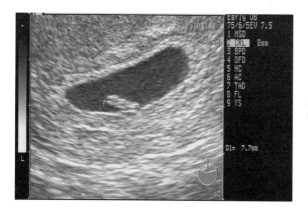

FIGURE 3. Method error of ± 3 days.

4. At what gestational age can the gestational sac view be reliably obtained?

At 5 menstrual weeks' gestation (5 mm mean sac diameter) (Fig. 4). The sac has been reported as early as 4½ weeks (2 mm). The echogenic rim should be at least 2 mm in thickness and brighter than the myometrium. The double rim should be visible once the sac reaches 10 mm in internal diameter.

5. When does the yolk sac normally become visible?

The yolk sac identified by ultrasound is actually the secondary yolk sac, which forms at 28 days, but is usually identified on the transvaginal scan at 5 weeks' gestation (mean gestational sac diameter 5 mm) (Fig. 5). The yolk sac should be visualized by 5.5 weeks (8 mm mean gestational sac diameter) at the latest in a viable pregnancy. By the transabdominal approach, the latter point is reached at 7 weeks, with a sac of 20 mm. The normal yolk sac rarely exceeds 6 mm in diameter at its maximum size. The structure cannot be visualized after the onset of the second trimester. The yolk sac is sometimes confused with the amnion in abnormal gestations when the embryo is not visible.

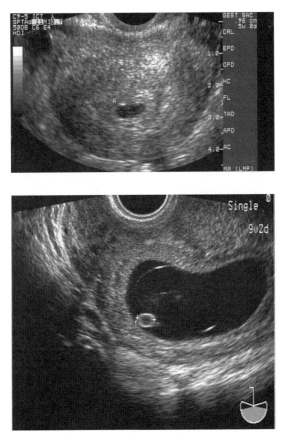

FIGURE 4. Five-week size gestational sac.

FIGURE 5. Transvaginal scan showing yolk sac at 5 weeks' gestation (mean gestational sac diameter 5 mm).

6. At what gestational sac size should the embryonic pole be visible?

The embryonic disc reaches 1–2 mm by the 6th gestational week, at a gestational sac size between 5 and 12 mm. Once ectopic gestation has been excluded, it is desirable but rarely medically urgent to establish that the pregnancy has implanted successfully and is "viable."

ULTRASOUND FINDING (TRANSVAGINAL)	NORMAL FOR EGA	HCG (3RD STANDARD IU)	DIFFERENTIAL DIAGNOSIS (NONHETEROTOPIC)	COMMENT/ACTION
Thickened uterine lining, normal stripe, eccentric sac	< 5 weeks	< 1200 (doubles every 48 hr)	Normal (< 5 wk) IUP, complete abortion, ectopic	Clinical evaluation; repeat hCG to confirm appropriate rise. Next scan timed for hCG ≥ 1200
Double sac, no pole, with or without YS	5.0–5.4 weeks	1000–2000 IU	Until YS present, normal early IUP, incomplete or missed abortion, less likely ectopic with decidual cast; if YS present, then normal IUP or missed abortion	The sac should grow by 0.6–1.0 mm daily. The hCG should be doubling appropriately. Multiple gestations may have higher hCG values without usual U/S findings.

Table continued on following page.

ULTRASOUND FINDING (TRANSVAGINAL)	NORMAL FOR EGA	HCG (3RD STANDARD IU)	DIFFERENTIAL DIAGNOSIS (NONHETEROTOPIC)	COMMENT/ACTION
Double sac 8–10 mm with YS, embryonic pole (2 mm) with or without cardiac motion	5.5 weeks	> 5000 IU	IUP, missed abortion	YS *always* present by 8 mm gestational sac size Embryo *always* present by 6 mm YS
Double sac, embryo, with or without cardiac motion	6 weeks	> 11,000 IU	IUP, missed abortion	Embryo and sac should grow 1 mm daily Cardiac activity always present by 5 mm embryo Rates < 80–100 bpm linked to high abortion risk
Sac, YS, pole, cardiac motion	6.5 weeks		IUP, missed abortion	Pole always present if sac > 18 mm Cardiac activity always present by this gestational age
Transabdominal approach feasible	7–8 weeks	> 35,000 IU	IUP, missed abortion	20 mm sac, 10 mm pole, FHT present, fetal movements

EGA = estimated gestational age; FHT = fetal heart tone; hCG = human chorionic gonadotropin; IUP = intrauterine pregnancy; U/S = ultrasound; YS = yolk sac.

7. In a viable pregnancy, what is the latest point by age and measurements at which cardiac activity should be identified?

Cardiac activity should be present 100% of the time by 6 weeks and 4 days (6.5 weeks) of gestation. At this point, the embryo has reached 5 mm in length within a gestational sac of 18 mm mean diameter (measured transvaginally). A missed abortion can also be confirmed transabdominally when the sac size measures 25 mm, or at 8 weeks confirmed gestational age.

8. With what ultrasound modality should cardiac activity be documented?

Because of its higher degree of resolution, the transvaginal approach is appropriate in questionable cases (Fig. 6). Real time B-mode cine or VCR clips can be used for documentation of cardiac activity at the extreme limits of early gestation; however, M-mode measurement is preferable (when feasible) because it permits quantification of the rate and comparison to the maternal rate. Either technique results in lower energy input to the embryo than Doppler interrogation.

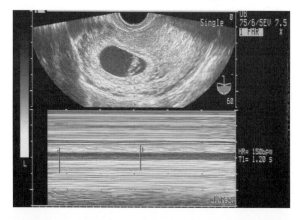

FIGURE 6. Transvaginal approach documenting cardiac activity.

9. What is the significance of the yolk sac number in multiple gestations?

For each amniotic sac, there should be a yolk sac. If two yolk sacs are visible, diamniotic twinning is virtually assured (Fig. 7), although there is a theoretic possibility of a rare exception. The converse is less reliable.

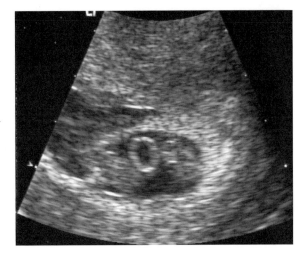

FIGURE 7. Monoamniotic twin pair in a triplet gestation.

10. What diagnosis does Figure 8 illustrate?

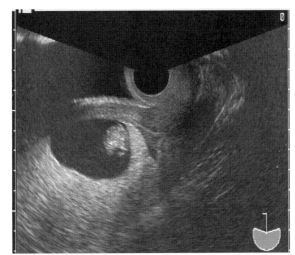

FIGURE 8

This is an intrauterine blood collection overlying the internal cervical os, with a complete posterior placenta previa. This image would not exclude a threatened or a missed abortion. Sixty percent of early studies will demonstrate a low-lying placenta or partial or complete previa. The majority of early lower segment placentation will resolve by the end of the second trimester secondary to both development of the lower segment and trophic placental growth away from the os. Central location and cord insertion near the cervix are ultrasonographic risk factors for persistence; anterior site in a patient with prior cesarean delivery is a clinical risk for both previa and accretion.

11. Does Figure 9 show a "blighted twin"?

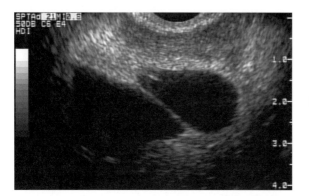

FIGURE 9

The sac has no evidence for either a yolk sac or embryonic pole, similar to a blighted gestation. The membrane and external decidual ring are thin and the latter is not well demarcated. However, unless previous scans had unequivocally identified a twin gestation, this image is more consistent with a synechium, a generally benign finding. Early pregnancy wastage of co-twins in multiple gestations is common, however. The "vanishing twin" may begin with similar or smaller measurements to the survivor but ceases to be viable in the first trimester. The sac is usually compressed and obscured by the surviving gestational elements, rather than resorbed or expelled. The differential diagnosis for a missed abortion of a co-twin also includes subchorionic hemorrhage and venous lakes, but these will not contain a fetal pole or yolk sac, requisite for the initial confirmation of a twin gestation.

12. What is the normal rate of growth for the embryonic pole?
The embryo and the amniotic sac increase in size by 1 mm/day and are similar to one another in size during the majority of the first trimester. These linear relationships permit simple estimations of the gestational age in days, by adding a constant of 30 or 42 to the mean sac diameter or the crown-rump length in millimeters, respectively. A valuable use for this feature is in timing a follow-up study to establish viability, based on critical thresholds for cardiac activity and sustained growth.

13. When does the placenta become localized to one portion of the uterine cavity?
The placenta rarely remains diffuse throughout gestation except in the condition known as *placenta membranacea* or *placenta diffusa*. Usually, the site of localization is signaled by thickened echogenic placental tissue, visible by the 10th week of gestation (Fig. 10). Localization of the placenta is essential in performing chorionic villus sampling.

14. What is the normal range for embryonic heart rates?
The relationship between gestational age and cardiac rates increases from initial identification until a plateau is reached at the 10th week. The rate of loss increases sharply for rates below 100 bpm; aneuploidy may be somewhat more frequent in embryos with rates above 160 bpm during the first trimester.

15. First trimester ultrasound is frequently performed on patients with excessive vomiting (hyperemesis gravidarum). Although an early viable pregnancy is the most common ultrasound diagnosis in these cases, what two conditions associated with hyperemesis are identified by ultrasound?
Multiple gestations and **gestational trophoblastic disease** frequently cause both high levels of hCG and hyperemesis gravidarum. Other conditions may have unusually high hCG values, including trisomy 21, intrauterine growth restriction, and poor obstetric outcome, but are less strongly linked to hyperemesis.

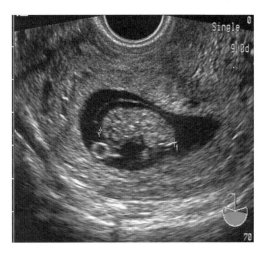

FIGURE 10. Thickened echogenic placental tissue.

16. What ovarian finding is associated with elevated hCG values?

Theca lutein cysts are often found in patients with molar pregnancies, multiple gestations, exogenous hCG, hydrops fetalis, and placentomegaly. The cysts are typically thin walled, bilateral, variable in size, and present risks for hemorrhage, necrosis, torsion and rupture; they generally regress within the puerperium.

17. What is the difference between molar degeneration, partial mole, and hydatidiform mole?

Molar degeneration is a pathologic descriptor for necrosis and hydropic swelling of villi, often found in abortion specimens. It is not a gestational trophoblastic disease. Because fluid-filled villi are more echogenic than normal, the ultrasound appearance may mimic early molar pregnancy. Hydatidiform moles and partial moles, on the other hand, have significant degrees of overlap, but are distinguished by the presence of fetal or amniotic elements in the latter. In addition to either a fetus or an amniotic sac, a partial mole is usually focal; genetically, it is found to have a high incidence (80%) of triploidy from paternal dispermy and nondysjunction. The hydatidiform mole is usually diploid but anembryonic, without an amniotic sac and characterized by hydropic, swollen, avascular villi with proliferation of the trophoblast. On ultrasound, the cavity may contain a "snow storm" of highly echogenic placental tissue interspersed with bizarre fluid collections reflecting areas of hemorrhage and fluid filled vesicles. Twenty percent of complete moles may develop trophoblastic tumors. Occasionally, a hydatidiform mole may occur in association with a viable co-twin, delaying diagnosis and producing a number of difficult management issues.

18. What is the most likely diagnosis for the ovarian finding in Figure 11?

FIGURE 11

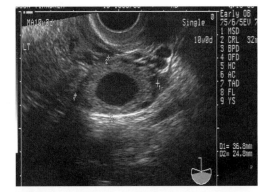

A thick-walled, simple, single ovarian cyst in pregnancy is consistent with a corpus luteum cyst. The cyst wall may be well vascularized, with low resistance, moderate-to-high velocity Doppler flow. The corpus luteum is hormonally essential for the maintenance of the pregnancy through the majority of the first trimester. A corpus luteum cyst may increase in size until 7–8 weeks' gestation, occasionally exceeding 6 cm in diameter. The cyst typically involutes by 14 weeks' gestation. In some cases, the corpus luteum may persist but without further growth until the puerperium. Less commonly, these cysts may undergo hemorrhagic changes, associated with pain, rupture and significant intraperitoneal bleeding, or torsion.

19. What proportion of first trimester pregnancies confirmed by ultrasound will abort?

The rate of spontaneous pregnancy loss is approximately 16% in low-risk patients. The finding of fetal cardiac activity reduces the likelihood of wastage to 5% at weeks 6–8 and to 2% after week 12. Patients with recurrent losses remain at high risk (in excess of 20%) in spite of documentation of cardiac activity, as do older gravidae.

20. What is the usual range of error for crown-rump length measurement?

Prior to 8 weeks' estimated gestational age (EGA), the crown-rump length measurement actually represents embryonic disc length (week 6) succeeded by a neck-tail length; it remains accurate to 8%, or 3–5 days through 11 weeks (Fig. 12).

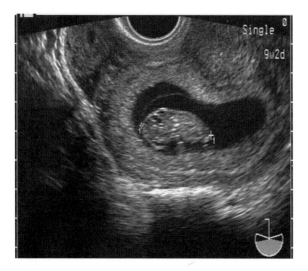

FIGURE 12. Crown-rump measurement at 9 weeks, 2 days.

21. What is the proper technique for measuring the nuchal translucency?

The measurement should be obtained between 11 and 14 weeks' gestation. The fetal neck should be in a neutral position (Fig. 13). The amnion should be separately visualized, distinct from the fetal tissues. The calipers should be placed from inner surface to inner surface of the fold. Measurements greater than 3 mm are associated with an increased risk of aneuploidy, particularly trisomy 13, other anomalies, and adverse outcomes. Median values by crown-rump length can be combined with serologic markers for 80% or greater sensitivity with a 5% false-positive rate.

22. At what gestational age is chorionic villus sampling for genetic diagnosis usually performed?

Current practice in the United States limits chorionic sampling to 10 weeks or later because of reports of oromandibular-limb hypogenesis defects from procedures at earlier gestational ages (Fig. 14). The transvaginal approach becomes more technically difficult after 13 weeks' gestation.

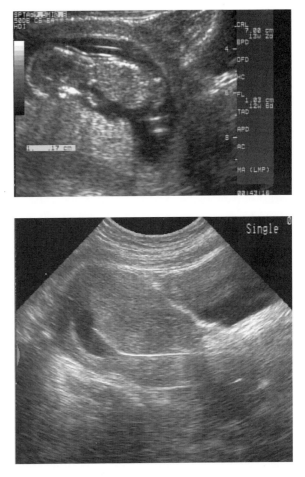

FIGURE 13. Fetal neck in neutral position.

FIGURE 14. An echogenic curved transvaginal chorionic villus sampling catheter within the uterine cavity. The villi are cultured to provide karyotypes and other genetic diagnostic information.

23. What is the most likely finding on karyotype at time of chorionic villus sampling of the pregnancy shown in Figure 15?

Approximately 75% of fetuses with cystic hygromas are aneuploid; of the aneuploidies, about 60% are monosomy X (Turner syndrome) (Fig. 15). Other chromosomal abnormalities include

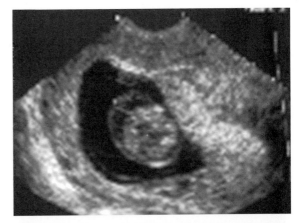

FIGURE 15. Transverse view of head and neck at 10 weeks' gestation.

trisomies 21 and 18 and triploidy. Fetuses with normal karyotypes may have Noonan's syndrome, multiple pterygia, Pena-Shokeir syndrome, or Roberts' syndrome. Cystic hygromas result from an interruption in the path of lymphatic return to the heart via the jugular vein, usually present by day 40 of life. Septate, massive cystic hygromas likely reflect one extreme of a spectrum of nuchal lucencies, with milder forms linked to trisomy 21. This is one of the most common, reliably identified, first trimester structural anomalies; the rate of spontaneous abortion and intrauterine demise may reach 90% when there are associated effusions or hydrops. Resolution to a webbed neck with neonatal survival is more common with isolated, nonseptate, small lucencies. Cardiac and renal abnormalities are frequent associations.

24. How can one alter the fetal position in the first trimester?
Wait for spontaneous movement, vary transducer pressure against the lower segment and cervix, or ask the patient to cough or laugh. The requisite first trimester views, including nuchal lucency, can be obtained within 10–20 minutes in the majority of normal singleton gestations.

25. Through what gestational age is the view in Figure 16 considered a normal finding?

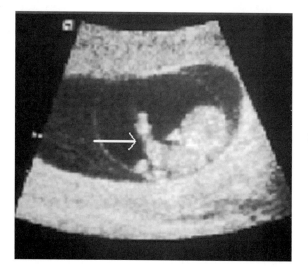

FIGURE 16

The arrow points to the physiologic herniation of the gut. Completion of the external rotation and closure of the anterior abdominal wall occurs by 11^{5}/$_{7}$ weeks (45 mm crown-rump length). The measurement at the base of the cord should not normally exceed 7 mm, and neither the stomach nor the liver should be identified in the cord at any point. Omphaloceles with liver involvement have been identified as early as 9 weeks' gestation.

26. Of cataracts, biliary atresia, transposition of the great arteries, and exencephaly, which has not been identified by ultrasound in the first trimester?
Biliary atresia. The normal fetal gallbladder is not usually visualized prior to 16–17 weeks' gestation. Exencephaly (Fig. 17) is more reliably identified in the first trimester than other neural tube defects because of the characteristic brain mass extruded above relatively normal facial bones. Routine use of first trimester screening for malformations complements, but does not replace, traditional midtrimester assessment for most lesions.

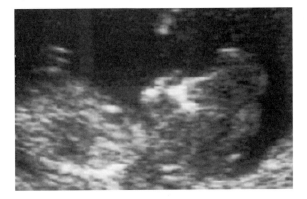

FIGURE 17. Exencephaly in a 13-week fetus.

27. What additional ultrasound concerns are raised by the finding in Figure 18?

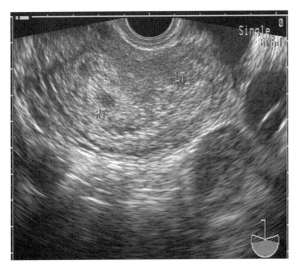

FIGURE 18. Transverse uterine view through transvaginal approach at 6 weeks' gestation.

A bicornuate uterus is a form of müllerian duplication. Maternal views should include renal and ureteral structures because of an increased rate of duplications and anomalies. An attempt should also be made to exclude cornual and extrauterine implantation of additional sacs. There may be duplication of the cervix or vagina in these patients; length of the cervix is also of concern because patients with müllerian anomalies may have an increased risk of cervical incompetence. Documentation of the placental site and fetal renal anatomy are features that should be included in later studies.

28. What proportion of unassisted conceptions will result in triplets?
The natural rate of twinning is approximately 1% (with variability across ethnicity, age, and hormonal therapy use), with triplets estimated at 1 in 1000 births. A factor of 10 is used to estimate the occurrence for each higher order of multiples; however, assisted reproductive techniques can dramatically alter the likelihood of both multiple and heterotopic gestations. The majority of multiple gestations are dizygotic with increased rates based on ethnicity, family history, maternal age, parity, and medication use. Uniquely, *in vitro* techniques also may increase the frequency of monozygotic multiple gestations.

29. What are the potential advantages to assigning chorionicity in multiple gestations?

Because 95% of the less common monozygotic twinning is monochorionic, a dichorionic placentation is generally dizygotic. The risk for one or the other of a dizygotic pair to be aneuploid is
effectively double the patient's age-related risk (although for both to be affected is the product of the
probabilities). In contrast, monochorionic twins (Fig. 19) share the age-related risk of aneuploidy, as
well as a markedly higher rate of malformations and perinatal mortality. In addition, the potentially
deadly twin-twin transfusion syndrome only affects diamniotic, monochorionic twins. Although the
appearance of the membrane and chorionic plate has been used effectively in identification of
dizygotic twins in later gestation, early gestational sac appearance is highly sensitive and specific.

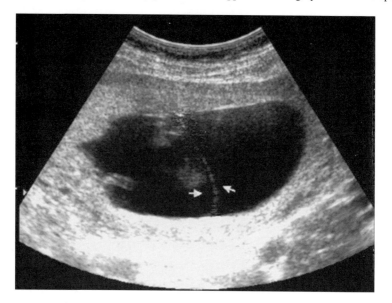

FIGURE 19. Monochorionic twins.

30. What complications have been reported with genetic amniocentesis prior to 15 weeks?

Early amniocentesis, performed between 10 and 14 weeks, is associated with a higher rate of
pregnancy loss (2–4%), failure to obtain samples, a higher rate of cell culture failure, clubbed foot
deformities, and amniotic band formation.

31. When can complete renal agenesis with anhydramnios be confirmed?

Although posterior urethral valves and megacystis have been described at 11 weeks' gestation, and the fetal kidneys and bladder (Fig. 20) are often identified by 12 weeks, anhydramnios

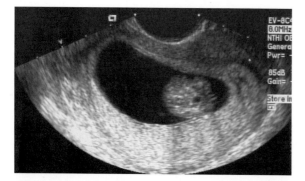

FIGURE 20. Oblique abdominal
view of fetal bladder.

is almost never present prior to 15 weeks' gestation because of amniotic fluid production by the fetal membranes.

32. Is the fluid-filled central nervous system structure shown in Figure 21 in an 8 weeks' gestation embryo evidence of abnormality?

FIGURE 21

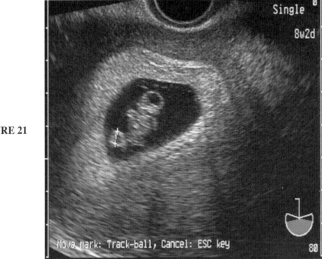

This view is consistent with a normal rhombencephalon. However, an unequivocal distinction between the rhombencephalon and mesencephalon would also require a sagittal projection.

33. What is the likely diagnosis for the uterine finding in Figure 22?

FIGURE 22

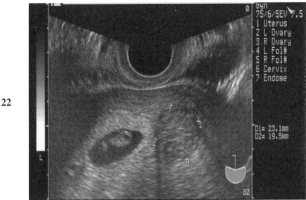

This well-demarcated, rounded, whorled region is consistent with a uterine myoma. The chief differential is with focal uterine contractures; the latter may persist for $\geq$ 45 minutes and are generally better vascularized.

34. A patient with a previously confirmed viable intrauterine gestation presents for ultrasound evaluation (Fig. 23) after vaginal passage of "some tissue" at home. Her physician wonders if she has had a complete abortion. How can ultrasound aid in this determination?
Clinical determination of a complete abortion relies on a cessation of symptoms, generally pain and bleeding, paired with physical examination confirming a closed cervix and a well-contracted uterus. Ultrasound findings that contradict the diagnosis include identification of a gestational sac or > 1 cm^3 of echogenic tissue within the cavity.

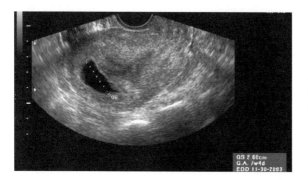

FIGURE 23. A longitudinal image from the patient's transvaginal ultrasound.

35. What is the difference between a threatened and an inevitable abortion?
A **threatened** abortion consists of bleeding with or without cramping in the first 20 weeks of gestation. Up to one third of pregnancies may have some bleeding, and about half abort. An **inevitable** abortion is defined by the rupture of membranes and cervical dilatation.

36. What is the difference between a missed abortion and blighted ovum?
A missed abortion occurs when a nonviable gestation remains within the uterus, generally without excessive bleeding or contractions. When no embryonic pole is identified in a nonviable pregnancy, the term *blighted ovum* is sometimes used. Missed abortions may lack both a yolk sac and embryonic material and may have a very small gestational sac. Clinical correlation with serial hCG levels and verification of dating may be needed to exclude ectopic gestations or early viable pregnancy with erroneous dates. Eventually, the majority of these gestations will abort spontaneously. Significant maternal coagulopathy may rarely occur with prolonged retention of dead midtrimester fetuses.

37. A patient undergoing treatment for infertility presents with decreased urinary output and painful abdominal distention; her qualitative hCG is positive. Her sonographic findings are shown in Figure 24; what do they indicate?
The finding of a large cystic structure in the cul de sac is consistent with ovarian hyperstimulation secondary to exogenous gonadotropins and early pregnancy. A large hydrosalpinx or other ovarian cysts including torsion would have a similar appearance. Doppler interrogation would be valuable in evaluation of torsion and neoplasia. Ascites or free cul de sac fluid might have a similar static appearance but would tend to layer around visceral structures. After clinical confirmation, the patient will benefit from fluid and electrolyte support.

BIBLIOGRAPHY

1. American College of Obstetricians and Gynecologists: ACOG practice bulletin. Clinical management guidelines for obstetrician-gynecologists. Prenatal diagnosis of fetal chromosomal abnormalities. Obstet Gynecol 97(5 pt 1):S1–S12, 2001.

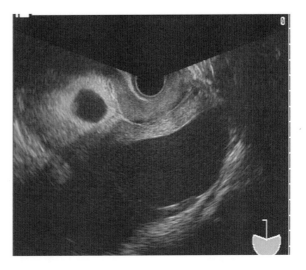

FIGURE 24. Sagittal transvaginal view showing a large cystic structure in the cul de sac.

2. Bromley B, Benacerraf B: Using the number of yolk sacs to determine amnionicity in early first trimester monochorionic twins. J Ultrasound Med 14:415–417, 1995.
3. Cunningham FG, Gant N, Leveno KJ, et al (eds): Williams Obstetrics, 21st ed. New York, McGraw-Hill, 2001.
4. Guidelines for performance of the antepartum obstetric ultrasound examination. J Ultrasound Med 15:185–188, 1996.
5. Laing FC, Frates MC: Ultrasound evaluation during the first trimester of pregnancy. In Callen PW (ed): Ultrasonography in Obstetrics and Gynecology, 4th ed. Philadelphia, W.B. Saunders, Philadelphia, 2000.
6. Lyons EA, Levi CS, Dashefsky SF: The first trimester. In Rumack CM, Wilson SR, Charboneau JW (eds): Diagnostic Ultrasound, vol. 2, 2nd ed. St. Louis, Mosby, 1998.
7. Nyberg DA, Hill LM, Bohm-Velez M, Mendelson EB (eds): Transvaginal Ultrasound. St. Louis, Mosby, 1992.
8. Sanders RC (ed): Structural Fetal Abnormalities: The Total Picture, 2nd ed. St. Louis, Mosby, 2002.
9. Timor-Tritsch IE, Monteagudo A, Cohen HL: Ultrasonography of the Prenatal and Neonatal Brain, 2nd ed. New York, McGraw-Hill, 2001.

7. SECOND AND THIRD TRIMESTER ULTRASOUND EVALUATION

Vernon D. Cook, M.D., and Dinesh M. Shah, M.D.

TRANSVAGINAL IMAGING

1. Can cervical length be reliably measured by transabdominal scanning?

No. Comparison of transabdominal and transvaginal images reveals that transvaginal evaluation of cervical length is significantly more accurate than transabdominal measurement (Fig. 1).

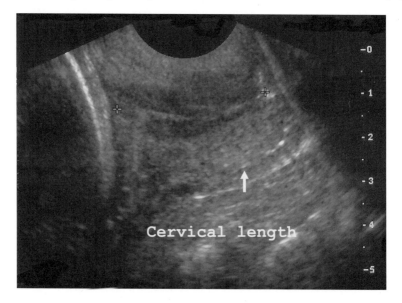

FIGURE 1. Endovaginal ultrasound demonstrates the cervical length (*within the calipers*) and arrow points to cervix.

2. What common factors adversely affect measurement of cervical length?

A partially distended or full bladder artificially elongates the cervical length. Thus, the bladder should be empty or nearly so when evaluating cervical length. Contraction of the lower uterine segment or a uterine myoma can obscure the location of the internal os, resulting in overestimation of cervical length.

3. In evaluating for the presence or absence of preterm labor, what signs may be sought during transvaginal imaging of the cervix?

Measurement of cervical length, cervical funneling (i.e., descent of membranes and amniotic fluid into the upper cervical canal), and cervical dynamicism may be evaluated as signs of preterm labor or cervical incompetence.

4. What is cervical dynamicism and when is it observed?

The term *cervical dynamicism* describes a cervix that exhibits marked funneling of membranes and amniotic fluid within the cervical canal only while a uterine contraction is present. In the absence of a uterine contraction or manual fundal pressure, such a cervix may appear normal.

5. What is the average (mean) length of a normal cervix on transvaginal ultrasound examination and what is an abnormally short cervical length?

The mean cervical length is 3.5 cm. An easy-to-remember clinical rule is that, by 0.5-cm increments, cervical length centiles are as follows: first centile, 1.5 cm; 5th centile, 2.0 cm; 10th centile, 2.5 cm; 25th centile, 3.0 cm, 50th centile (mean) 3.5 cm, and 75th centile, 4.0 cm. A cervical length of 2.5 cm or less may be considered abnormally short, depending on the clinical circumstances.

6. Describe the measurement technique of a cervix that exhibits funneling.

A cervix that exhibits funneling may be described by the following three measurements:

1. The length of the cervical canal that remains closed
2. The length of the funnel as measured along the cervix to the estimated location of the internal os
3. The dilation at the internal os

7. What ultrasonographic signs suggest cervical incompetence (CI)?

During the second or early third trimester, a cervical length < 2.5 cm with funneling is suggestive, but not diagnostic, of CI. CI is a clinical rather than sonographic diagnosis.

8. What are some causes of CI?

CI may be caused by congenital factors (water diethylstilbestrol exposure), cervical trauma from procedures or childbirth, hormonal factors, or a combination of influences.

COMPLICATIONS, ANOMALIES, AND ANEUPLOIDY

9. How do marginal, partial, complete, and central placenta previa differ?

A **marginal placenta previa** lies within 2–3 cm of the internal cervical os but does not overlie the internal os. A **partial placenta previa** partially overlies but does not overlap (i.e., go across) the internal os. A **complete previa** completely covers (i.e., goes across) the internal cervical os. In a **central placenta previa,** the placenta is approximately centered over the internal os and covers both the anterior and posterior and the lateral lower uterine segments.

10. What are the optimal imaging routes to differentiate these entities?

The optimal imaging route to evaluate placenta previa is determined by the presence or absence of vaginal bleeding. In the absence of vaginal bleeding, the relationship of the inferior placental margin to the internal cervical os is optimally evaluated by transvaginal sonography. In the presence of vaginal bleeding, transabdominal imaging should be initially performed because transvaginal examination might disturb the uteroplacental interface and exacerbate the bleeding. If the cervical-placental relationship is not clearly defined on transabdominal examination, transvaginal examination may be performed to further assess the cervical-placental relationship, pending clinical assessment of the amount of bleeding, anatomic factors, and patient consent. On occasion, transperineal (also called translabial) sonography may be helpful in evaluating the relationship of the placenta to the internal cervical os.

11. Describe a placental abruption.

A placental abruption refers to separation of the placental-decidual interface by active bleeding, fresh clot, or a resolving clot in the process of autolysis. Small abruptions frequently do not involve retention of a sufficiently large quantity of blood or clot within the uterine cavity to be evident on ultrasound examination.

Usually a placental abruption is accompanied by vaginal bleeding. However, a placental abruption may be concealed, such that a large collection of blood and clot may be contained within the uterine cavity that has not yet dissected a path between the amniotic membranes and decidua to the cervical canal, to become evident as vaginal bleeding.

12. In a pregnant patient with a prior cesarean section and placental implantation directly underlying the cesarean section scar, what abnormality of the placenta might ultrasound examination detect and what are the ultrasonic signs of this condition?

Placenta accreta is present in up to 25% of pregnancies in which the placental site underlies a prior cesarean section scar. Signs of placenta accreta include irregularly shaped sonolucent areas within the placenta and areas of placental invasion through the uterus into the bladder including loss of the normal, thin sonolucent area between the placenta and uterus. Large venous sinuses and an increased arterial network, especially on the outer surface of the uterus, suggest a high risk for severe hemorrhage.

13. What structures in the fetal brain should be routinely and adequately imaged on a second or third trimester sonogram? What views include these structures? What measurements does each view provide?

The lateral ventricles, choroid plexus, cerebellum, cisterna magna, cerebellar vermis, cavum septum pellucidum, and thalami with a normal third ventricle are components of a normal examination in a second or third trimester sonogram.

The transthalamic view depicts the thalamus. The biparietal diameter, head circumference, and occipital-frontal diameters are measured in this view.

The transcerebellar view includes the configuration of the cerebellum (including the vermis and fourth ventricle) and the cisterna magna. The cerebellar diameter, the nuchal thickness (before 21 weeks), and occasionally the cisterna magna are measured on this view.

The transventricular view depicts the lateral ventricles and the choroid plexus. The ventricular diameter is measured if enlargement is suspected (Fig. 2).

14. What is the optimal gestational age at which to evaluate a fetus for congenital anomalies?

The optimal timing of ultrasound examination varies among practitioners and is based on the patient's medical concern. Women desiring evaluation for fetal aneuploidy or other abnormalities often have examinations performed at 15–18 weeks, which may coincide with amniocentesis or maternal serum screen. However, follow-up examination at later gestational age may be required for optimal evaluation of some structures (e.g., heart). Low-risk patients often have a single ultrasound examination at 18–22 weeks for anatomic survey of the fetus.

15. What documentation is required by the American Institute of Ultrasound Medicine (AIUM) criteria for fetal anatomy survey in the second trimester?
- Fetal life, number, presentation, and activity
- Amniotic fluid volume
- Placental location
- Assessment of gestational age
- Fetal weight

The study should include, but not necessarily be limited to, the following:
- Cerebral ventricles
- Posterior fossa (including cerebellar hemispheres and cisterna magna)
- Four-chamber view of the heart
- Views of spine, stomach, kidneys, and urinary bladder
- Fetal umbilical cord insertion site
- Determination of intactness of the anterior abdominal wall

Suspected anomalies may require targeted evaluation of the area of concern.

16. What measurements are used to calculate the cephalic ratio and of what practical use is it? When is the cephalic ratio commonly abnormal?

The cephalic ratio (CI) equals the biparietal diameter (BPD) divided by the occipital frontal diameter. *Brachycephaly* is defined as a CI less than 0.70 and *dolicocephaly* is defined as a CI greater

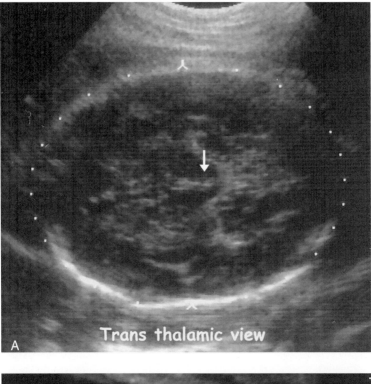

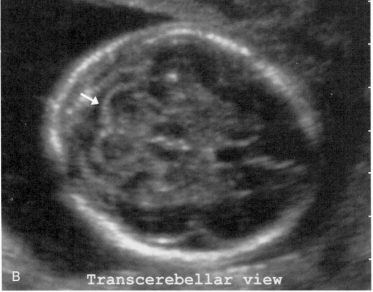

FIGURE 2. *A*, Transthalamic view (*arrow* points to thalamus). The head circumference and biparietal diameter should be measured at this level. *B*, Transcerebellar view. The cisterna magna is measured at this level (*arrow*).

than 0.86. When either brachycephaly or dolicocephaly is present, then the BPD is not a reliable indicator of the gestational age and it must then be excluded in calculating the gestational age.

The CI is commonly abnormal whenever marked molding of the fetal head is present, such as may occur with breech presentation.

17. The standard views of the fetal face include which structures? Which additional views of the face do many centers commonly document?

The 1994 AIUM standards for obstetric sonography do not mention examination of the fetal face. However, most centers routinely image the lips, the anterior maxilla, the nose, the orbits, and a profile view of the mandible (Fig. 3).

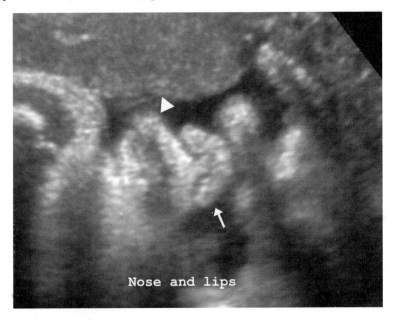

FIGURE 3. Coronal view of the nose (*arrow*) and lips (*arrowhead*).

18. Describe two criteria that define ventriculomegaly.

Ventriculomegaly is present if the atrium of the lateral ventricle measures ≥ 10 mm in transverse diameter. Normally the medial margin of the choroid plexus lies immediately adjacent to the medial wall of the lateral ventricle. Another criteria of ventriculomegaly is a dangling choroid plexus sign that consists of two observations. The initial sign of mild ventriculomegaly is a narrow wedge of cerebrospinal fluid between the medial side of the choroid plexus and the medial wall of the lateral ventricle. When ventriculomegaly is more pronounced, the free-floating portion of the choroid plexus (which is heavier than cerebrospinal fluid) sinks or dangles within the dilated ventricle (Fig. 4).

19. What is nuchal thickness and what is the role of nuchal thickness in screening for congenital anomalies?

The terms *nuchal thickness* and *nuchal fold* are synonymous. They refer to measurement of the tissue (including the skin) that overlies the occipital bone in the plane that includes the cavum septum pellucidum and the cerebellum. From the 15th through the 20th week of gestation, nuchal thickness measurements should be less than 5–6 mm. Before 15 weeks, nuchal sonolucency technique is used rather than nuchal thickness technique. Evaluation of nuchal thickness after 20 weeks' gestation has not been widely addressed in the literature.

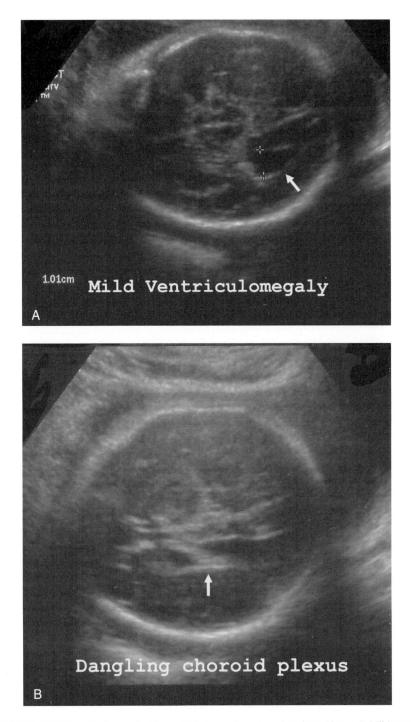

FIGURE 4. *A,* Mild ventriculomegaly. The ventricle (*arrow*) measures just above 10 mm. *B,* Mild ventriculomegaly depicting dangling choroids. The arrow points to the choroid plexus.

20. What is the differential diagnosis of increased nuchal thickness?

Although most fetuses with increased nuchal thickness are normal, the differential diagnosis of increased nuchal thickness includes an increased risk of fetal aneuploidy, particularly trisomy 21. Improper image plane is a potential etiology of factitiously increased nuchal thickness.

21. What is nuchal translucency?

The terms *nuchal translucency* and *nuchal sonolucency* are synonymous. They refer to measurement of the posterior nuchal sonolucent region between the skin and neck musculature. It is measured in sagittal section while the crown-rump length is 45–84 mm (i.e., at approximately 10–14 weeks' gestation).

22. What is a choroid plexus cyst and what is its significance?

A choroid plexus cyst is an oval or round sonolucent collection of cerebral spinal fluid (CSF) area within the choroid plexus. Even though they are most frequently single and unilateral, they can also be bilateral or multiple. Approximately 1% of fetuses have a choroid plexus cyst. They thus constitute the most common intracranial "abnormality" observed prenatally.

Choroid plexus cysts have a weak (less than 1% incidence) association with trisomy 18. Further evaluation and counseling regarding this finding may be desired by the patient.

23. What is cystic hygroma?

A cystic hygroma represents bilateral dilation of the jugular lymph sacs. It is usually readily distinguishable from increased nuchal thickness based on the presence of large, bilaterally symmetrical, posterior nuchal cysts with a midline septum.

24. According to the most recent (1994) AIUM guidelines for a basic examination, is measurement of the nuchal thickness a routine component of the basic examination?

When the AIUM guidelines were written, nuchal thickness measurements were not widely used, and thus were not specified as a component of the basic examination.

25. Of the three planes in which the spinal column is usually imaged, which is most helpful to evaluate subtle defects of the spine?

The spine can be imaged in sagittal, coronal, and transverse (or axial) planes. The transverse plane is most sensitive for evaluating subtle defects of individual vertebral segments in that it evaluates the vertebral pedicles of each vertebral segment. Sagittal or parasagittal and coronal views can image large portions of the spinal column in a single view.

26. What is the sensitivity of cranial signs in screening for spina bifida?

Greater than 99% of fetuses with spina bifida have cranial abnormalities observable on ultrasound examination.

27. Name the three most common cranial abnormalities associated with spina bifida.

The lemon sign, the banana sign, and ventriculomegaly are strongly associated with spina bifida.

28. Describe the lemon sign.

The lemon sign consists of flattening or slight indentation of the frontal bones and slight angulation of the frontal-parietal suture, such that, on axial view, the calvarium has a lemon shape.

29. What is the Arnold-Chiari type II malformation? Describe its ultrasonic appearance.

The Arnold-Chiari malformation represents herniation of the brain stem through the foramen magnum with compression of the cerebellum in the posterior fossa and consequent obliteration of the cisterna magna. It is from this compression that the cerebellum has a banana shape rather than a normal bulbar appearance on ultrasound examination.

30. In the normal population, what is the false-positive incidence of the lemon and banana signs?

Approximately 1% of normal fetuses have a (false-positive) mild lemon sign. False-positive cerebellar signs of spina bifida are virtually nonexistent.

31. If the cerebellum cannot be visualized because of fetal position or attenuation, what else might be done to evaluate the cerebellum?

If the posterior fossa cannot be satisfactorily visualized on transabdominal examination, at least three methods of further evaluation may be performed:

1. If the fetus is in cephalic presentation, transvaginal examination often provides satisfactory visualization of the posterior fossa throughout the second and into the third trimesters.

2. Follow-up evaluation of the posterior fossa may successfully image the posterior fossa.

3. Maternal serum alpha fetoprotein screening for spina bifida can be offered when the posterior fossa cannot be visualized.

32. In the second trimester, which is more readily apparent, the cranial signs of spina bifida or a spinal defect itself?

The cranial signs of spina bifida are often more readily apparent and more easily observed than direct images of a spina bifida defect.

33. A basic examination of the fetal heart includes which views and structures?

A basic examination of the heart would optimally include a four-chamber view, a view of the left outflow tract, and the right outflow tract. The four-chamber view includes the following structures: the right and left atria and ventricles and the symmetrical size thereof, the tricuspid and mitral valves, the foramen ovale, the atrial septum, the interventricular septum, the thickness of the cardiac muscles, and the pericardial space. Views of the left and right outflow tracts depict the origin, the approximately equivalent diameter of the two great vessels, and their anatomic relation as they cross at approximately a right angle.

34. Describe the cardiac axis in the fetal chest and its significance.

The mean cardiac axis is approximately 45° to the left of the midline but may vary from about 30–60° in normal fetuses. An abnormal cardiac axis is a strong sign that congenital heart disease or a mass in the pleural cavity may be present.

35. What percent of heart abnormalities can be anticipated to be discovered by a four-chamber view alone as compared to a four-chamber view with views of the outflow tracts?

An optimal four-chamber view alone detects approximately 60% of congenital heart disease, whereas a four-chamber view in combination with views of the outflow tracts may detect approximately 80% of congenital heart disease.

36. Name the limiting factors that frequently result in a suboptimal examination of the fetal heart.

Factors that may limit the examination of the heart commonly include early gestational age, fetal position, shadowing from overlying structures, and attenuation related to maternal size.

37. What does an echogenic intracardiac focus (EIF) represent and what is the frequency of this finding?

An EIF is a bright specular echo from the papillary muscles or chordae tendinae that may correlate with foci of mineralization in these structures. EIF are observed in 3–4% of fetuses and may vary in frequency by ethnic group, possibly being more frequent in Asians. In women with risk factors for fetal aneuploidy (e.g., age, other ultrasound findings), an EIF has been considered a possible additional risk factor for aneuploidy (Fig. 5).

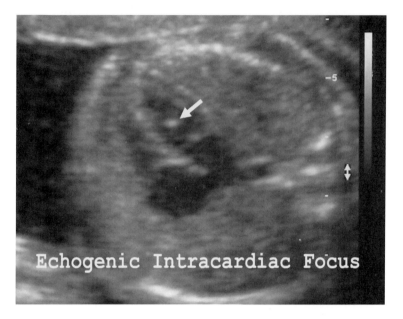

FIGURE 5. Four-chamber view of the heart demonstrates intracardiac echogenic focus (*arrow*).

38. Why and how should the fetal diaphragm be examined?

The diaphragm should be carefully examined to evaluate for diaphragmatic hernia. The diaphragm is examined both directly and indirectly, based on position of adjacent organs, particularly the stomach. The diaphragm is imaged in coronal and parasagittal planes. On transverse plane, the diaphragm should *not* be adjacent to the fetal heart. On coronal section, the stomach should be below the diaphragm. On direct examination of the diaphragm, the hemidiaphragms appear as thin, relatively sonolucent lines between the pleural and abdominal compartments (Fig. 6).

39. Describe a diaphragmatic hernia.

A diaphragmatic hernia consists of a diaphragmatic defect with herniation of abdominal viscera into a hemithorax. The most common ultrasonic signs of diaphragmatic hernia include a mass in the chest cavity, rotation of the cardiac axis, and, in an axial view of the chest, presence of the stomach bubble adjacent to the heart.

40. Landmarks that indicate correct position to measure the abdominal circumference include what organs?

The abdominal circumference is measured on transverse section at the level of the fetal stomach and the umbilical vein (Fig. 7).

41. At what gestational age should the stomach be readily observable?

If the stomach is not apparent by 14 weeks' gestation, congenital anomaly should be suspected.

42. Describe some technical factors that may cause apparent echogenic fetal bowel.

During the second trimester, the mildly hyperechoic echo texture of normal fetal bowel (as compared to liver) may be accentuated by use of a high-frequency transducer. One should also account for time-gain compensation curve and location of the focal zone to evaluate bowel for echogenicity. A good rule of thumb is that for bowel to be considered echogenic, it should be of similar echogenicity to bone as also viewed in the same image.

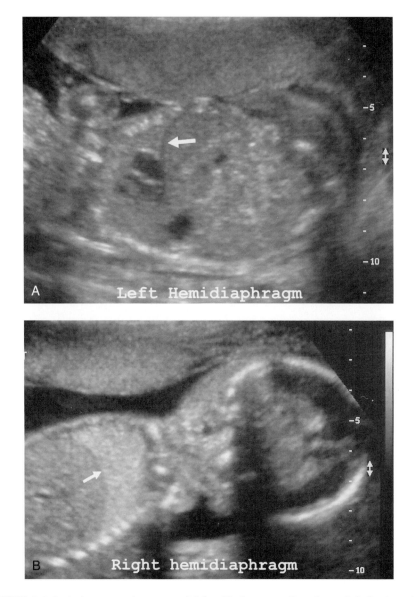

FIGURE 6. *A,* Sagittal sonogram demonstrates left hemidiaphragm as a linear hypoechoic line (*arrow*). *B,* Sagittal sonogram demonstrates right hemidiaphragm as a linear hypoechoic line (*arrow*).

43. What is the differential diagnosis of echogenic fetal bowel? When echogenic bowel is present, what percent of fetuses have a normal outcome?

Of fetuses with echogenic bowel, approximately 85% are normal and approximately 15% have an abnormal outcome. Abnormal outcomes associated with echogenic bowel include aneuploidy (e.g., trisomy 21), cystic fibrosis, congenital infection (including cytomegalovirus, herpes virus, varicella-zoster virus, parvovirus), bowel complications such as obstruction or perforation, fetal growth restriction, and an increased incidence of fetal demise.

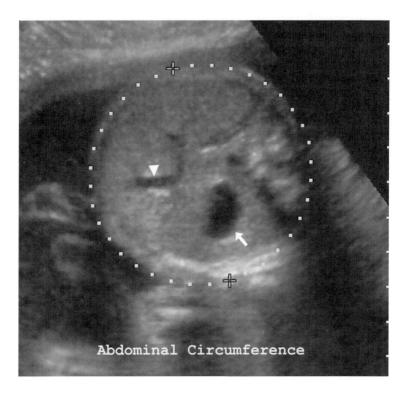

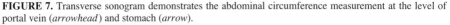

FIGURE 7. Transverse sonogram demonstrates the abdominal circumference measurement at the level of portal vein (*arrowhead*) and stomach (*arrow*).

44. Does measurement of the femur length include or exclude the epiphysis of the femoral head and the distal condyles?
The femoral head and the distal condyles are cartilaginous structures that are not yet ossified and therefore are not measured as part of the femoral length.

45. Which extremities are included in the routine examination of a normal fetus?
Even though the 1994 AIUM guidelines do not address documenting each extremity, it has become common practice to do so.

46. What are rocker bottom feet?
Rocker bottom feet refer to feet in which the arch of the foot is not only absent, but rather everts, similar to the curved rocker on a rocking chair. Frequently, a protuberant heel accompanies rocker bottom feet. Rocker bottom feet are a sign of trisomy 18.

47. During the second trimester, if the fetal bladder is not initially apparent because of voiding, how soon should it be visible?
If the fetal bladder does not fill and become apparent within 1 hour, abnormality should be suspected.

48. In performing a biophysical profile (BPP), what must be observed to document each of the following: tone, movement, adequate amniotic fluid, and fetal breathing?
Tone: At least one episode of active extension and flexion of one limb, or one hand opening and closing.
Movement: At least three movements of fetal trunk or limbs.

Adequate amniotic fluid: At least one vertical pool greater than 2 cm in two perpendicular planes.

Fetal breathing: Sustained breathing motions for at least 30 seconds.

Each of these parameters gets 2 points for a total of 8 of 8 points on a sonographic BPP scale.

49. Cite two measurement criteria commonly used to define oligohydramnios.

Common definitions of oligohydramnios include an amniotic fluid index (AFI) $\leq$ 5 cm and the largest pocket of amniotic fluid measuring < 2 by 2 cm.

50. What are the most common causes of oligohydramnios?

Some of the most common etiologies of oligohydramnios include fetal death, bilateral renal agenesis, intrauterine growth restriction, and premature rupture of membranes (PRIP).

51. What are common ultrasonic criteria used to define polyhydramnios?

Polyhydramnios is often defined as an AFI > 24 cm or a single pocket of fluid $\geq$ 8 cm in depth. Polyhydramnios can also be diagnosed by subjective impression or "gestalt."

52. What are the common causes of polyhydramnios?

Multiple gestations, esophageal atresia (usually associated with a tracheoesophageal fistula), tracheal agenesis, duodenal atresia and other intestinal atresias, CNS abnormalities, congenital cardiac rhythm anomalies, maternal type 2 diabetes mellitus, and chromosomal abnormalities, most commonly trisomy 21, followed by trisomy 18 and trisomy 13.

53. Describe the sonographic characteristics of subchorionic hemorrhage.

The sonographic appearance of subchorionic hemorrhage depends on the age, location, and size of the hemorrhage. On grayscale examination, acute hemorrhage may be difficult to distinguish from placental tissue because the echo texture is similar. However, color Doppler examination demonstrates absence of normal placental flow in an area of acute hemorrhage. As an area of hemorrhage resolves, it is initially hypoechoic and subsequently sonolucent.

54. At what gestational age does bowel normally herniate into the umbilical cord and at what age is migration back into the abdominal cavity completed?

At 8 weeks' gestational age by menstrual weeks, the midgut herniates into the base of the umbilical cord. By 12 weeks' gestation it has returned into the abdomen.

55. What is an omphalocele?

An omphalocele is a congenital midline defect of the anterior abdominal wall that results in herniation of intra-abdominal structures (usually intestine or liner) into the base of the umbilical cord. The herniated structures are covered by a membrane consisting of the peritoneum and amniotic membrane.

56. An omphalocele is associated with what other anomalies?

Approximately 50–70% of omphaloceles are associated with other anomalies and 30–40% of omphaloceles are associated with aneuploidy, with trisomy 18 being the most common aneuploidy. The most frequent anomaly is congenital heart defects (30–50%); others include CNS anomalies, gastrointestinal anomalies, and genitourinary anomalies.

57. What is pentalogy of Cantrell?

Pentalogy of Cantrell consists of lower chest and upper abdominal wall malformations including cleft sternum, ectopia cordis, other cardiac defects, anterior midline diaphragmatic defects, and a large upper abdominal omphalocele.

58. What is gastroschisis?

Gastroschisis consists of a congenital defect in the right lower quadrant of the abdominal wall through which the intestines protrude and float freely in the amniotic fluid. In gastroschisis (compared with omphalocele), a hernia sac is not present and the abdominal wall insertion of the umbilical cord is normal. It can usually be observed as distinct from the intestines.

59. What is the most common complication of gastroschisis?

Intrauterine growth restriction is the most common complication of gastroschisis. Approximately 10% of fetuses with gastroschisis may also have other bowel abnormalities such as atresia.

60. Which two common prenatal screening tests have a high sensitivity for gastroschisis?

Maternal serum alpha fetoprotein, which also screens for spina bifida, is usually elevated in pregnancies with gastroschisis. Ultrasound examination of the fetus can reveal eviscerated bowel suspended in the amniotic fluid, without a surrounding membrane (as is present in gastroschisis).

61. What is the limb-body wall complex?

The limb-body wall complex is also called the body-stalk abnormality. It may include extensive defects of the abdominal and thoracic wall, large cranial defects, facial clefts, extremity defects, and marked kyphoscoliosis.

62. The most common ultrasonic abnormalities in fetuses with trisomy 18 are in which organ systems?

Manifestations of trisomy 18 can occur in virtually any organ system. Of fetuses with trisomy 18, approximately 90% have congenital heart disease, 50% have a single umbilical artery, 40% have skeletal anomalies such as clubbed feet or overlapping digits, choroid plexus cyst, or spina bifida, and 10% have omphalocele.

63. Ultrasound examination is most sensitive for which common aneuploidy? What are the most common ultrasonic findings in this condition?

Some studies report greater than 90% sensitivity of ultrasound examination for trisomy 13 and approximately 80% sensitivity for trisomy 18. The most common ultrasonic findings of trisomy 13 include cleft lip and palate (60–70%), postaxial polydactyly (70%), cardiovascular malformations (80% or greater), microcephaly, micro-ophthalmia, CNS malformations (including holoprosencephaly and cerebellar anomalies), and anomalies in most other organ systems.

64. Regarding cystic hygroma, what percentage of fetuses with cystic hygroma have this karyotype and what is the differential diagnosis of cystic hygroma?

Approximately 50% of fetuses with large cystic hygroma have Turner syndrome (45XO). The differential diagnosis includes Noonan's syndrome, Roberts' syndrome, and other types of aneuploidy including trisomy 18, trisomy 21, and 47XXX.

65. What are the characteristic ultrasonic features of a fetus with Turner syndrome?

Other conditions frequently observed by ultrasound examination of a fetus with Turner syndrome include hydrops fetalis and renal anomalies such as horseshoe kidney and hydronephrosis. Congenital heart disease is present in approximately 25% of fetuses with Turner syndrome. Whereas aortic coarctation is the most common congenital heart abnormality of fetuses with Turner syndrome, it may not be readily diagnosable prenatally.

66. What are the typical ultrasonographic anomalies in a fetus with triploidy?

Severe fetal growth restriction is one of the most common ultrasonographic signs of triploidy. Microphthalmia, cleft lip and palate, CNS anomalies including myelomeningocele, cardiac anomalies, omphalocele, and genitourinary anomalies (e.g., renal cystic dysplasia) are also commonly seen with triploidy. In addition, cystic placental changes are commonly seen with triploidy.

67. What is Down syndrome?

Down syndrome is the eponym for trisomy 21. It was first described by John Langdon Down in 1866. It is the most common chromosomal abnormality among newborns, with an incidence of 1 in 700 births.

68. How is trisomy 21 diagnosed?

Prenatal screening tests including the maternal serum alpha fetoprotein triple or quad test (including estriol, beta human chorionic gonadotropin, and alpha-inhibin) and ultrasound examination are not diagnostic for trisomy 21; they are only screening tests. An invasive diagnostic test such as amniocentesis or chorionic villus sampling to permit tissue karyotype or, alternatively, awaiting evaluation after delivery is required to diagnose trisomy 21.

69. What are the ultrasonic markers for trisomy 21?

The single most predictive second trimester sign of trisomy 21 is increased nuchal thickness, which has a relative risk for trisomy 21 of approximately 11. The other ultrasonic markers for trisomy 21 have much lower relative risks, which usually range between 1.5 and 3.0. The most commonly sought markers are short femur or short humerus (approximately 0.9 of expected length based on observed BPD), congenital heart abnormalities, clinodactyly, absent second phalanx of the fifth digit, a wide gap between the first and second toes, wide angle of the hips, and echogenic bowel. Occasionally, a fetus with trisomy 21 has major anomalies.

70. What is Meckel-Gruber syndrome?

It is characterized by omphalocele, encephalocele, and multicystic dysplastic kidney.

71. What is hydrops fetalis?

Hydrops fetalis (i.e., fetal hydrops) is defined as the presence of fetal subcutaneous tissue edema accompanied by serous effusions in one or more body cavities.

72. What are the two types of hydrops fetalis?

- Immune hydrops fetalis (due to rhesus isoimmunization)
- Nonimmune hydrops fetalis. There are many causes of nonimmune hydrops fetalis, including cardiovascular diseases, infections, chorioangioma, diabetes mellitus, and chromosomal abnormalities.

73. Describe the sonographic features of hydrops fetalis.

Sonographic findings include ascites, pericardial effusion, pleural effusion, subcutaneous edema, polyhydramnios, and placental thickness > 4 cm..

74. What is anencephaly?

This neural tube defect is characterized by absence of the calvarium. It is incompatible with life. It has an incidence of 1 in 1000 live births. Sonographically, anencephaly is seen as absence of cranial vault and cerebral hemispheres.

75. Describe the S/D ratio and its significance.

The S/D ratio refers to the systolic to diastolic ratio of blood flow velocity in an arterial vessel, such as the umbilical artery. During pregnancy, its primary significance is when fetal growth restriction is present. In the presence of growth restriction, absent or reversed end-diastolic flow is associated with an increased risk of fetal demise. To avoid misleading results, proper technique is crucial in measuring the umbilical artery S/D ratio. An S/D ratio of > 3 after 30 weeks is abnormal.

76. What is the normal umbilical Doppler flow pattern?

The normal flow pattern of the umbilical artery depends on gestational age. Diastolic flow is present in normal umbilical artery flow studies.

The normal flow pattern of the umbilical vein is smooth, laminar flow. The presence of pulsatile venous flow (a venous pulse in association with each arterial pulse) may be pathologic and indicates that further fetal evaluation may be required.

BIBLIOGRAPHY

1. Benacerraf BR: Ultrasound of Fetal Syndromes. New York, Churchill Livingstone, 1998.
2. Callen PW: Ultrasonography in Obstetrics and Gynecology, 4th ed. Philadelphia, W.B. Saunders, 2000.
3. Nyberg DA, McGahan JP, Pretorius DH, Pilu G: Diagnostic Imaging of Fetal Anomalies. Philadelphia, Lippincott Williams & Wilkins, 2003.

8. DOPPLER EVALUATION IN INTRAUTERINE GROWTH RESTRICTED FETUSES

Noam Lazebnik, M.D., and Roee S. Lazebnik, Ph.D.

1. What is the definition of intrauterine growth restriction (IUGR)?

In the United States, IUGR is defined as being below the 10th percentile of mean weight for gestation. In Europe, it is defined as two standard deviations below the mean estimated fetal weight for gestation.

2. What is the definition of small for gestational age (SGA) fetus?

Two important components define an SGA fetus: a birth weight of less than the 10th percentile and an absence of pathologic process (i.e., no abnormal Doppler findings). The SGA fetus reaches its potential of growth, is normal but small, and is not at risk for an adverse perinatal outcome.

3. What abnormalities are found in the maternal vascular response in pregnancies complicated by IUGR?

Preeclampsia and IUGR are associated with an inadequate quality and quantity of the maternal vascular placentation response. Both conditions have characteristic pathologic findings of the placental bed. In pregnancies with IUGR, irrespective of coexistent preeclampsia, atheromatous-like lesions completely or partially occlude the spiral arteries; these changes are not present in pregnancies with preeclampsia in the absence of IUGR.

4. What are symmetric and asymmetric IUGR?

In **symmetric** IUGR, fetuses tend to have impaired growth of the whole body, including the head, and are often found to have infection or genetic and anatomic defects. In **asymmetric** IUGR fetuses, the head normally is spared, and other parts of the body show growth retardation. This division into two types is somewhat artificial, because growth-retarded fetuses fall in a continuum with respect to the degree of asymmetry versus symmetry of their body parts.

5. What is the prevalence of IUGR fetuses?

The prevalence of IUGR is 10% by definition, because fetuses with an estimated weight of less than 10% are defined as growth restricted.

6. Why is it important to diagnose IUGR fetuses *in utero*?

The perinatal mortality for infants with IUGR is six to ten times greater than that of a normal growth population. IUGR is a major cause of intrapartum fetal distress, intrapartum asphyxia, hypoglycemia, hypocalcemia, meconium aspiration, and intrauterine demise.

7. What risk factors are associated with IUGR?

FETAL FACTORS	PLACENTAL FACTORS	MATERNAL FACTORS
Chromosomal	Abnormal trophoblast invasion	Constitutional
Congenital	Abnormal cord insertion	Nutrition
abnormalities	Abnormal placental disc	Genetic (i.e., PKU)
Infection	Placental location (i.e., previa)	Cardiovascular disease including cardiac
Multiple gestation	Tumors	disease and hypertension
	Infarcts	Autoimmune disease
		Diabetes
		Renal disease
		Environmental (e.g., smoking, alcohol and
		drug abuse, high altitude, toxin exposure)

8. Could IUGR be suspected in advance?

Pregnancies at risk for IUGR may be diagnosed on the basis of previous history (low fetal birth weight in earlier pregnancies), associated disorders (autoimmune diseases, high blood pressure), and toxic habits (smoking, drug abuse). Positive history of a prior pregnancy complicated by IUGR is the most important risk factor.

9. What options are available for diagnosing size–date discrepancy?

To diagnose size–date discrepancy, it is important to diagnose the gestational age. The first trimester ultrasound is the preferred method. Once gestational age is known, one can use the clinical parameter of *symphysis fundal height* (SFH) or an ultrasound study to assess fetal growth. The fundal height is often used as a gross screen for IUGR. Uterine size–date discrepancy, using a cutoff of > 3 cm in the SFH, detects about 50% of affected pregnancies. This clinical judgment is made difficult by maternal obesity, uterine anomalies, and fibroids. Ultrasound screening of fetuses at risk at 32–36 weeks detects fetuses with weight assessment below the 10th percentile with a sensitivity of 72% and a 68% positive predictive value.

10. What should be routinely studied using ultrasound to detect IUGR?

The most common determination of fetal growth restriction is based on the estimated fetal weight (EFW), measured using a combination of biometric data. Fetal measurements using formulas incorporating more than one body part, such as biparietal diameter (BPD), head circumference (HC), abdominal circumference (AC), and femur length (FL), have the highest accuracy for *in utero* weight estimation. Nonetheless, weight estimates will usually fall within 15–18% of the actual newborn weight in 95% of cases. Whenever possible, it is prudent to use a gender- and fetal number–specific growth curve. The best interval for serial scanning is 2–3 weeks because of normal dynamics of fetal growth and limitations of the technical components of the measurements. Ultrasonographically, AC is the single best biometric value in detecting suboptimal fetal weight.

11. Are there additional ultrasound parameters used to diagnose suboptimal fetal growth?

Other ultrasound parameters for diagnosis of IUGR include ratios of various measurements such as HC to AC. This ratio normally exceeds 1.0 before 32 weeks, is approximately 1.0 at 32–34 weeks, and falls below 1.0 after 34 weeks. In asymmetric IUGR, the HC remains larger compared to the AC because of the brain sparing growth phenomenon. In symmetric IUGR, the HC and AC are both reduced, and, therefore, the HC-to-AC ratio is not helpful. Another potentially useful ratio is FL to AC. In asymmetric IUGR, the FL is spared in comparison to the AC measurements from 21 weeks on, and therefore, a ratio > 24.0 suggests the presence of IUGR.

12. What is the fetal arterial blood flow redistribution?

In fetal hypoxemia, there is an increase in the blood supply to the brain, myocardium, and adrenal glands and a reduction in the perfusion of the kidneys, gastrointestinal tract, and lower extremities.

13. What is the fetal brain sparing effect?

Animal and human experiments show increased blood flow to the brain in IUGR fetuses. This increase can be shown by Doppler ultrasound of the middle cerebral artery. This effect has been called the *brain sparing effect* and is demonstrated by a lower value of the pulsatility index.

14. What are the indices used to evaluate vascular resistance and flow?

Doppler ultrasound provides information on vascular resistance and, indirectly, blood flow. Three indices are related to vascular resistance: the systolic-to-diastolic ratio (S/D ratio), the resistance index (RI = systolic velocity − diastolic velocity/systolic velocity), and the pulsatility index (PI = systolic velocity − diastolic velocity/mean velocity).

15. What is the cerebroplacental ratio?

Fetal arterial Doppler studies are useful in the differential diagnosis of IUGR fetuses. In the hypoxemic group, the PI in the umbilical artery is increased, due to impaired placental perfusion, and the PI in the fetal middle cerebral artery is decreased; consequently, the ratio of PI between the umbilical artery and middle cerebral artery (UA/MCA) is increased. This is known as the cerebroplacental ratio. It was shown that an abnormally low cerebroplacental ratio is associated with increased perinatal morbidity and mortality and that the use of this ratio improves prediction of perinatal outcome compared with umbilical artery PI alone.

16. Which vessels are studied in pregnancies complicated by IUGR?

Uterine arteries   Inferior vena cava
Umbilical artery   Umbilical vein
Fetal middle cerebral artery   Fetal aorta
Ductus venosus

17. Describe the technique to study the maternal uterine arteries.

The uterine artery Doppler waveform is best imaged by first identifying the maternal internal iliac artery. The transducer is then moved slightly cephalad and medial until uterine vessels are seen in the myometrium through color mapping. The Doppler gate is then placed over the artery to obtain the Doppler waveform, which is easily recognized by its shape and the slower rate consistent with the maternal pulse (Fig 1).

Color flow imaging is used to visualize flow through the main uterine artery medial to the external iliac artery, and the Doppler sample gate is placed at the point of maximal color brightness. Color flow imaging allows a greater number of reliable recordings to be obtained, shortens the observation time, and reduces the intra- and interobserver coefficients of variation.

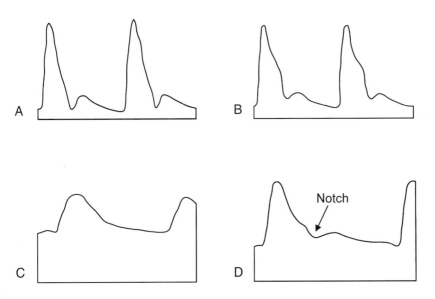

FIGURE 1. *A,* Normal wave flow of the uterine artery in the first trimester. *B,* Normal wave flow of the uterine artery in the early second trimester (< 18 weeks). *C,* Normal wave flow of the uterine artery in the third trimester. *D,* Abnormal wave flow of the uterine artery at 24 weeks' gestation showing low diastolic flow and a notch, which is indicative of high resistance to flow.

18. What is the normal impedance to flow in the uterine artery?

In normal pregnancy, impedance to flow in uterine arteries decreases with gestation. This is reflected in the PI, RI, and S/D ratio, which significantly decrease with advancing gestation. The initial decrease until 24–26 weeks is thought to be caused by trophoblastic invasion of the spiral arteries, but a continuing decrease in impedance may be partially explained by a persistent hormonal effect on elasticity of arterial walls.

19. What is the significance of the protodiastolic notch?

The protodiastolic notch is seen in the uterine arterial Doppler waveform in patients with IUGR or preeclampsia (see Figure 1D).

20. Describe the technique to image and Doppler study the umbilical artery.

The umbilical artery was the first fetal vessel evaluated through Doppler velocimetry. Flow velocity waveforms from the umbilical cord have a characteristic saw-tooth appearance of arterial flow in one direction and continuous umbilical venous blood flow in the other (Figs. 2 and 3). With a pulsed wave Doppler system, first an ultrasound scan is performed, a free-floating portion of the cord is identified, and finally the Doppler sample volume is placed over an artery and the vein.

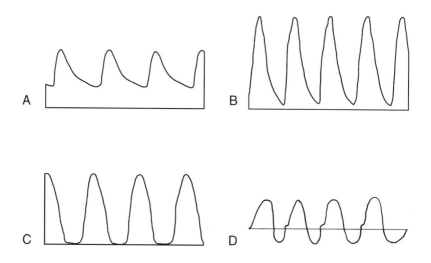

FIGURE 2. *A,* Normal wave flow of the umbilical artery in the third trimester. *B,* High resistance to flow in the umbilical artery with very low flow during diastole. *C,* Very high resistance to umbilical arterial blood flow with absent diastolic flow. *D,* Reversal of diastolic flow in the umbilical artery.

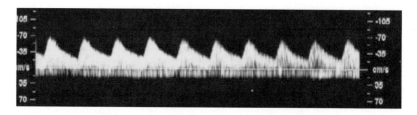

FIGURE 3. Normal waveforms of the umbilical artery and vein.

21. Is it important to study the waveforms of a specific location in the umbilical cord?

Yes. The location of the Doppler sampling site in the umbilical cord affects the Doppler wave-form because impedance indices are significantly higher at the fetal end of the cord compared with the placental end. Preferably, it should be measured toward the placental insertion of the cord.

22. How do the umbilical artery waveforms differ between normal pregnancies and pregnancies complicated by IUGR?

In the normal fetus, the pulsatility index decreases with advancing gestation. In fetuses with IUGR, the pulsatility index is increased secondary to the decrease, absence, or reversal of end-diastolic flow. The absent or reversed end-diastolic flows represent the extreme end of the spectrum. Such cases are associated with a high perinatal mortality and an increased incidence of lethal fetal structural and chromosomal defects.

23. Could an obstetrician use umbilical Doppler studies in the clinical management of pregnancies complicated by IUGR?

Yes. In terms of monitoring growth-restricted pregnancies, abnormal waveforms in the umbilical artery are an early sign of fetal impairment. When growth-restricted fetuses longitudinally are followed up, the abnormalities in the umbilical artery preceded the occurrence of cardiotocographic (nonstress test) signs of fetal hypoxemia in more than 90% of cases.

24. Describe the normal umbilical vein waveform pattern. How does it differ in compromised fetuses?

The normal umbilical vein exhibits a continuous forward flow without any pulsations. This pattern can be identified in most pregnancies after the first trimester (Fig. 4).

Presence of pulsations in the umbilical vein waveform between 8 and 12 weeks is normal, but their persistence after that time is abnormal. The presence of umbilical vein pulsations is associated with an increased risk of adverse perinatal outcome.

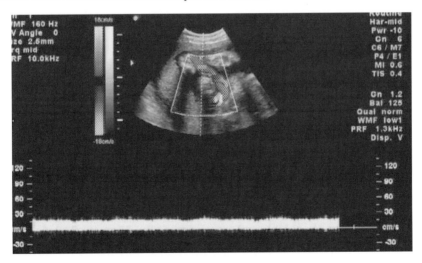

FIGURE 4. Normal waveforms of the fetal umbilical vein.

25. Describe the normal waveforms in the fetal aorta.

Velocity waveforms of the fetal descending aorta are usually recorded at the lower thoracic level just above the diaphragm. Diastolic velocities are always present during the second and third trimesters of normal pregnancy, and the pulsatility index remains constant (Fig. 5).

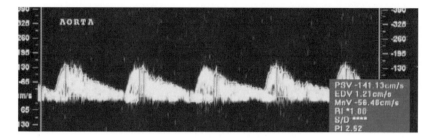

FIGURE 5. Normal waveforms of the fetal aorta.

26. What is the physiologic function of the ductus venosus?

The ductus venosus plays a central role in the return of venous blood from the placenta. Well-oxygenated blood from the umbilical vein is shunted via the ductus venosus into the inferior vena cava toward the heart. Approximately 40% of umbilical vein blood enters the ductus venosus and accounts for 98% of blood flow through the ductus venosus, because portal blood is directed almost exclusively to the right lobe of the liver.

27. How does the normal waveform in the ductus venosus look?

The typical waveform for blood flow in venous vessels consists of three phases. The highest pressure gradient between the venous vessels and the right atrium occurs during ventricular systole (S), which results in the highest blood flow velocities toward the fetal heart during that part of the cardiac cycle (Figs. 6 and 7). Early diastole (D), with the opening of the atrioventricular valves and passive early filling of the ventricles (E-wave of the biphasic atrioventricular flow waveform), is associated with a second peak of forward flow. The nadir of flow velocities coin-

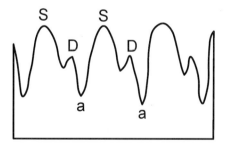

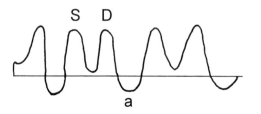

FIGURE 6. *Top,* Normal ductus venosus waveform in late second trimester showing positive flow during atrial contraction. *Bottom,* Abnormal waveform with reversal of flow during atrial contraction in the ductus venosus. S = ventricular systole; D = early diastole; a = atrial contraction.

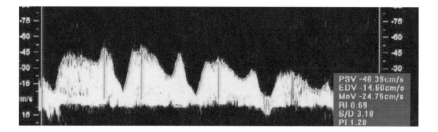

FIGURE 7. Normal waveforms of the fetal ductus venosus.

cides with atrial contraction (A) during late diastole (A-wave of the atrioventricular flow waveform). During atrial contraction, the foramen ovale flap and the crista dividens meet, thereby preventing direct blood flow from the ductus venosus to the left atrium during that short period of closure of the foramen ovale.

28. Describe the technique of ductus venosus sampling.

The ductus venosus is best identified in a sagittal section or an oblique section through the upper fetal abdomen. It is seen as a continuation of the intra-abdominal umbilical vein with a narrow inlet and a wider outlet, and connects to the inferior vena cava (IVC). Once identified, color Doppler imaging can confirm its location. A blood flow velocity recording can be made with the gate placed above the inlet of the ductus venosus. These measurements should not be taken during fetal breathing.

29. Describe the site of IVC sampling and the normal IVC waveform.

The highest reproducibility of IVC waveforms is achieved by recording the waveform between the entrance of the renal vein and the ductus venosus. Normal and abnormal waveforms are shown in Figure 8.

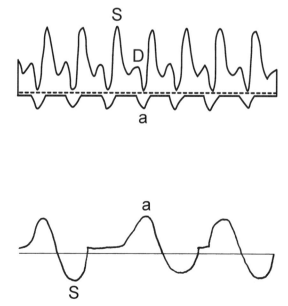

FIGURE 8. *Top,* Normal waveform flow in the inferior vena cava. *Bottom,* Abnormal waveform with reversed flow during atrial contraction in the inferior vena cava. S = ventricular systole; D = early diastole; a = atrial contraction.

30. What is the significance of an abnormal waveform in the ductus venosus?

In IUGR, abnormalities in the ductus venosus waveform have been associated with worsening fetal hypoxemia and acidemia. The abnormal waveform is seen as reversal of flow in ductus venosus.

31. Describe the temporal sequence of Doppler abnormalities in IUGR.

The temporal sequence of Doppler abnormalities is as follows:
- Abnormal uterine arterial
- Middle cerebral artery and the umbilical artery.
- Ductus venosus—reversal of flow

At this time, a nonstress test would be abnormally low. Doppler study of the umbilical vein is very likely to show venous pulsations. Intervention at this point, through delivery of the fetus, may result in a live birth, although long-term, severe dysfunction of the brain and other organs abnormalities is very likely. The frequency of the mentioned fetal studies should be determined based on the entire clinical impression.

32. What are the best predictors of IUGR?

The fetal weight (< 10th percentile), amniotic fluid volume (oligohydramnios), and abnormal Doppler waveforms are the best predictors of IUGR.

33. What measurement is the single best predictor of fetal weight?

Abdominal circumference measurement is the single best predictor of fetal weight and growth.

34. What are long-term sequelae of IUGR?

These fetuses have higher rates of cardiovascular disease and diabetes mellitus. Severe neurologic abnormalities are seen in at least 10% of fetuses with IUGR, and minor abnormalities can be observed in 32% of these fetuses.

BIBLIOGRAPHY

1. Al-Ghazali W, Chita SK, Chapman MG, Allan LD: Evidence of redistribution of cardiac output in asymmetrical growth retardation. Br J Obstet Gynaecol 96:697–704, 1989.
2. Arduini D, Rizzo G, Boccolini MR, et al: Functional assessment of uteroplacental and fetal circulations by means of color Doppler ultrasonography. J Ultrasound Med 9:249–253, 1990.
3. Campbell S, Diaz-Recasens J, Griffin DR, et al: New Doppler technique for assessing uteroplacental blood inflow. Lancet i:675–677, 1983.
4. Hecher K, Campbell S, Snijders R, Nicolaides K: Reference ranges for fetal venous and atrioventricular blood flow parameters. Ultrasound Obstet Gynecol 4:381–90, 1994.
5. Kiserud T, Eik-Nes SH, Blaas HG, Hellevik LR: Foramen ovale: An ultrasonographic study of its relation to the inferior vena cava, ductus venosus and hepatic veins. Ultrasound Obstet Gynecol 2:389–396, 1992.
6. Reed KL, Appleton CP, Anderson CF, et al: Doppler studies of vena cava flows in human fetuses. Insights into normal and abnormal cardiac physiology. Circulation 81:498–450, 1990.
7. Rizzo G, Arduini D, Romanini C: Inferior vena cava flow velocity waveforms in appropriate- and small-for-gestational-age fetuses. Am J Obstet Gynecol 166:1271–1280, 1992.
8. Rizzo G, Capponi A, Arduini D, Romanini C: Ductus venosus velocity waveforms in appropriate and small for gestational age fetuses. Early Hum Dev 39:15–26, 1994.
9. Schmidt KG, Silverman NH, Rudolph AM: Assessment of flow events at the ductus venosus-inferior vena cava junction and at the foramen ovale in fetal sheep by use of multimodal ultrasound. Circulation 93:826–833, 1996.
10. Vyas S, Nicolaides KH, Bower S, Campbell S: Middle cerebral artery flow velocity waveforms in fetal hypoxemia. Br J Obstet Gynaecol 97:797–803, 1990.

9. ECTOPIC PREGNANCY

Raj Mohan Paspulati, M.D., and Tara Maria McElroy, M.D.

1. In the United States, what is the leading cause of death in reproductive age women in the first trimester of pregnancy?
Ectopic pregnancy is the most common, accounting for 9% of pregnancy-related deaths.

2. What is the most important risk factor for ectopic pregnancy?
Prior history of pelvic inflammatory disease (PID) is the most important factor. The most common organism responsible for PID is *Chlamydia trachomatis*.

3. In addition to pelvic inflammatory disease, list other risk factors for ectopic pregnancy.
- Prior tubal reconstructive surgery
- Intrauterine device (IUD)
- Use of ovulation-inducing agents
- History of prior ectopic pregnancy
- In vitro fertilization
- Advanced maternal age
- Endometriosis

4. Describe the locations of ectopic pregnancies.
Ninety-five percent of ectopic pregnancies occur in the fallopian tube, most commonly in the ampulla (80%), followed by the isthmic portion (10–15%) and the interstitial or cornual region (< 2%). The other 5% may be found in the ovary, cervix, and abdomen.

5. What is the clinical presentation of ectopic pregnancy?
The classic presentation is pain, vaginal bleeding, and an adnexal mass. This triad is present in 45% of women with an ectopic pregnancy.

6. What other conditions mimic ectopic pregnancy on clinical presentation?
- Spontaneous abortion
- Symptomatic ovarian cysts
- Pelvic inflammatory disease
- Dysfunctional uterine bleeding

7. What is the prognosis of a patient with an ectopic pregnancy?
Nine percent of maternal deaths are due to ectopic pregnancy. There is also an increased risk of future ectopic pregnancy, and 40% of women who have had an ectopic pregnancy have infertility problems.

8. Is the location of pain experienced by the patient specific for identifying the ectopic pregnancy?
No. The pain in ectopic pregnancy patients is nonspecific. Patients with ectopic pregnancies may experience pain generalized to the abdomen, shoulder, lower abdomen, lower quadrant ipsilateral or contralateral to the ectopic gestation, back, and vagina.

9. How is the diagnosis of ectopic pregnancy determined?
Ultrasound findings correlated with serum beta human chorionic gonadotropin (hCG) and clinical presentation are the mainstay of diagnosis. A negative serum beta-hCG essentially excludes ectopic pregnancy. Urine pregnancy test is negative in 50% of patients with ectopic pregnancy.

10. What is the normal rate of elevation in serum beta-hCG in a normal intrauterine pregnancy (IUP) and how may this be altered in an ectopic pregnancy?

Beta-hCG should double or at least increase 66% in 48 hours in a normal IUP. In ectopic pregnancy, the elevation in beta-hCG is significantly less in most cases. However, approximately 15% of normal IUPs have a less than 66% increase or doubling time and 17% of ectopic pregnancies have a normal doubling time. Approximately 90% of women with an ectopic pregnancy have a beta-hCG that is less than 6500 IU/ml (IRP).

11. What is the discriminatory zone for confirming an IUP with endovaginal ultrasound?

In most laboratories, the presence of a gestational sac (a sonographic term), which is defined as a fluid collection with an echogenic rim, can be seen when the beta-hCG is between 1000 and 2000 mIU/ml (IRP). This is often referred to as the *discriminatory zone*.

12. What is the discriminatory zone for confirming an IUP by transabdominal ultrasound?

An IUP should be visualized when the beta-hCG is > 6500 mIU/ml (IRP).

13. Name conditions in which the beta-hCG value can be markedly elevated.

Molar pregnancies have markedly elevated beta-hCG values. These can occur in patients with ectopic pregnancy.

14. What are the limiting factors in performing endovaginal ultrasound?

Obesity, uterine fibroids, and position of the uterus may compromise the study and result in suboptimal evaluation.

15. Describe the attributes of double decidual sac (DDS) sign.

The DDS sign is defined by an inner rim of chorionic villi surrounded by a wedge of fluid in the endometrial cavity and further encased by a rim of decidua vera that is echogenic (Fig. 1). This is considered a reliable indicator of an IUP; however, its presence does not exclude ectopic pregnancy.

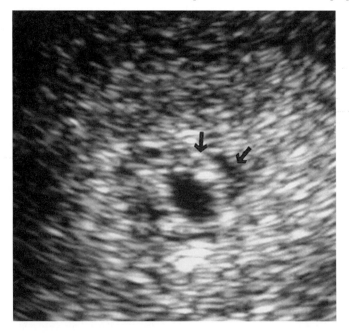

FIGURE 1. Double decidual sac sign. The decidua capsularis overlying the gestational sac is separated from the deciduas parietalis by a wedge-shaped fluid (*between two arrows*).

16. What is a pseudogestational sac?
Pseudogestational sacs are usually ovoid in shape and central in the endometrial cavity, have poorly defined margins, do not demonstrate decidual reaction, and usually have a single decidual layer. It usually consists of decidual cast or hemorrhage (Fig. 2). Gestational sacs are round and often eccentrically located in the endometrium, and have well-defined margins. The outline of the gestational sac is hyperechoic.

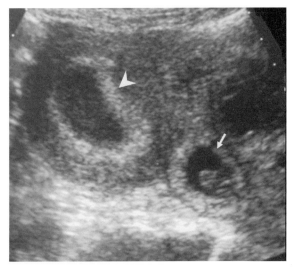

FIGURE 2. Ectopic pregnancy. Transabdominal sonogram demonstrates an extrauterine gestational sac with embryo (*arrow*) and a pseudogestational sac (*arrowhead*).

17. Describe the sonographic findings in ectopic pregnancy.
- Live embryo outside the uterus is 100% specific.
- Nonovarian adnexal mass containing a yolk sac or nonliving embryo has a 100% positive predictive value (PPV).
- Tubal ring sign—echogenic rim around a fluid collection or mass—has 50% sensitivity and 95% PPV.

18. What is a tubal ring and what might its presence suggest?
A tubal ring, or echogenic ring, is defined as an extrauterine, nonovarian, hypoechoic ring-like mass usually 1–3 cm in diameter that may be surrounded by free fluid. Its presence is specific for an ectopic pregnancy.

19. What is the most sensitive and specific ultrasound finding in a patient suspected of having an ectopic pregnancy?
The presence of a nonovarian complex adnexal mass is the most sensitive and specific ultrasound finding (Fig. 3). The finding is due to the bleeding and clotting of blood in the wall and lumen of the fallopian tube as the tube distends to accommodate the enlarging products of conception. This has 92% PPV for diagnosing ectopic pregnancy.

20. What is the significance of fluid in the cul de sac in a patient with an ectopic pregnancy?
Approximately 40–83% of patients with a complicated ectopic pregnancy have hemorrhage or hemoperitoneum. This has 90% PPV for ectopic pregnancy.

21. How often can a fetal heartbeat be detected in an ectopic pregnancy?
The presence of a fetal heartbeat outside the uterine cavity is pathognomonic for an ectopic pregnancy. It is speculated that an extrauterine heartbeat is present in approximately 6–28% of cases of ectopic pregnancy. If an extrauterine gestational sac with an embryo (with or without a heartbeat) or a yolk sac is identified, this is 100% specific for an ectopic pregnancy.

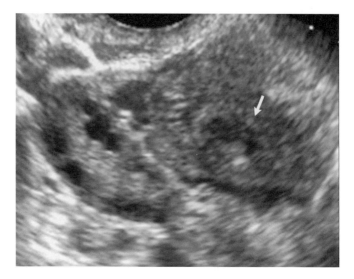

FIGURE 3. Ectopic pregnancy. Non-ovarian adnexal mass. Endovaginal sonogram demonstrates a non-ovarian adnexal mass (*arrow*).

22. Can an ectopic pregnancy be excluded if no extrauterine mass is seen?
No. In 15–35% of cases, no mass is seen. Up to 26% of patients with an ectopic pregnancy may have a completely normal ultrasound evaluation.

23. What is the role of color and pulsed Doppler analysis in the diagnosis of ectopic pregnancy?
The role of Doppler sonography is somewhat controversial in the diagnosis of ectopic pregnancy. A normal IUP has low-impedance, high diastolic flow, which is not visualized in the pseudogestational sac of the ectopic pregnancy. However, ectopic pregnancies in the fallopian tube have also been found to have low-impedance, high diastolic flow. Use of Doppler is usually limited to situations in which the finding of flow will determine the medical management.

24. What are the chances of having a subsequent ectopic pregnancy?
There is a 7–15% risk of recurrent ectopic gestation.

25. What conditions may mimic an ectopic pregnancy?
Several conditions may visually mimic findings seen with an ectopic pregnancy or hematosalpinx. These include pedunculated fibroid, retrograde blood flow from a spontaneous abortion, exophytic corpus luteum cyst, tubovarian abscess, tubal cyst or adjacent bowel.

26. Can sonography distinguish a corpus luteum cyst from an ectopic gestation sac?
Yes. The corpus luteal cyst is of ovarian origin and the ectopic sac is outside the ovary. Color Doppler evaluation does not play a role in their discrimination, because they both have a peripheral low-impedance, high diastolic flow, which is seen as "ring of fire." It is more important to demonstrate the extraovarian location of the adnexal mass to diagnose ectopic gestation. An ectopic gestation in the ovary is rare (0.5–1.0%).

27. Even though abdominal ectopic pregnancies occur rarely, what are potential life-threatening complications of this condition?
The complications of abdominal ectopic pregnancies include bowel obstruction, hemorrhage, bowel perforation, and erosion of the pregnancy through the abdominal wall.

28. What is a lithopedion?

In an abdominal pregnancy, a calcified, mummified dead fetus is called a *lithopedion*.

29. What are risk factors for a cervical ectopic pregnancy and what findings may be seen on ultrasound?

Women who have had multiple pregnancies or cervical manipulation such as dilation and curettage are at greater risk for having a pregnancy implant within the cervix. Ultrasound findings may be a live embryo or gestational sac with peritrophoblastic flow found within the cervix. It is important to distinguish cases of spontaneous abortion, which occurs much more frequently from cervical ectopic pregnancy.

30. What is a cornual pregnancy?

An ectopic pregnancy at the cornua is called cornual pregnancy. It is rare and the incidence is less than 2%. Sonographically, it is identified by the presence of an ectopic pregnancy that is eccentric in location to the endometrial stripe (Fig. 4), and usually an echogenic band can be seen connecting the ectopic pregnancy with the endometrial stripe, called interstitial line (sign). It is important to recognize this pregnancy because it has the greatest incidence of fatal hemorrhage. This pregnancy can grow with no warning sign, but once the placenta outgrows the available myometrium, patients present with ruptured uterus.

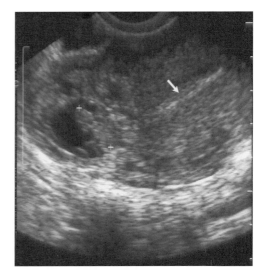

FIGURE 4. Cornual pregnancy. Endovaginal sonogram in longitudinal view reveals a gestational sac with live embryo (*within calipers*) lying eccentric to the endometrial stripe (*arrow*).

31. What is heterotopic pregnancy?

A pregnancy in which both an IUP and ectopic pregnancy coexist is a heterotopic pregnancy. In 1948, this was estimated to occur in 1 in 30,000 pregnancies. The current estimate is approximately 1 in 7000, secondary to the greater use of fertility drugs. The rate is estimated to be 1 in 100 in cases of in vitro fertilization (IVF), particularly when multiple embryos are transferred to the uterus.

32. How are cases of ectopic pregnancy managed?

If an ectopic pregnancy is suspected and the patient is hemodynamically unstable, then an immediate laparotomy or laparoscopic surgery is performed. If the patient is hemodynamically stable, then the treatment is usually methotrexate injection.

33. What are absolute indications for systemic methotrexate therapy?
- Hemodynamically stable patient
- No evidence of hemoperitoneum
- Nonlaparoscopic diagnosis of ectopic
- Patient desire for future fertility
- Significant risk posed by use of general anesthesia
- Ectopic size < 3 cm
- Stable or increasing hCG levels with peak values < 15,000 IU/ml (IRP)
- No cardiac activity in the gestational sac
- Ability of patient to return for follow-up
- No contraindications to methotrexate

34. What are absolute contraindications to methotrexate therapy?
- Breastfeeding
- Alcoholism
- Liver disease
- Immunodeficiency
- Blood dyscrasia
- Known sensitivity to methotrexate
- Active pulmonary disease or peptic ulcer disease
- Renal dysfunction

35. What are signs and symptoms of methotrexate failure and tubal rupture?
Patients may experience significantly worsening abdominal discomfort, hemodynamic instability, a beta-hCG that increases or plateaus but does not decrease, or a beta-hCG level that does not decrease between postmethotrexate injection days 4–7. A decrease of 15% is considered satisfactory response. If the beta-hCG does not decrease between days 4–7, then a second injection of methotrexate is usually indicated.

36. Describe the role of ultrasound in a patient after methotrexate treatment?
Ultrasound can be performed 2 weeks after the methotrexate treatment and not before. In the first 2 weeks after the methotrexate treatment, the ectopic size increases because of edema and hemorrhage and sometimes is falsely presumed to be indicative of methotrexate treatment failure; after 2 weeks of treatment, the ectopic size decreases.

BIBLIOGRAPHY

1. Atri M, Leduc C, Gillet P, et al: Role of endovaginal sonography in the diagnosis and management of ectopic pregnancy. Radiographics 16:755–774, 1996.
2. Bateman BG, Nunley WCJ, Kolp LA, et al: Vaginal sonography findings and hCG dynamics of early intrauterine and tubal pregnancies. Obstet Gynecol 75:421–427, 1990.
3. Brown DL, Felker RE, Stovall TG, et al: Serial endovaginal sonography of ectopic pregnancies treated with methotrexate. Obstet Gynecol 77:406–409, 1991.
4. Callen P: Ultrasonography in Obstetrics and Gynecology, 4th ed. Philadelphia, W.B. Saunders, 2000, pp 912–933.
5. Emerson DS, Cartier MS, Altieri LA, et al: Diagnostic efficacy of endovaginal color Doppler flow imaging in an ectopic pregnancy screening program. Radiology 183:413–420, 1992.
6. Gabrielli S, Romero R, Pilu G, et al: Accuracy of transvaginal ultrasound and serum hCG in the diagnosis of ectopic pregnancy. Ultrasound Obstet Gynecol 2:110–115, 1992.
7. Jurkovic D, Hacket E, Campbell S: Diagnosis and treatment of early cervical pregnancy: A review and report of two cases treated conservatively. Ultrasound Obstet Gynecol 8:373–380, 1996.
8. Nyberg DA, Mack LA, Jeffrey RB Jr, et al: Endovaginal sonographic evaluation of ectopic pregnancy: A prospective study. Am J Roentgenol 149:1181–1186, 1987.

10. THE POSTPARTUM UTERUS

Stephen W. Tamarkin, M.D.

1. What are the common causes of postpartum fever?
Most persistent fevers are caused by genital tract infections. Other causes include atelectasis or pneumonia, pyelonephritis, intense breast engorgement, bacterial mastitis, thrombophlebitis, and wound infection.

2. What entities comprise the spectrum of postpartum pelvic infectious or inflammatory complications?
- Endometritis
- Pelvic cellulitis
- Ovarian vein thrombophlebitis
- Pelvic vein thrombophlebitis
- Pelvic abscess

3. Is the presence of air within the uterus normal in the postpartum period?
A small quantity of air within the uterus is a normal finding after a cesarean section or a vaginal delivery.

4. What are the typical symptoms of endometritis?
Pelvic pain and fever.

5. What factors increase the likelihood of postpartum endometritis?
Endometritis is more common after cesarean section. It is also associated with prolonged labor, premature rupture of membranes, retained products of conception, multiple cervical examinations, and internal fetal monitoring.

6. Is there a specific ultrasound appearance of postpartum endometritis?
No. Possible findings include thickened endometrium, fluid in the uterine canal, and air in the canal, all nonspecific findings in the postpartum setting (Fig. 1).

7. What is postpartum pelvic cellulitis and what are the common clinical symptoms?
Parauterine inflammatory changes of varying severity may occur as a result of the introduction of vaginal flora into the parauterine veins and lymphatics, or via direct extension from surgical or birth trauma. The severity of the inflammatory changes depends on a combination of pathogen inoculum and virulence, and other factors such as degree of venous stasis and preexisting hematomas. Pelvic cellulitis commonly presents as postpartum pain and fever.

8. What are the imaging options and appearances of postpartum pelvic cellulitis?
Imaging with ultrasound, computed tomography (CT), or magnetic resonance imaging (MRI) may be performed in this setting to differentiate indistinct changes of parauterine cellulitis from *focal* fluid collections including abscesses or hematomas, or ovarian or pelvic vein thrombophlebitis. Ultrasound shows nonspecific findings with an enlarged uterus and possibly some prominence of the parauterine structures and small amounts of fluid, but no large focal collections. Similarly, CT shows an enlarged uterus and prominent adnexal region tissue with indistinct tissue margins. The inflammatory changes are seen as increased T_2 signal on MRI.

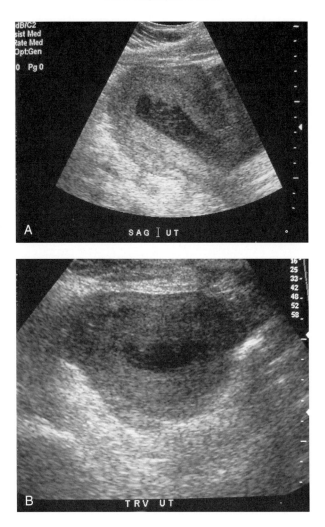

FIGURE 1. Endometritis. Sagittal and transverse sonogram of a woman with pain and fever 10 days after cesarean section. The complex fluid in the uterine cavity and thick irregular endometrium are suggestive of, but not specific for, endometritis.

9. What is the relationship between pelvic cellulitis and ovarian vein thrombophlebitis?

The combination of pelvic cellulitis and pelvic venous stasis together increase the risk for thrombophlebitis of the ovarian or other pelvic veins. Thus, thrombophlebitis often coexists in cases of severe postpartum pelvic cellulitis.

10. What are the risk factors for pelvic cellulitis and ovarian vein thrombophlebitis?

Similar to endometritis risk factors, these inflammatory processes are much more common following cesarean sections than vaginal deliveries, and they are more common after difficult, prolonged vaginal deliveries than following uncomplicated vaginal births.

11. What is the typical clinical presentation of ovarian vein thrombophlebitis?

Fever, lower abdominal pain, and possibly a palpable mass typically manifest 48–96 hours postpartum.

12. Are the right and left ovarian veins involved equally as often?
No. Ninety percent of cases of ovarian vein thrombophlebitis involve the right ovarian vein. Experimental studies have shown differences in the patterns of flow and stasis between the right and left ovarian veins during pregnancy and postpartum.

13. What is the best imaging method or modality to diagnose ovarian vein thrombophlebitis?
Contrast-enhanced CT or MRI are about equivalent, and both are more sensitive than ultrasound. This diagnosis should be considered, and specifically evaluated for, with any imaging performed in the setting of postpartum pain and fever.

14. Can ovarian vein thrombophlebitis be detected with ultrasound and if so, how?
Yes. The sonologist must consider this diagnosis in the proper clinical setting (i.e., postpartum pain and fever). The expected course of the ovarian veins should be evaluated, extending from the adnexal regions, anterior to the psoas muscles, to the site of the confluence of the right ovarian vein with the inferior vena cava (IVC) or left vein with the left renal vein. Acute clot is typically hypoechoic and distends the vein (Fig. 2), and then becomes more heterogeneous and echogenic with time. The enlarged postpartum uterus and abdomen, patient discomfort, and possibly ileus can add to the difficulty of this interrogation.

15. Can postpartum abscesses be drained percutaneously?
Yes. A safe access route for catheter placement can usually be found with ultrasound or CT guidance using an anterior or trans-sciatic approach. Transvaginal or transrectal approaches can also be used.

16. What are common causes of postpartum hemorrhage?
- Uterine atony or failure to involute
- Unrecognized lacerations of the vagina or cervix
- Retained placental tissue
- Endometritis
- Uterine artery injury

17. What are the meanings of *primary* and *secondary* postpartum hemorrhage?
Primary refers to excessive vaginal bleeding within the first 24 hours postpartum. **Secondary** refers to abnormal bleeding > 24 hours and < 6 weeks postpartum.

18. How do CT and ultrasound compare in assessing postpartum hemorrhagic complications?
CT is superior for assessing large internal hematomas and can demonstrate sites of active hemorrhage. Ultrasound should be used to detect retained products of conception, and it demonstrates "bladder flap" hematomas better than CT.

19. What is a bladder flap hematoma?
During a cesarean section, the obstetric surgeon dissects a *plane* into the extraperitoneal space between the anterior aspect of the lower uterine segment and the posterior aspect of the bladder to allow access for a lower uterine transverse incision. This created space is a common site for varying sized hematomas (bladder flap hematoma), which can be seen as characteristic heterogeneous collections on either ultrasound or CT scan (Fig. 3). It can extend subserosally around the uterus, along the broad ligament, and into the retroperitoneum.

20. What are other possible locations for postpartum hematomas or hemorrhages?
- Broad ligament hematomas
- Prevesical (space of Retzius) or superficial abdominal wall hematomas
- Hemoperitoneum

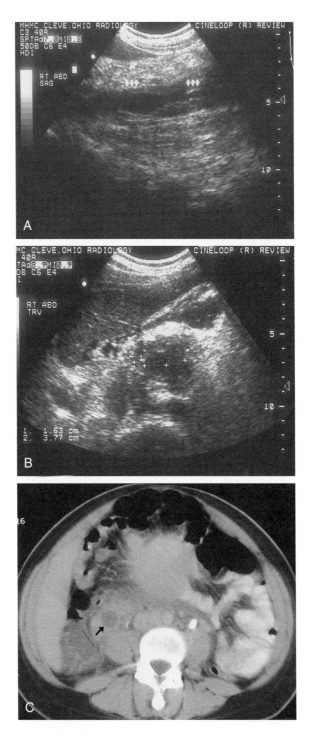

FIGURE 2. Ovarian vein thrombophlebitis. Sagittal (*A*) and transverse (B) sonogram of distended right ovarian vein with hypoechoic thrombus (*arrows*). Corresponding CT (*C*) further confirms the thrombus in right ovarian vein (*arrow*).

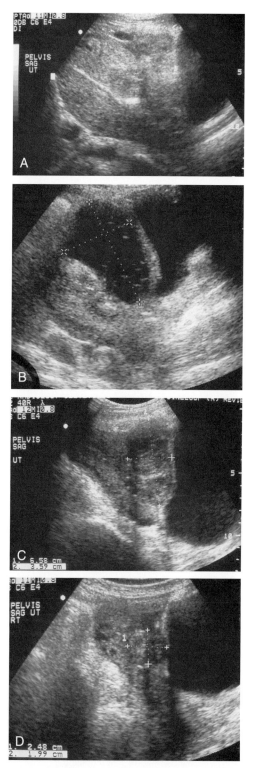

FIGURE 3. Bladder flap hematoma. *A*, Sagittal sonogram reveals a heterogeneous collection between the lower uterine segment and bladder in a patient 3 days after cesarean section. *B*, Follow-up at 5 weeks shows further resolution of this hematoma. *C*, Patient at 3-month follow-up. *D*, Patient at 6-month follow-up.

21. What is the incidence of and what are the risk factors for secondary postpartum hemorrhage?

Secondary hemorrhage has an incidence of about 1%. The risk factors include primary hemorrhage and manual removal of retained placenta.

22. What ultrasound appearances are more or less suggestive of retained products of conception (RPOC)?

RPOC typically consists of retained placental tissue. An echogenic mass in the uterine cavity is the most suggestive ultrasound finding. A heterogeneous mass or collection in the central cavity may represent blood clot or some combination of retained placenta, necrotic debris, and clot (Fig. 4). Color Doppler may help differentiate vascularized from nonvascularized tissue, which may help distinguish vascularized retained placental tissue; however, retained nonvascularized placental tissue may not have flow. A normal-appearing endometrial stripe or punctate echogenic foci not associated with a discrete mass make RPOC unlikely.

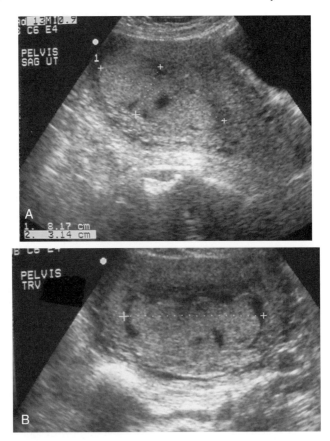

FIGURE 4. Retained products of conception. Sagittal (*A*) and transverse (*B*) sonogram demonstrates a hyperechoic mass within the uterus (*within calipers*) typical of retained products of conception.

23. Why is it important to diagnose or exclude RPOC in the setting of excessive postpartum bleeding?

Excessive bleeding not due to RPOC may resolve with conservative measures, and curettage is indicated to evacuate RPOC. Curettage has potential complications including uterine perforation and synechiae formation, and thus should not be performed unless there is high suspicion for RPOC.

24. What types of uterine artery injuries can occur and what is the proper treatment?

Uterine artery pseudoaneurysms, acquired arteriovenous malformations, arteriovenous fistulas, vessel rupture, or various combinations of injuries may occur secondary to curettage or other surgical obstetric trauma. Color Doppler should be used when assessing a postpartum or postcurettage uterus in the setting of excessive bleeding. If a vascular injury is suspected, angiography should be performed for further diagnosis and possibly embolization therapy.

25. What is the expected time course for a postpartum uterus to return to its nongravid size?

The uterus usually returns to its prepregnancy size in 5–6 weeks, possibly faster in nursing mothers because of increased oxytocin release. Partial involution is usually rapid during the first hours after delivery. Increased postpartum uterine tone tends to be more constant following first pregnancies and more intermittent in multiparous women.

26. What are other possible postpartum maternal complications?
- Uterine rupture (Fig. 5)
- Neurologic events such as cerebral ischemia or sagittal sinus thrombosis
- Breast pathology
- Miscellaneous entities such as appendicitis and pyelonephritis

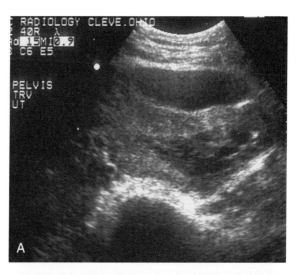

FIGURE 5. Uterus rupture. *A,* Transverse sonogram shows a complex collection in the expected location of uterus in a patient 7 days after vaginal delivery. *B,* Corresponding computed tomography confirms the uterus rupture.

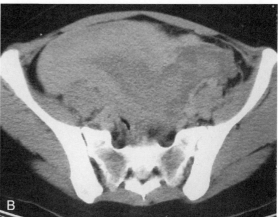

BIBLIOGRAPHY

1. Cunningham FG, Gant NF, Leveno KJ, et al (eds): Williams Obstetrics, 21st ed. New York, McGraw-Hill, 2001.
2. Edwards A, Ellwood DA: Ultrasonographic evaluation of the postpartum uterus. Ultrasound Obstet Gynecol 16:640–643, 2000.
3. Grant TH, Schoettle BW, Buchsbaum MS: Postpartum ovarian vein thrombosis: Diagnosis by clot protrusion into the inferior vena cava at sonography. Am J Roentgenol 160:551–552, 1993.
4. Hertzberg BS, Bowie JC: Ultrasound of the postpartum uterus: Prediction of retained placental tissue. J Ultrasound Med 10:451–456, 1991.
5. Hoveyda F, MacKenzie IZ: Secondary postpartum haemorrhage: Incidence, morbidity and current management. Br J Obstet Gynaecol 108:927–930, 2001.
6. Kubik-Huch RA, Hebisch G, Huch R, et al: Role of duplex color Doppler ultrasound, computed tomography, and MR angiography in the diagnosis of septic puerperal ovarian vein thrombosis. Abdom Imaging 24:85–91, 1999.
7. Kwon JH, Kim GS: Obstetric iatrogenic arterial injuries of the uterus: Diagnosis with US and treatment with transcatheter arterial embolization. Radiographics 22:35–46, 2002.
8. Maldjian C, Adam R, Maldjian J, Smith R: MRI appearance of the pelvis in the post-cesarean-section patient. Magn Reson Imaging 17:223–227, 1999.
9. Pelage JP, Soyer P, Repiquet D, et al: Secondary postpartum hemorrhage: Treatment with selective arterial embolization. Radiology 212:385–389, 1999.
10. Salem S: The uterus and adnexa. In Rumack CM, Wilson SR, Charboneau JW (eds): Diagnostic Ultrasound, 4th ed. St. Louis, Mosby, 1998.
11. Twickler DM, Setiawan AT, Evans RS, et al: Imaging of puerperal septic thrombophlebitis: Prospective comparison of MR imaging, CT, and sonography. Am J Roentgenol 169:1039–1043, 1997.

III. Gynecology

11. PELVIC SONOGRAPHY

Amy R. Harrow, M.D.

1. What are the three layers that compose the uterus?

The outer serosal layer is followed by the central muscular layer (the myometrium) followed by the inner layer of endometrium.

2. What are the three layers that comprise the myometrium (the muscular layer of the uterus) that can be distinguished sonographically?

The outermost layer is composed of longitudinally oriented muscle fibers and is more hypoechoic than the intermediate layer. The intermediate layer, the thickest of the three layers, consists of spiral muscle bands and is echogenic with respect to the innermost layer and is slightly more echogenic than the outermost layer. The innermost layer is comprised of longitudinal and circular fibers and provides the appearance of a thin hypoechoic rim around the endometrium.

3. What is the endometrium?

The endometrium is a mucosal layer that is continuous with the vaginal epithelium inferiorly and with the fallopian tubes and peritoneum superolaterally.

4. What is the endometrial stripe?

The endometrium appears as an interface whose thickness and appearance vary cyclically with menstruation. The superficial layer of the endometrium, or stratum functionale, fluctuates with the menstrual cycle. The stratum basale, or basal layer, varies little with the menstrual phase. The superficial layer is relatively hypoechoic, whereas the basal layer is echogenic as a result of specular reflections from retained mucus-containing glands. These central opposing surfaces result in the appearance of a thin midline echogenic stripe called the "endometrial stripe."

5. When is the optimal time to evaluate the endometrium?

It is optimal to image patients during days 7–10. It is best to image when the endometrium is "layered," because echogenic pathology may best stand out in the hypoechoic background.

6. How does the endometrial thickness vary with menstruation?

During the early proliferative phase (days 5–9) the endometrium is a thin echogenic line. In the later proliferative phase (days 10–14), the endometrial thickness increases as a result of the effects of estrogen. During this time the functional layer appears hypoechoic with respect to the basal layer and typically ranges from 4–8 mm. During the secretory phase (days 15–28), the functional layer also becomes thick and increases in echogenicity (isoechoic to the basal layer) as a result of the effects of progesterone, typically ranging from 7–14 mm. During the menstrual phase, it appears as a thin interrupted echogenic line.

7. What is "double-layer" thickness?

Endometrial thickness is measured in the true sagittal plane of the uterus and includes both the anterior and posterior portions of the endometrium. The endometrial layers, both anterior and posterior to the endometrial canal, are thus referred to as double-layer thickness.

8. What is considered a "normal" endometrial thickness?

Normal endometrial thickness is 4–8 mm in the proliferative phase, 6–10 mm in the peri-ovulatory period, and 7–14 mm in the secretory phase. Marked variability, however, can be noted.

9. What is considered an abnormal postmenopausal endometrial thickness in an asymptomatic patient?

The endometrium in a postmenopausal female should be less than 5 mm in an asymptomatic individual (Fig. 1).

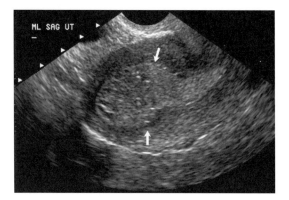

FIGURE 1. Longitudinal ultrasound demonstrates a uniformly thickened hyperechoic endometrium (*arrows*) measuring 2.0 cm in a postmenopausal asymptomatic woman. The differential diagnoses include endometrial polyp, endometrial hyperplasia, and endometrial carcinoma.

10. What is considered an abnormal postmenopausal endometrial thickness in a symptomatic (postmenopausal bleeding) patient?

Any symptomatic postmenopausal female with an endometrial double-layer thickness of ≥ 5 mm should be referred for further evaluation. *Note:* Patients undergoing hormone replacement therapy (HRT) may demonstrate a wider range of endometrial thicknesses than those not receiving HRT.

11. What is endometriosis?

Ectopic endometrial glands and stroma undergo hormonally influenced cyclic change.

12. What is adenomyosis?

The term adenomyosis is applied when ectopic endometrium invades the myometrium by at least 2.5 mm into the basalis layer. Patients can present with dysmenorrhea or hypermenorrhea.

13. What are the sonographic features of adenomyosis?

Most commonly, invasion of the myometrium by endometrial tissue results in diffuse uterine enlargement without disruption of uterine echotexture or contour. Focal adenomyosis may be diagnosed when a focal area of either increased or decreased echotexture is identified within the myometrium. Sonographic cysts at the endometrial-myometrial junction are considered pathognomonic.

14. What is another modality that can be useful in aiding the diagnosis of adenomyosis?

Magnetic resonance imaging (MRI).

15. What entity can appear as a focal area of endometrial thickening and be a source of vaginal bleeding?

Endometrial polyps, either pedunculated or sessile, typically occur in symptomatic females with vaginal bleeding or mucous discharge (Fig. 2). These are most commonly located in the fundus and are multiple in 20% of patients.

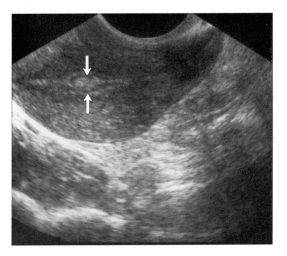

FIGURE 2. Transvaginal longitudinal ultrasound reveals a focal hyperechoic lesion surrounded by a hypoechoic rim in the endometrium (*arrows*) consistent with a polyp.

16. What is the differential diagnosis for postmenopausal vaginal bleeding?
- Endometrial hyperplasia
- Submucosal fibroids
- Endometrial carcinoma (less commonly)
- Polyps
- Atrophy (the most common cause of postmenopausal bleeding)

17. What is an appropriate algorithm for handling female postmenopausal bleeding?
Pelvic ultrasound is the first test of choice. If the endometrium is ≤ to 4 mm, the source of the bleeding is likely due to atrophy. If the endometrium is ≥ 4 mm, a sonohysterogram should be performed. If the sonohysterogram demonstrates diffuse thickening, it is likely that a dilation and curettage is the next step. If focal thickening is discovered by sonohysterogram, hysteroscopy is the next logical step with directed biopsy.

18. What is the most common pelvic tumor?
Leiomyomas are benign tumors of smooth muscle arising from the uterine wall. They vary greatly in size and are more often multiple than solitary. Their clinical significance depends on their size and location. They may be submucosal (5–10%), intramural (most common), or subserous in location. They are believed to demonstrate estrogen dependence and therefore can increase in size and number during pregnancy. Leiomyomas are discrete myometrial masses that can be shelled out surgically.

19. With what symptoms can individuals with "fibroids" present?
Submucosal fibroids tend to be most symptomatic. These lesions can produce menorrhagia, metrorrhagia, infertility, or postmenopausal bleeding. If large enough, leiomyomas can undergo torsion and necrosis.

20. What is the pitfall of Doppler analysis with regard to leiomyomas?
Myomas can significantly affect blood flow velocity in the uterine arteries such that Doppler measurements cannot be used to distinguish benign from malignant lesions.

21. What is the sonographic appearance of a leiomyoma?
The sonographic appearance of these lesions varies greatly with respect to the size, site, age, and individual patient hormonal influences. They can often be mistaken for polyps, adnexal masses, and even adjacent large bowel loops, and vice versa. In one third of cases, leiomyomas

present as a hypoechoic solid mass with poor through transmission resulting from their predominant muscular component. Fibrous degeneration of these lesions results in increasing echogenicity caused by the development of cystic spaces with increasing through transmission. Cystic degeneration of the mass produces an anechoic mass with through transmission. These can also calcify (Fig. 3).

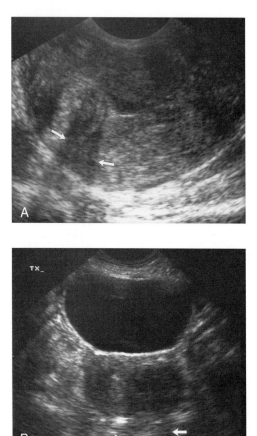

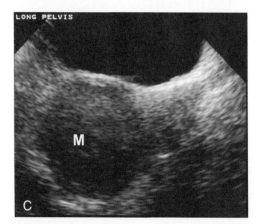

FIGURE 3. *A,* Transvaginal longitudinal ultrasound reveals a discrete isoechoic to hypoechoic mass in the myometrium with posterior acoustic shadowing (*arrows*) resulting from calcification within the fibroid. *B,* Transvaginal transverse ultrasound of the uterus demonstrates a focal hyperechoic lesion with a punctate area of hyperechogenicity with posterior shadowing (*arrows*) consistent with a leiomyoma with focal calcification. *C,* Transvaginal longitudinal ultrasound reveals a fundal mass (*M*) of mixed echogenicity with central areas of necrosis, which at pathology was deemed a leiomyosarcoma.

22. What other modality can be used to further characterize a leiomyoma?

Leiomyomas can have a varied appearance by MRI and usually demonstrate low signal. However, degenerated fibroids typically display moderate to high T_2-weighted signal.

23. What entity should be considered when ultrasonography demonstrates endometrial thickening and irregularity in the postpartum period?

Endometritis, or retained products of conception, demonstrates these nonspecific features but should be considered particularly in the postpartum or postinstrumentation period. These findings should be correlated with clinical history and could also include fluid, debris, or gas within the endometrial cavity (Fig. 4).

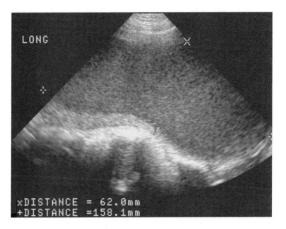

FIGURE 4. Longitudinal ultrasound reveals a dilated uterus expanded by homogenous echogenic material. This represents hematometra in a postpartum patient with known cervical stenosis.

24. What is Asherman syndrome and what is its characteristic sonographic presentation?

Following dilation and curettage, intrauterine fibrous adhesions of the uterine synechiae cross the endometrial cavity and calcify. Small foci of calcification within the uterine cavity may be identified.

25. What is the most common gynecologic malignancy?

Endometrial carcinoma is the most common gynecologic malignancy. Risk factors include unopposed estrogen effect, tamoxifen, nulliparity, diabetes, and obesity. Endometrial carcinoma is only seen in less than 1% of postmenopausal females with abnormal vaginal bleeding (Fig. 5).

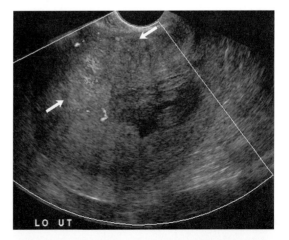

FIGURE 5. Longitudinal ultrasound of the uterus reveals a large fundal mass, complex in echo texture, with ill-defined margins of the myometrium and endometrium. Color Doppler evaluation reveals the vascularity of the large hyperechoic component (*arrows*) of this endometrial carcinoma.

26. What sonographic feature of endometrial carcinoma helps distinguish it from other uterine entities?

Beyond simple thickening of the endometrium, usually there is focal irregularity and myometrial invasion that is often echogenic (Fig. 6).

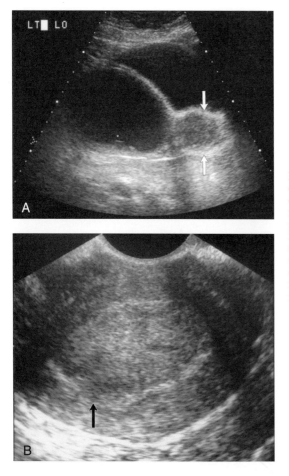

FIGURE 6. *A,* Longitudinal ultrasound demonstrates an expanded uterine cavity containing hypoechoic to anoechoic material caused by an obstructing homogenous hypoechoic tumor (*arrows*). Histologically, it was revealed to be an adenosquamous carcinoma. *B,* Transverse transvaginal ultrasound shows a thickened hyperechoic endometrium with irregularity (*arrow*) consistent with endometrial carcinoma.

27. How is endometrial carcinoma staged?
- Stage 0: Carcinoma in situ
- Stage 1A: No myometrial invasion
- Stage 1B: Less than half the myometrium is invaded
- Stage 1C: More than half the myometrium is invaded

Note: MRI is more accurate than ultrasound for detecting myometrial invasion of endometrial carcinoma.
- Stage 2A: Tumor invades cervical mucosa
- Stage 2B: Tumor invades cervical mucosa and stroma
- Stage 3: Tumor invades uterine serosa, parametrium, adnexa, or para-aortic lymph nodes
- Stage 4: Tumor invades mucosa of bladder or rectum and extends beyond the true pelvis or distant metastases

28. What are guidelines to help distinguish benign from malignant conditions in women with postmenopausal bleeding?

Malignant uterine tumors tend to demonstrate a thickened echogenic endometrium, are enlarged, and lack the characteristic subendometrial halo. Benign and malignant uterine diseases do not possess distinguishing Doppler features.

29. What are two modalities that can be employed to detect uterine diseases such as polyps, endometrial hyperplasia, carcinoma, adhesions, and submucosal fibroids?

Transvaginal ultrasound and hysterosonography can be used to detect uterine diseases. Hysterosonography may better depict the contents of the uterine cavity.

30. What are some causes of infertility that can be diagnosed by ultrasound?

Uterine, tubal, and adnexal abnormalities can often be detected such as endometriosis, pelvic inflammatory disease, endometrial adhesions (Asherman's syndrome), ovarian endometriosis, or fibroids and polyps.

31. How does HRT affect sonographic appearances?

Most sources indicate that HRT will result in an increase in postmenopausal endometrial thickness but not myometrial thickness. In general this increase is typically observed soon after initiation of therapy but thickness does not continue to increase with continued duration of therapy. The effect, however, varies with different regimens. Although some use an endometrial stripe thickness of 8 mm as the cut-off of normal range, many use less than 5 mm even with HRT.

32. How does tamoxifen affect sonographic evaluation?

Tamoxifen is a partial estrogen receptor agonist often used in postmenopausal women with breast cancer. The effect of tamoxifen on the uterus includes epithelial metaplasia, hyperplasia, and potentially carcinoma. Ultimately, this may result in a thickened, irregular, and even cystic endometrium. An increased endometrial thickness in the setting of a woman on tamoxifen with endometrial cancer is of uncertain significance. Regimens for follow-up remain unclear.

33. What is the differential diagnosis of a cystic endometrial stripe?

- Tamoxifen effect (Fig. 7)
- Endometrial polyps

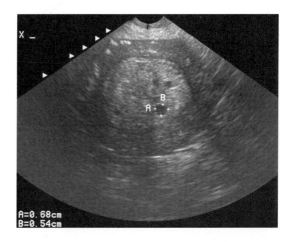

FIGURE 7. Transverse ultrasound of the uterus reveals a thickened echogenic endometrium with cystic components (*cursors*) compatible with tamoxifen hyperplasia.

34. What are the most common sites of endometriosis?

Endometrial tissue outside the endometrium and myometrium is most commonly encountered on the following:

- Ovaries
- Uterine ligaments
- Rectovaginal septum
- Cul-de-sac
- Pelvic peritoneum

35. Endometriomas have what kind of sonographic appearance?

The appearance of endometriomas range from anechoic cysts with few or no internal echoes to a solid mass. Classically a cystic pelvic mass with homogenous hypoechoic low-level internal echoes is described. They are avascular and can have thick walls and be multiple. Linear or punctate calcification of the wall of the lesion is also a good indicator of an endometrioma. Microcalcification within the lesion can result in acoustic shadowing. These often need to be differentiated from a hemorrhagic cyst that should demonstrate regression with time.

36. What are the classic symptoms of endometriosis?

- Dysmenorrhea
- Dyspareunia
- Lower abdominal, pelvic, and back pain
- Irregular vaginal bleeding
- Infertility

BIBLIOGRAPHY

1. Callen PW: Ultrasonography in Obstetrics and Gynecology, 4th ed. Philadelphia, WB Saunders, 2000.
2. Rumack CM, Wilson SR, Charboneau JW (eds): Diagnostic Ultrasound, 4th ed. St. Louis, Mosby, 1998.
3. Woodward P: Imaging of uterine disorders. In Radiologic Pathology. Washington, DC, Armed Forces Institute of Pathology, 2002, pp 401–412.

12. BENIGN AND MALIGNANT ADNEXAL LESIONS

Stephen W. Tamarkin, M.D., and Vikram Dogra, M.D.

1. How is an ovary measured?

Ovarian size is evaluated by assessing the volume. The three dimensions (length [L], height [H], width [W]) or (anteroposterior [AP], transverse, craniocaudad) are multiplied, then the product is multiplied by 0.543. This estimation is based on the mathematical formula for volume of a prolate ellipse: $L \times W \times H \times 0.543$.

2. What is the normal size of an ovary?

The normal ranges for ovarian volumes vary with a woman's age. The upper limit for normal ovarian volume is highest in young adult women (9.8–14 ml) and declines with increasing age. The decrease in size progresses more rapidly after menopause.

3. What are some common structures normally seen within an ovary with ultrasound?

Multiple follicles are typically visualized as small anechoic cysts within each ovary (Fig. 1). More follicles are visible with transvaginal scanning or with high-quality transabdominal (TA) scanning, particularly in thin women. With each menstrual cycle, one follicle enlarges and becomes the dominant follicle. A normal dominant follicle can measure up to 2.5 cm. The dominant follicle releases the oocyte (ovulation) and then becomes a corpus luteum. If no pregnancy has occurred, the corpus luteum gradually involutes. On ultrasound, this normal structure is cystic, possibly with wall irregularity or internal echoes. These detailed findings are also more commonly appreciated with transvaginal imaging.

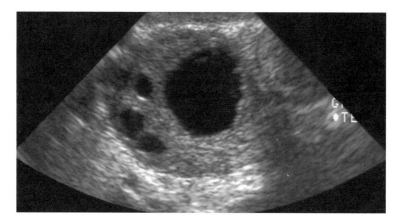

FIGURE 1. Longitudinal view of the ovary shows follicles as anechoic.

4. How are ovaries identified with ultrasound?

Ovaries can usually be identified by scanning the adnexal regions lateral to and sometimes superior, posterior, or anterior to the uterus. They are often anterior to the internal iliac vessels. The uterine size and position also affects ovarian position. The combination of typical ovarian size and shape, presence of follicles, and subtle echo texture difference compared with the background allows the ovaries to be discretely visualized with ultrasound in most women.

5. What is the size of the postmenopausal ovary?

Normal postmenopausal ovaries are between 6 and 15 cc but may be as large as 20 cc, as long as the remaining stromal tissue is normal.

6. What percentage of postmenopausal ovaries are identified by ultrasound?

At best, < 80% of postmenopausal ovaries are identified by ultrasound.

7. What are some causes of nonvisualization of ovaries?

Anything that obscures visualization of portions of the pelvis can prevent ovary visualization. Common causes include acoustic shadowing from uterine leiomyomas or bowel loops, patient obesity, and inadequate bladder distention (for transabdominal scanning). Small ovaries, commonly in postmenopausal women, are more difficult to identify.

8. Can other structures simulate ovaries on ultrasound?

Yes. Pelvic structures, including the broad ligament and exophytic leiomyomas, may be mistaken for the ovary, limiting additional search. Evaluation of the structure's echo texture, confirming ovarian morphology in transverse and sagittal planes, differentiating follicles from vessels with color Doppler, and experience are all helpful. The entire adnexal region should be examined in every pelvic examination, with particular emphasis given when ovarian identification is questionable.

9. Are the terms *follicle* and *follicular cyst* synonymous?

No. Follicles are normal ovarian structures and normally visible with good quality ultrasound examination of premenopausal women. One relatively larger follicle, the dominant follicle, is commonly visible before ovulation and is visible after ovulation as the corpus luteum. A follicular cyst is an abnormal structure, due either to a stimulated (mature) dominant follicle that does not release its oocyte or a nondominant follicle that retains fluid.

10. Are the terms *corpus luteum* and corpus *luteum cyst* synonymous?

Whereas a corpus luteum is a normal structure, a corpus luteum cyst or hemorrhagic corpus luteum refers to a corpus luteum that has either retained fluid or had internal hemorrhage. Follicular and corpus luteum cysts and hemorrhagic corpus luteum are common causes of nonneoplastic ovarian cysts on ultrasound study and together can be referred to as *physiologic* cysts. They resolve with time and are the reason follow-up ultrasounds are commonly recommended for indeterminate ovarian cysts.

11. What are some common causes of cystic adnexal masses?

Physiologic ovarian cysts such as hemorrhagic, follicular, or corpus luteal cysts, ovarian neoplasms, or endometriomas are relatively common. Tubal ectopic pregnancies or tuboovarian abscesses may be partially cystic complex masses. Parovarian or paratubal cysts or dilated fallopian tubes (hydrosalpinx) are also possible.

12. How do hemorrhagic ovarian cysts occur?

At the time of ovulation, the granulosa layer along the margin of the follicle becomes more vascular. These vessels are fragile and susceptible to rupture, leading to hemorrhage into the cyst.

13. What are the common appearances of a hemorrhagic cyst?

The most common appearance is a thin-walled cyst measuring 2.5–8.5 cm with innumerable internal septations. This pattern has been referred to as "cobweb" or "fishnet weave" pattern (Fig. 2). These septations do not have flow on color Doppler because they represent fibrin strands. A cystic mass with a retracting peripheral clot, cyst with fluid-fluid level, or cyst with thick or irregular wall is less commonly seen.

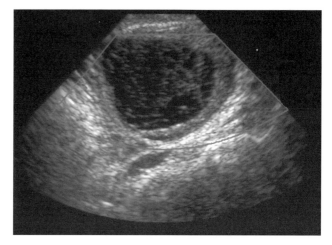

FIGURE 2. Sonogram of the ovary demonstrates classic fishnet appearance in a hemorrhagic cyst. These cysts show minimal through transmission as opposed to endometriomas.

14. What are some additional uncommon adnexal region cystic masses?

Pedunculated fibroid with cystic degeneration, lymphoceles, theca lutein cysts, perineural cysts, varicose ovarian veins, arterial aneurysms or other vascular malformations, loculated ascites, and peritoneal or mesenteric cysts are among the many possible uncommon causes of adnexal region cysts.

15. What are endometriomas?

Endometriosis refers to the ectopic presence of endometrial tissue outside the uterus. It may occur as endometrial implants along various peritoneal surfaces, or it may have a focal cystic collection, referred to as an *endometrioma*. Endometriomas are also known as "chocolate cysts" and are usually asymptomatic. Endometrial implants not associated with a larger mass or cyst are not typically visualized with ultrasound.

16. What are the typical ultrasound characteristics of endometriomas?

Endometriomas are usually cystic, masslike collections, often containing low-level echoes. Small echogenic foci along the wall (Fig. 3) and multiple loculations are common.

17. What is the most common site of endometriosis?

Ovarian involvement accounts for 80% of cases of endometriosis

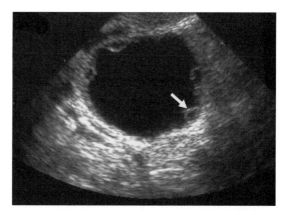

FIGURE 3. Sonogram of an endometrioma reveals hyperechoic wall foci (*arrow*), presumed to be cholesterol deposits, characteristic of endometrioma seen in 10% of cases.

18. What are the extraovarian sites of endometriotic implants?

Extraovarian involvement includes pleural surfaces, peritoneum, rectosigmoid, urinary bladder, and soft tissue.

19. What is catamenial pneumothorax?

In patients with pleural surface involvement, repeated pneumothoraces correspond to the woman's menstrual period. This pleural involvement is exclusively right sided.

20. What are some of the common histologic types of ovarian neoplasms?

There are numerous different histologic types of ovarian neoplasms. The most common are neoplasms arising from ovarian epithelium including benign serous and mucinous cystadenoma, and malignant serous and mucinous cystadenocarcinomas. Dermoids are also common and are the most common of the germ cell neoplasms, with malignant teratomas being much less common. Benign neoplasms arising from the ovarian stroma such as fibromas and thecomas are rare. Metastatic disease can involve the ovaries.

21. What do ovarian neoplasms look like with ultrasound?

Ovarian neoplasms may be cystic, cystic and solid, or solid masses causing overall ovarian enlargement.

22. What ultrasound features of an ovarian mass increase the likelihood for malignancy?

The greater the solid component, the greater the likelihood the lesion is malignant. And, malignant masses tend to be larger. Thick or irregular septations, mural nodules, and papillary projections all increase the probability that a cystic mass is malignant.

23. Does color Doppler have any role in evaluation of ovarian masses?

Yes. Color Doppler flow within the central aspect of the solid component of a mass is a feature that increases the suspicion that a mass is malignant. Malignant masses may have low-resistance spectral Doppler flow because of neovascularity, but this is a nonspecific finding that may also be seen in benign neoplasms and non-neoplastic entities such as corpus luteum cysts or ectopic pregnancies.

24. What is the significance of resistive index (RI) and pulsatility index (PI) when assessing arterial flow within an ovarian mass?

An RI of < 0.4 and PI of > 1 are suggestive of malignancy (due to neovascularity).

25. Does the ovarian mass size help in determining its benignity?

Yes. Ovarian masses < 5 cm (in long axis) are more likely to be benign; ovarian masses > 10 cm are more likely to be malignant.

26. Can any of the histologic neoplasm types be determined sonographically?

Mature cystic teratoma (MCT) can have a characteristic appearance allowing accurate histologic diagnosis based on ultrasound in some cases. Some mixed cystic and solid masses may be suggestive of the various epithelial neoplasms, but in general they do not have specific appearances. Metastatic disease can be suggested in the right clinical setting with a solid ovarian mass.

27. What is the ultrasound appearance of MCT?

MCT often has a highly characteristic echogenic component called the *dermoid plug*. This varying sized echogenic component is usually part of a complex mass that often also has cystic components and sometimes focal calcifications. Fat is the main content. The MCT may cause sound attenuation obscuring the deeper portions of the mass. The old and commonly used clinical terminology for MCT is dermoid (Fig. 4).

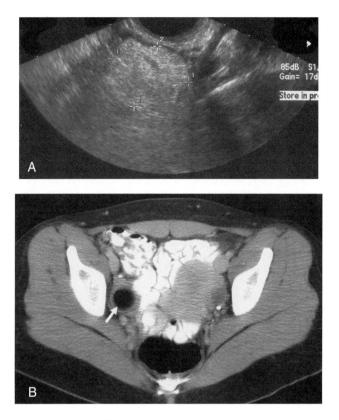

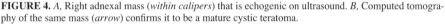

FIGURE 4. *A,* Right adnexal mass (*within calipers*) that is echogenic on ultrasound. *B,* Computed tomography of the same mass (*arrow*) confirms it to be a mature cystic teratoma.

28. Describe an immature cystic teratoma.

Immature teratomas are composed of tissues derived from the three germ layers. Immature teratomas differ from mature cystic teratomas in that they demonstrate clinically malignant behavior, are much less common (< 1% of ovarian teratomas), affect a younger age group (usually during the first 2 decades of life), and are histologically distinguished by the presence of immature or embryonic tissues. These are of large size at presentation.

29. How often are MCTs bilateral?

Ten to fifteen percent of dermoids are bilateral.

30. What types of malignancies metastasize to the ovaries?

Breast and gastrointestinal malignancies are most common. Metastatic spread from endometrial carcinoma may be difficult to differentiate from primary endometroid neoplasm of the ovary. Lymphoma may also involve the ovaries.

31. What is the common appearance of metastasis to the ovary?

Bilateral solid masses are commonly seen in ovarian metastasis.

32. What is Krukenberg's tumor?

This is a rare type of ovarian tumor that is usually secondary to metastatic disease from a gastrointestinal primary, especially from the stomach.

33. What is Meigs' syndrome?

This refers to ascites and pleural effusion related to an ovarian fibroma, which is a rare mass. This is sometimes also used to describe pleural effusion and ascites secondary to other ovarian tumors. In cases of Meigs' syndrome, removal of fibroma results in resolution of ascites and pleural effusion.

34. What is struma ovarii?

Presence of thyroid tissue in ovary is called struma ovarii. Struma ovarii accounts for approximately 3% of all mature teratomas.

35. Does ultrasound have role in ovarian cancer screening?

Yes. However, screening ultrasound has not been proven to be sensitive and specific enough in detecting early stage ovarian malignancies to warrant mass population screening. Current recommendations limit screening to women with increased risk for development of ovarian cancer, particularly those with a family history of ovarian malignancy. Correlation with the serologic marker Ca-125 can also be performed.

36. If ovarian screening is performed, should a transabdominal or transvaginal approach be used?

A transvaginal approach allows more detailed evaluation of the ovary.

37. What is the appearance of the ovaries with polycystic ovarian disease?

The ovaries are typically enlarged and contain multiple follicles. However, these findings are not universal and the ovarian volumes are normal in 30% of cases. Increased ovarian stromal echogenicity on transvaginal scanning is also characteristic.

38. What is the relationship between pelvic inflammatory disease (PID) and tubo-ovarian abscess?

PID is a general term referring to an inflammatory condition involving to varying degrees the fallopian tubes, ovaries, and surrounding tissues. A thickened, inflamed tube (salpingitis), an inflamed, dilated, pus-filled tube (pyosalpinx), or an abscess involving the tube and ovary (tubo-ovarian abscess), are all within this spectrum.

39. What causes PID?

PID is usually an ascending infection from the vagina and uterus, often caused by a sexually transmitted infection such as *Chlamydia* or gonorrhea. Rarely direct spread of an adjacent pelvic inflammatory process such as diverticulitis, appendicitis, or inflammatory bowel disease may secondarily involve the ovaries and adnexa.

40. What are sonographic findings in PID?

The findings fall in a wide spectrum. They range from endometritis manifested as endometrial thickening or fluid within the endometrial cavity (Fig. 5) to tubo-ovarian abscess, including pyosalpinx, hydrosalpinx, and particulate fluid in the cul de sac. Sometimes the particulate fluid in the cul de sac may appear as a solid mass surrounding the pelvic structures with variable echo texture. Patients with PID have extreme pain and tenderness in the adnexa at the time of endovaginal examination.

41. Are normal fallopian tubes visible with ultrasound?

No. The broad ligaments including the tubes may be visualized, but normal caliber tubes are not discretely identified. The broad ligaments are most easily visualized when surrounded by ascites.

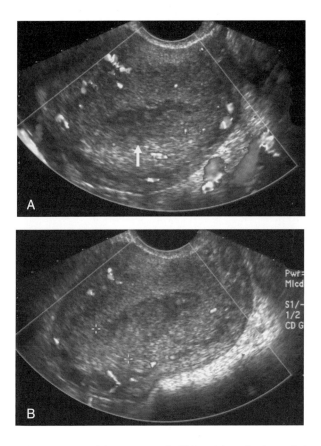

FIGURE 5. Longitudinal sonogram of the uterus reveals thickened, irregular, hypoechoic endometrium by arrow in (*A*) and within calipers in (*B*) in a patient with confirmed endometritis.

42. Can dilated tubes be seen with ultrasound?

Yes. Abnormally dilated fallopian tubes may be identified as tubular, serpiginous, aperistaltic, fluid-filled structures in the adnexal region, with one end often closely related to the ovary. When the dilated tube is filled with anechoic fluid (hydrosalpinx), a definable wall is usually visible. The wall may have small irregularities, which have a spacing pattern similar to that of colonic haustra.

43. What can cause complex fluid in a dilated tube?

A dilated pus-filled tube is called a pyosalpinx, which is usually a component of pelvic inflammatory disease. Hematosalpinx is a blood-filled fallopian tube, often caused by a tubal ectopic pregnancy.

44. Describe the sonographic features of hydrosalpinx?

- Convoluted cystic structures
- Echogenic wall
- Fluid debris level (Fig. 6)
- Small polypoid excrescences

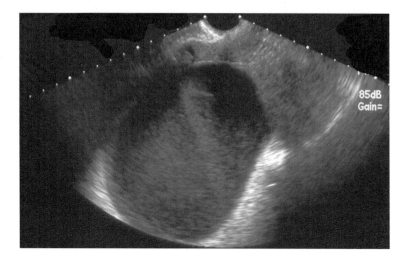

FIGURE 6. Adnexal mass reveals fluid-debris level, consistent with hydrosalpinx.

BIBLIOGRAPHY

1. Albayram F, Hamper UM: Ovarian and adnexal torsion: Spectrum of sonographic findings with pathologic correlation. J Ultrasound Med 20:10, 2001.
2. Brown DL, Doubilet PM, Miller FH, et al: Benign and malignant ovarian masses: Selection of the most discriminating gray-scale and Doppler sonographic features. Radiology 208:103–110, 1998.
3. Cohen HL, Tice HM, Mandel FS: Ovarian volumes measured by US: Bigger than we think. Radiology 177:189–192, 1990.
4. Hensley ML, Castiel M, Robson ME: Screening for ovarian cancer: What we know, what we need to know. Oncology (Huntingt) 14:1601–1607, 2000.
5. Jain KA: Sonographic spectrum of hemorrhagic ovarian cysts. J Ultrasound Med 21:879–886, 2002.
6. National Institutes of Health Consensus Development Conference Statement: Ovarian cancer: Screening, treatment, and follow-up. Gynecol Oncol 55(3 pt 2):S4–S14, 1994.
7. Patel MD, Feldstein VA, Chen DC, et al: Endometriomas: Diagnostic performance of US. Radiology 210:739–745, 1999.
8. Salem S: The Uterus and adnexa. In Rumack CM, Wilson SR, Charboneau JW (eds): Diagnostic Ultrasound, 2nd ed. St. Louis, Mosby, 1998, pp 519–573.

13. OVARIAN TORSION

Raj Mohan Paspulati, M.D.

1. What is the incidence of ovarian torsion?
Ovarian torsion accounts for 2.7% of all gynecologic emergencies.

2. Which ovary is commonly involved in torsion?
It is more common on the right side because the sigmoid colon occupies the left lower quadrant.

3. What are the predisposing factors for ovarian torsion?
An ovarian mass is the most common predisposing factor and is present in 50–81% of patients. These are usually benign. Mature cystic teratoma is the most common mass. Other causes of ovarian enlargement are ovarian hyperstimulation syndrome, paraovarian cysts, follicular cysts, and benign ovarian tumors such as fibromas, thecomas, and cystadenomas.

4. Can ovarian torsion occur without an underlying mass?
Yes. Torsion of a normal ovary without a predisposing mass can occur in prepubertal females because of adnexal mobility.

5. What is the pathogenesis of ovarian torsion?
Torsion of the ovarian pedicle produces circulatory stasis, which is initially venous but becomes arterial as the torsion and resultant edema progress. The vascularity depends on the degree of torsion, which varies from an incomplete twist of 180° to multiple twists. If torsion is complete and arterial supply is obstructed, hemorrhagic necrosis and gangrene of the ovary occurs. If torsion is partial and intermittent with spontaneous untwisting, blood flow to the ovary is preserved.

6. What is the clinical picture of adnexal torsion?
Patients present with lower abdominal pain of acute onset, which can mimic other causes of acute abdomen such as acute appendicitis. Symptoms can be intermittent, and a palpable adnexal mass may be present.

7. Which is the first imaging modality to be used for diagnosis of ovarian torsion?
Transabdominal and transvaginal ultrasonography is the first examination to be performed in an emergency setting.

8. Is there any role of CT and MRI in a patient with suspected ovarian torsion?
When the sonographic features are inconclusive of ovarian torsion and an alternative diagnosis is suspected, computed tomography (CT) and magnetic resonance imaging (MRI) are useful ancillary modalities to confirm the diagnosis (Fig. 1).

9. What determines the sonographic features of ovarian torsion?
- Duration and degree of torsion
- Complete or incomplete torsion
- Presence or absence of an underlying ovarian mass or hemorrhage

10. What are the grayscale ultrasound findings of ovarian torsion?
The following grayscale findings in ovarian torsion are nonspecific (see Figure 1):
- Enlarged ovary
- Enlarged ovary with multiple peripheral follicles has been described in about 64% of patients with ovarian torsion

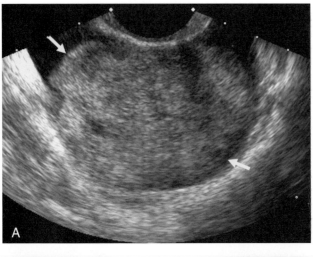

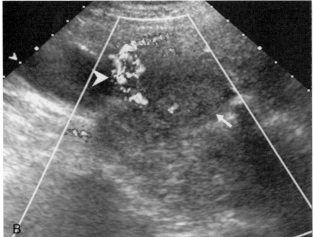

FIGURE 1. *A,* Surgically confirmed infracted right ovary. Sonogram demonstrates a large right ovary (*within arrows*). *B,* Color Doppler demonstrates vascularity of the twisted pedicle (*arrowhead*) and absence of vascular flow in the infracted right ovary (*arrow*) (see also Color Plates, Figure 4). *C,* CT of the pelvis showing enlarged ovary (*arrow*) with multiple small hypodensities and an enlarged pedicle extending medially. There is no significant central enhancement consistent with infracted ovary.

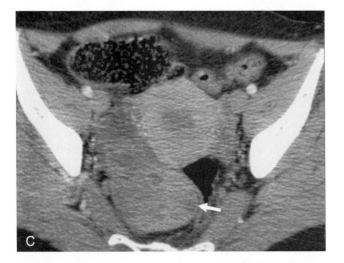

- Cystic, solid, or complex mass
- Cyst with hemorrhage
- Cyst with eccentric wall thickening
- Free fluid in the pelvis, which can be anechoic or hemorrhagic

11. What are the color Doppler findings of ovarian torsion?
The main finding is an enlarged ovary with absent or markedly diminished blood flow as compared to the contralateral ovary. Demonstration of blood flow depends on the degree of torsion. In the early stages of torsion, there will be absence of venous flow and arterial flow can be demonstrated with diminished or absent diastolic component. With further progression of torsion, there is no demonstrable arterial flow.

12. Does the presence of arterial flow on Doppler ultrasound excludes ovarian torsion?
No. In early stages of torsion and partial torsion, arterial flow may be demonstrated. Persistent arterial flow in a torsed ovary is attributed to the dual arterial supply of ovary from the ovarian artery and uterine artery.

13. What is the twisted vascular pedicle sign on sonography?
The twisted vascular pedicle corresponds to the broad ligament, fallopian tube, and adnexal and ovarian branches of the uterine artery and vein. This is a definite sign of ovarian torsion. On ultrasound, it appears as a round, hyperechoic structure with multiple concentric hypoechoic stripes, giving it a target appearance. It can also appear as an ellipsoid or tubular structure with internal heterogeneous echoes. On color Doppler, flow within the twisted vessels of the pedicle can be demonstrated; this is known as the whirlpool sign of ovarian torsion.

14. What other adnexal masses can mimic ovarian torsion?
The nonspecific grayscale ultrasonographic features of ovarian torsion are indistinguishable from:
- Ectopic pregnancy
- Pelvic inflammatory disease
- Endometriosis
- Hemorrhagic ovarian cyst

15. What is the treatment of ovarian torsion?
Adnexectomy is performed when the ovary is not viable on gross examination and is avascular on Doppler ultrasound. Untwisting of the vascular pedicle is performed when the ovary is viable and has demonstrable vascularity. This conserves ovarian function but does raise concern for thromboembolism from the thrombosed ovarian vein.

BIBLIOGRAPHY

1. Desai SK, Allahbadia GN, Dalal AK: Ovarian torsion: Diagnosis by color Doppler ultrasonography. Obstet Gynecol 84:699–701, 1994.
2. Fleischer AC, Stein SM, Cullinan JA, et al: Color Doppler sonography of adnexal torsion. J Ultrasound Med 14:523–528, 1995.
3. Helvie MA, Silver TM: Ovarian torsion: Sonographic evaluation. J Clin Ultrasound 17:327–332, 1989.
4. Lee EJ, Kwon HC, Joo HJ, et al: Diagnosis of ovarian torsion by color Doppler sonography: Depiction of twisted vascular pedicle. J Ultrasound Med 17:83–89, 1998.
5. Rosado WM Jr, Trambert MA, Gosink BB, Pretorius DH: Adnexal torsion: Diagnosis by using Doppler sonography. AJR Am J Roentgenol 159:1251–1253, 1992.
6. Sommerville M, Grimes DA, Koonings PP, et al: Ovarian neoplasms and the risk of adnexal torsion. Am J Obstet Gynecol 164:577–578, 1991.

14. SONOHYSTEROGRAPHY

Jeanne A. Cullinan, M.D.

1. What is sonohysterography?

Sonohysterography (SHG) is a technique whereby saline enhancement is provided for transvaginal sonography.

2. Who should have this examination?

Patients with abnormal vaginal bleeding or infertility patients may benefit from this examination. It is used in the evaluation of an abnormal endometrial interface seen on a baseline pelvic examination.

3. What if the baseline examination is abnormal?

SHG is useful if the endometrium is noted to be "out of phase" with expected menses. A thick echogenic endometrium would not be expected in the preovulatory period. Demonstration of this finding significantly increases the yield of SHG. Failure to demonstrate a layered endometrium in days 7–10 of a menstrual cycle may suggest underlying pathology.

4. How is the examination performed?

The initial evaluation includes a baseline transvaginal examination. The uterine orientation, bilayer thickness of the endometrium, and size and location of pelvic pathology are noted. It is performed in the first part of the menstrual cycle to minimize the possibility of an unrecognized pregnancy.

5. How is SHG performed?

The catheter is introduced into the uterus under aseptic conditions. The transvaginal probe is reinserted. Sterile saline is injected under continuous sonographic visualization. Endometrial thickness with particular attention to asymmetry is undertaken, and the presence of any intraluminal masses is documented. Fluid in the posterior cul-de-sac at the termination of the procedure is presumed to be evidence of patency of at least one fallopian tube.

6. What type of catheter should be used?

Even though a 5-French pediatric feeding tube provides adequate distention, it may be difficult to insert. Its major advantage is that it is inexpensive. A compromise for cost and placement is an intrauterine insemination catheter. The slightly more rigid construction may aid in its placement. Alternatively, a plastic hysterosalpingogram catheter with an occluding balloon may be used.

7. Are there any contraindications to SHG?

Contraindications include acute pelvic inflammatory disease. A relative contraindication is a history of pelvic inflammatory disease.

8. Is premedication necessary?

Although no premedication is necessary for most patients, nonsteroidal anti-inflammatory agents may be useful in reducing symptoms of cramping. Prophylactic antibiotics are not used in our institution. The choice of specific medications is dictated by local practice. The institutional protocol for hysterosalpingography may serve as a reasonable guideline.

9. Will SHG lead to intraperitoneal seeding of endometrial carcinoma?

Prior clinical experience with hysterosalpingography makes this unlikely. All forms of endometrial sampling, dilatation and curettage, or hysteroscopy may result in spillage of endometrial cells into the peritoneal cavity. The theoretical risk of seeding is similar to that posed by these techniques.

10. What are the sonohysterographic findings in common conditions?

Normal appearance: A baseline endometrium shows a layered symmetric endometrial interface. It is important to examine the uterus in both sagittal and coronal planes to exclude subtle abnormalities (Fig. 1).

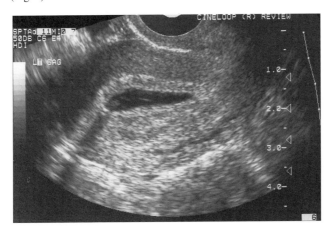

FIGURE 1. Normal. The uterine cavity is distended with saline. A symmetrical endometrial interface is seen.

Polyps: The baseline evaluation may show a thickened, often complex interface. As fluid is instilled, the polyp is identified as an intraluminal mass completely surrounded by fluid except at its point of attachment (Fig. 2).

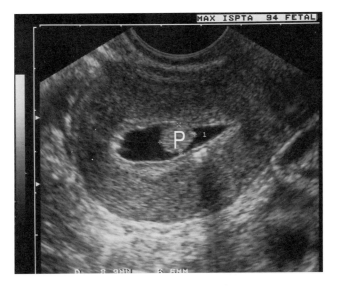

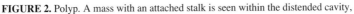

FIGURE 2. Polyp. A mass with an attached stalk is seen within the distended cavity,

Leiomyoma: The size and presumed location of leiomyomata are documented on the baseline evaluation. Fluid instillation allows precise determination as to the site of the fibroid (Fig. 3). A submucosal fibroid impinges on the cavity, but has a layer of endometrium overlying it. The size of the fibroid and its depth into the myometrium are important clinical findings. Intramural fibroids do not cause distortion of the endometrial cavity.

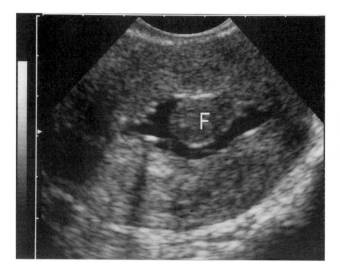

FIGURE 3. Fibroid. A submucosal fibroid is seen impinging on the endometrial cavity.

Intrauterine adhesions: The baseline evaluation is usually normal, although small echogenic foci may be seen at the endometrial-myometrial junction. Many patients have a history of prior instrumentation. With fluid instillation, fibrotic strands of tissue tether the cavity. The degree of distortion is determined by the extent of the adhesions. Extreme cases show no distention of the cavity, whereas less severe cases may show coaptation of portions of the wall with evidence of bridging adhesions. SHG may show minor changes with fragments of tissue seen undulating in the cavity as fluid is instilled. Minor findings on SHG may be clinically significant in patients with infertility because the adhesions are often more extensive at the time of hysteroscopy (Fig. 4).

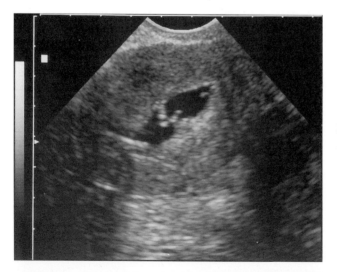

FIGURE 4. Adhesions. There is tethering of the endometrial cavity by thick intrauterine adhesions.

Endometrial hyperplasia or carcinoma: The baseline evaluation may show a complex endometrial interface. The installation of fluid allows assessment of the single-layer thickness. Because endometrial pathology may not be a global process initially, it is important to document asymmetry of the endometrium to direct the clinician to areas of possible pathology (Fig. 5).

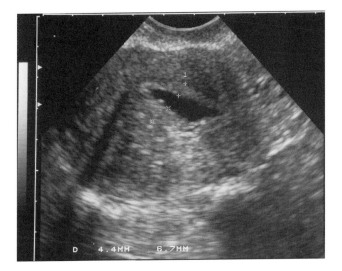

FIGURE 5. Endometrial hyperplasia. An asymmetric endometrial interface is noted.

Uterine anomalies: The baseline evaluation often suggests this finding. The serosal surface is examined to differentiate a septate from a bicornuate uterus. The installation of fluid helps document the size of the cavities as well as the thickness and extent of the septum. An occluding catheter improves the distention of the cavities.

Other abnormalities: SHG has been used to evaluate for retained products of conception and foreign bodies. The site of a prior cesarean scar can also be assessed by this technique.

11. Are there certain situations in which this test cannot be performed?

Entry of the cavity may be difficult in patients with cervical stenosis. The cervix can usually be dilated sufficiently to allow the placement of a 5-French catheter. Other situations limiting this technique include the presence of large uterine fibroids, which may limit distention of the cavity. A false-positive diagnosis may result if the patient is examined in postovulatory phase of the cycle because of wrinkling of the endometrial surface, presumably due to hormonal effects on the endometrium.

12. What is expected in a patient with abnormal vaginal bleeding?

SHG may demonstrate the cause of the bleeding. It differentiates between fibroids and polyps, and provides assessment for an abnormal endometrial thickening. This serves as a triage technique in women in whom further intervention is necessary.

13. What can be expected in women with infertility?

SHG is especially sensitive in evaluating the endometrial cavity, particularly in women with secondary infertility. It allows one to differentiate uterine polyps, abnormal endometrial interfaces, adhesions, and intramural fibroids. Its use is limited in the assessment of tubal patency because of the difficulty in assessing the fallopian tubes.

BIBLIOGRAPHY

1. Bree RL,Carlos RC: US for postmenopausal bleeding: Consensus development and patient-centered outcomes. Radiology 222:595–598, 2002.
2. Carlos RC, Bree RL, Abrahamse PA, et al: Cost-effectiveness of saline-assisted hysterosonography and office hysteroscopy in the evaluation of post-menopausal bleeding: A decision analysis. Acad Radiol 8:835–844, 2001.
3. Cullinan JA, Fleischer AC, Kepple DM, et al: Sonohysterography: A technique for endometrial evaluation. Radiographics 15:501–514, 1995.
4. Devore GR, Schwartz PE, Morris JM: Hysterography: A 5-year follow-up in patients with endometrial carcinoma. Obstet Gynecol 60:369–372, 1982.
5. Medverd JR, Dubinsky TJ: Cost analysis model to compare US versus endometrial biopsy in the evaluation of peri- and post-menopausal abnormal vaginal bleeding. Radiology 222:619–627, 2002.
6. Neele SJM, Van Baal M, Van Der Morren MJ, et al: Ultrasound assessment of the endometrium in healthy, asymptomatic early post-menopausal women: Saline infusion sonohysterography versus transvaginal ultrasound. Ultrasound Obstet Gynecol 16:254–259, 2000.
7. Smith RP, Bradley LD, Ke RW, Strickland JL (eds): Clinical Management of Abnormal Uterine Bleeding. Association of Professors of Gynecology and Obstetrics Educational Series. Boston, MA, Jespersen & Associates LLC, 2002.
8. Tak WK, Anderson B, Vardi JR, et al: Myometrial invasion and hysterography in endometrial carcinoma. Obstet Gynecol 50:159–165, 1977.

IV. General Abdomen

15. THE GALLBLADDER AND BILIARY TREE
Amy R. Harrow, M.D.

1. What are common indications for performing sonography of the gallbladder and biliary system?
- Jaundice
- Abnormal liver function tests
- Clinically suspected cholecystitis (right upper quadrant pain, fever, leukocytosis)
- Suspected gallstones as etiology of pancreatitis

2. What are the advantages of imaging the gallbladder and bile ducts with ultrasound rather than other modalities?
- Lack of ionizing radiation
- No need for administration of intravenous contrast material; noninvasive
- Speed and portability
- Independent of organ physiologic function regarding gastrointestinal and hepatobiliary systems

3. When is the best time to image the gallbladder?
Optimal examination of the gallbladder can be obtained after 6 hours of fasting. When possible, it is desirable to perform the gallbladder ultrasound examination after the patient has fasted overnight. Overlying distended or gas-containing bowel loops can obscure visualization. Physiologic gallbladder contraction results in the gallbladder having a small, thick-walled appearance. In an emergency study, gallbladder ultrasound can be performed without fasting because most of these patients have had little or nothing to eat.

4. What anatomic structure can be used to identify the gallbladder?
The neck of the gallbladder has a fixed relationship to the main interlobar hepatic fissure and the undivided right portal vein (Fig. 1). This relationship helps identify the gallbladder. Anomalous gallbladder location is highly unusual.

5. What are the anatomic parts of the gallbladder?
The gallbladder is divided into the neck, which is narrow, and connects to the cystic duct, the body, which has fairly parallel walls, and the fundus, which may dilate slightly and is the cup- or bowl-shaped end of the gallbladder. (The cystic duct contains the valves of Heister.)

6. What is a Hartmann's pouch?
Hartmann's pouch or diverticulum is located at the junction of the neck and cystic duct (stones collect in it). It may be present not as a normal anatomic feature, but rather as a result of chronic inflammation.

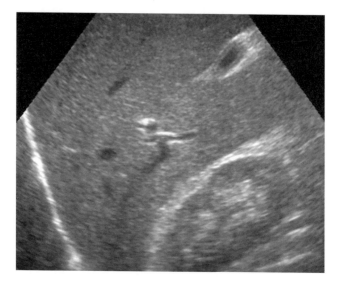

FIGURE 1. Longitudinal ultrasound shows a contracted gallbladder in the main interlobar fissure.

7. What is the normal size and shape of the gallbladder?

There can be considerable variation in size and shape of the normal gallbladder. However, the gallbladder is considered to be hydropic if it measures greater than 5 cm in transverse diameter and is not ovoid in shape. If the diameter is less than 2 cm despite appropriate fasting, it is considered abnormally contracted.

8. What is a Phrygian cap deformity?

This normal anatomic variant is present in approximately 4% of patients and is the result of folding of the gallbladder fundus on the body, creating a thick fold, which mimics a septation (Fig. 2).

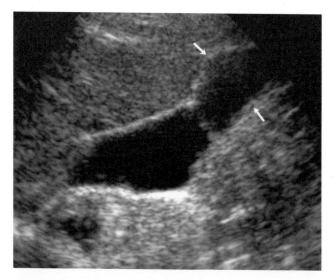

FIGURE 2. Longitudinal ultrasound shows a normal variant, a Phrygian cap deformity (*arrows*).

9. What is the normal gallbladder wall thickness?

The normal gallbladder wall is 3 mm or less. Diffuse gallbladder wall thickening is the most frequently encountered gallbladder wall abnormality detected by sonography. Abnormal wall edema appears as a hypoechoic band between two echogenic lines and may even be striated or septated.

10. What conditions besides cholecystitis cause a diffusely thickened gallbladder wall?

- Hepatitis (Fig. 3)
- Other viral etiologies—acquired immunodeficiency syndrome (AIDS), mononucleosis
- Hypoalbuminemia (due to renal or hepatic failure)
- Hepatic congestion (congestive heart failure)
- Pancreatitis
- Peptic ulcer disease
- Right-sided pyelonephritis
- Sepsis

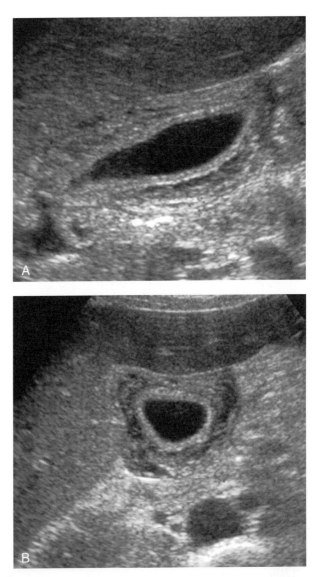

FIGURE 3. Longitudinal (*A*) and transverse (*B*) image of a diffusely thickened gallbladder wall demonstrates the characteristic hypoechoic wall edema sandwiched between echogenic striations. Gallbladder wall thickening is a nonspecific finding. This particular case was caused by hepatitis C.

11. What are less commonly encountered reasons for gallbladder wall thickening?
- Leukemic infiltration
- Interleukin-2 chemotherapy
- Gallbladder wall varices, postprandial state

12. What scanning techniques should be implemented to best visualize the gallbladder?

The patient should be placed supine or in a left posterior oblique position and scanned from a subcostal or an intercostal approach. The gallbladder should be scanned in a minimum of two positions, supine and decubitus, and from two planes, long axis and transverse. A patient may also be positioned upright or prone to demonstrate gallstone mobility (Fig. 4). The highest frequency transducer enabling penetration of the right upper quadrant should be used. Typically a 3.5-MHz or higher frequency is selected. Harmonics should be used, if available (Fig. 5).

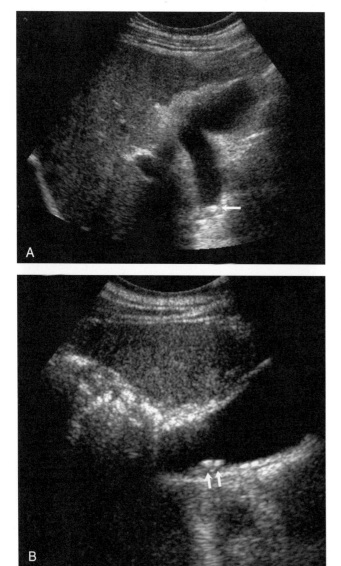

FIGURE 4. Cholelithiasis. *A,* Longitudinal supine ultrasound reveals a subtle echogenic nonshadowing focus in the gallbladder neck *(arrow)*. *B,* Decubitus view permits visualization of the stones *(arrows)*.

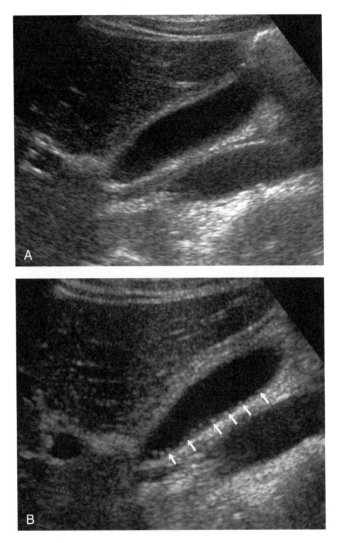

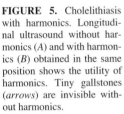

FIGURE 5. Cholelithiasis with harmonics. Longitudinal ultrasound without harmonics (*A*) and with harmonics (*B*) obtained in the same position shows the utility of harmonics. Tiny gallstones (*arrows*) are invisible without harmonics.

13. What is the sensitivity of ultrasound in detecting gallstones?
   Greater than 95%.

14. How do gallstones appear on ultrasound?
   Gallstones appear highly echogenic with posterior acoustic shadow (Fig. 6). Because the stone both absorbs and reflects the ultrasound beam, gallstones appear highly echogenic and an anechoic acoustic shadow results posteriorly. The posterior acoustic shadow is important because echogenic densities with posterior acoustic shadowing are associated with cholelithiasis nearly 100% of the time. Gallstones should also be mobile, except if they are impacted in the neck or are adherent to the gallbladder wall.

15. What echogenic masses can mimic cholelithiasis?
   Sludge balls and tumefactive biliary sludge (parasites, blood clot, aggregated pus, or contrast) can both present as mobile masses in the gallbladder and mimic gallstones. Polyps can also mimic cholelithiasis, but they are not mobile and are less likely to cause an acoustic shadow.

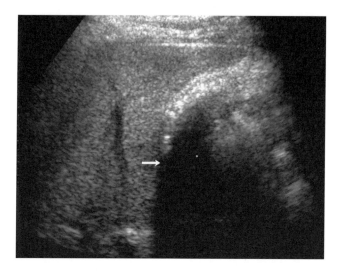

FIGURE 6. The gallbladder is filled with numerous stones resulting in marked posterior acoustic shadowing (*arrow*).

16. What is the wall-echo-shadow (WES) triad?

The WES triad or double arc shadow sign are two parallel curved echogenic lines separated by a thin anechoic space with distal acoustic shadowing (Fig. 7). The proximal echogenic line represents the gallbladder wall. The deeper echogenic line represents the anterior surface of the gallstone that produces the acoustic shadow. The WES triad is encountered in a contracted gallbladder containing numerous stones.

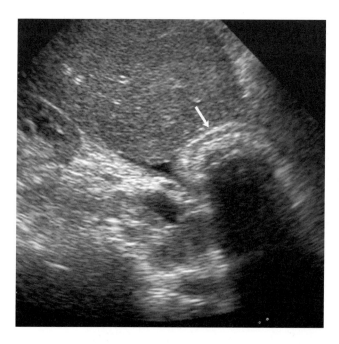

FIGURE 7. This transverse image shows an arrow demonstrating the anterior gallbladder wall in the setting of a wall-echo-shadow triad or double arc shadow sign. The sign is a hallmark of a contracted gallbladder containing multiple gallstones.

17. What is the differential diagnosis of focal gallbladder wall thickening?

The differential diagnosis is extensive:

- Cholecystitis
- Adenomyomatosis
- Pancreatitis
- Heart failure

- Cancer
- AIDS cholangiopathy
- Sclerosing cholangitis
- Hepatitis

- Hypoproteinemia
- Cirrhosis
- Portal hypertension
- Lymphatic obstruction

18. What are the hyperplastic cholecystoses?

The most common form is adenomyomatosis. The other form is cholesterolosis (strawberry gallbladder). Triglycerides and cholesterol are deposited in macrophages within the gallbladder wall. The cholesterol nodules give the wall a studded or seeded appearance contributing to the "strawberry" name. The echogenic deposits are typically less than 1 mm and there is no posterior acoustic shadowing. Sonography cannot differentiate these two entities with great confidence. *Hyperplastic cholecystosis* is a preferred term.

19. What are adenomyomatosis and its sonographic findings?

Adenomyomatosis is a benign condition characterized by hyperplastic changes of unknown etiology involving the gallbladder wall and results in overgrowth of the mucosa, thickening of the muscular wall, and formation of intramural diverticula or sinus tracts into the gallbladder wall muscular layer, termed Rokitansky-Aschoff sinuses (Fig. 8). These sinuses may contain cholesterol, bile, or calculi. The presence of cholesterol crystals in these sinuses can result in "ring down," "V-shape," or "comet tail" artifacts. Focal adenomyomatosis may be present as a focal mass or a septation, most commonly in the fundus (Fig. 9). The entity has no malignant potential.

20. What particulate matter makes up sludge?

Calcium bilirubinate and cholesterol crystals in bile result in mid-level echoes, which are viscous in nature and mobile. Bile stasis (encountered in hyperalimentation, biliary obstruction at the level of the gallbladder, cystic duct, or common bile duct) predisposes one to sludge formation. The presence of sludge suggests an underlying abnormality but is nonspecific.

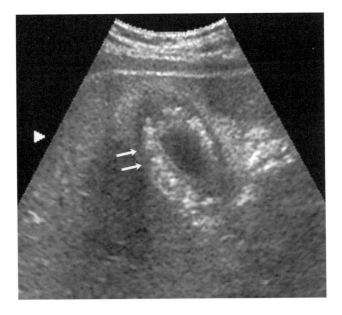

FIGURE 8. Transverse ultrasound shows highly echogenic cholesterol crystals (*arrows*) contained in Rokitansky-Aschoff sinuses, a benign condition known as adenomyomatosis.

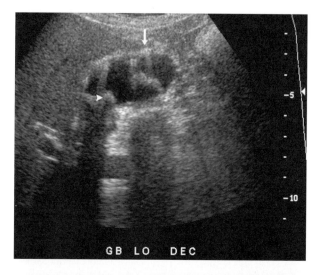

FIGURE 9. Longitudinal ultrasound shows multiple large echogenic stones (*arrowhead*) with posterior acoustic shadowing. Multiple hyperechoic foci (*arrows*) in the gallbladder wall with prominent ring down artifact are consistent with adenomyomatosis.

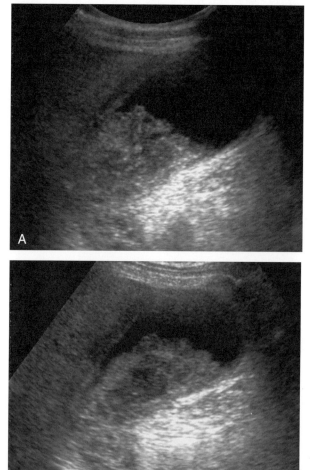

FIGURE 10. Longitudinal supine (*A*) and decubitus (*B*) views demonstrate the presence of mobile echogenic sludge, which changes in shape with change in patient position.

21. In what conditions can pericholecystic fluid be present?
Fluid may accompany acute cholecystitis with or without gallbladder perforation and abscess formation, pancreatitis, and peptic ulcer disease. The fluid tracks along the hepatoduodenal ligament. Trauma and other cause of ascites also result in pericholecystic fluid.

22. What are the sonographic features of acute cholecystitis?
Primary findings include the following (Fig. 11):
- Gallstones (acute cholecystitis is associated with cholelithiasis in approximately 90–95% of patients)
- Focally tender gallbladder (sonographic Murphy's sign)
- Impacted gallstone (stone does not change with patient positioning)

Secondary findings include the following:
- Gallbladder wall thickening (> 3 mm)
- Pericholecystic fluid
- Sludge
- Gallbladder dilatation

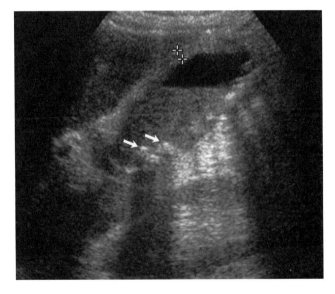

FIGURE 11. Longitudinal ultrasound in a patient with a positive Murphy sign demonstrates a thick gallbladder wall (*cursors*) with sludge and echogenic shadowing stones (*arrows*). All of these findings are consistent with acute cholecystitis.

23. What is a sonographic Murphy's sign?
A sonographic Murphy's sign is present when maximal tenderness is elicited with the transducer over the sonographically localized gallbladder (with that level of pain nowhere else).

24. What is emphysematous cholecystitis?
This entity is a surgical emergency wherein gas-producing bacteria invade the gallbladder wall (Fig. 12). The characteristic ultrasound appearance is that of a nondependent (hyperechoic) focus with accompanying reverberation artifact. Intramural gas released by the organism takes on a semicircular configuration and can mimic calcification of the gallbladder wall. Forty percent of cases are detected in diabetic patients.

25. What is the significance of gangrenous cholecystitis?
This has a mortality rate of 20% and should be suspected when a patient presents with history consistent with cholecystitis and irregular thickening of the gallbladder wall. Sixty-five percent of patients do not have a sonographic Murphy's sign, because the wall is necrotic and has no residual sensation.

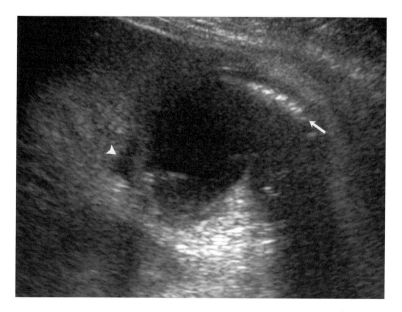

FIGURE 12. Transverse ultrasound shows nondependent echogenic foci (*arrow*) along the anterior gall-bladder wall consistent with air. Pericholecystic fluid (*arrowhead*) is evident. These findings are indicative of acute emphysematous cholecystitis.

26. What percentage of patients with acute cholecystitis have gallbladder perforation?

Gallbladder perforation occurs in 5–10% of cases. This should be suspected when sonography demonstrates complex pericholecystic fluid collections with or without septations. This usually occurs at the fundus of the gallbladder.

27. What is a porcelain gallbladder?

Extensive calcification of the gallbladder wall results in a brittle blue gallbladder suggesting a porcelain-like appearance (at surgery), hence the name. It is associated with chronic gallbladder inflammation and has an increased risk of carcinoma (13–61%). Therefore, prophylactic cholecystectomy is recommended. By ultrasound the gallbladder appears as an echogenic arc with posterior acoustic shadowing (due to extensive calcification). Differential diagnosis includes a gallbladder completely filled with stones or emphysematous cholecystitis. Plain radiograph or noncontrast CT can be used to confirm the diagnosis.

28. How does ultrasonography play a role in the clinical management of patients who are candidates for laparoscopic cholecystectomy?

- If small stones are detected, endoscopic retrograde cholangiopancreatography (ERCP) or intraoperative cholangiopancreatography should be considered.
- If the bile ducts are dilated or if choledocholithiasis is observed, preoperative ERCP or operative bile duct exploration may be indicated.
- If a large gallstone is detected, the conventional 1-cm umbilical incision may require extension to facilitate stone removal.
- If gangrenous cholecystitis is suspected, open cholecystectomy should be considered.
- Ultrasound-guided percutaneous cholecystostomy may be considered in critically ill patients (calculous and acalculous) who are poor surgical candidates in cases of suspected acute cholecystitis.

29. What is pseudolithiasis?

This is a precipitate formed when a third generation antibiotic, ceftriaxone, combines with calcium bile salts, mimicking the presence of cholelithiasis.

30. What entities should be considered when the gallbladder is not visualized?

Physiologic contraction, contraction associated with hepatitis, congenital absence of the gallbladder, anomalous anatomic gallbladder location, operator error, or gallbladder previously removed by surgery should be considered.

31. What is milk of calcium?

Also known as "limey bile," it is the result of concentrated intravesicular bile salts in the setting of long-standing common bile duct obstruction. Its sonographic appearance varies and can appear as an echogenic fluid level or a convex shadow.

32. How are gallbladder polyps distinguished from gallstones and sludge?

Gallbladder polyps, typically less than 5 mm in size, can be distinguished from stones and sludge by their lack of mobility with change in patient position, although some are on stalks and can move slightly. If the patient is positioned so that the polyp is on the antidependent wall, the polyp does not fall to the dependent surface, whereas a stone does. Polyps also usually lack the posterior acoustic shadowing seen with stones.

33. What is the current recommendation for management of gallbladder polyps based on size?

If the gallbladder polyp is less than 5 mm, no further work-up is required. If the gallbladder polyp is 5–10 mm in size, interval sonographic monitoring is recommended to ensure stability of the lesion. If the gallbladder polyp is greater than 10 mm, surgical removal is indicated because it is indistinguishable from a cancer.

34. What are the sonographic features of gallbladder carcinoma?

The most common appearance (40–65%) of gallbladder carcinoma is that of an echogenic mass contained in the gallbladder fossa with associated gallstones (Fig. 13). (Gallbladder cancer may be due to chronic irritation of the gallbladder wall from stones.) This mass extends extraluminally into the liver. Other less common appearances include focal or diffuse gallbladder wall thickening (20–30% of cases), and single or multiple intraluminal masses (15–25%). Associated findings include bile duct obstruction, liver metastases, and peripancreatic lymphadenopathy. Gallbladder cancer is the fifth most common gastrointestinal malignancy and is more common in women than men.

35. What is the main differential diagnosis of gallbladder carcinoma?

In patients with diffuse or focal wall thickening, adenomyomatosis should be considered in the differential. The other entity that deserves consideration is xanthogranulomatous cholecystitis. The differential diagnosis for a mass replacing the gallbladder fossa includes hepatocellular carcinoma, cholangiocarcinoma, and metastatic disease to the gallbladder fossa.

36. What is xanthogranulomatous cholecystitis?

Xanthogranulomatous cholecystitis is a pseudotumoral inflammatory condition of the gallbladder that radiologically simulates gallbladder carcinoma. Sonograpghic appearance of xanthogranulomatous cholecystitis includes hypoechoic bands or nodules within the thickened gallbladder wall. The hypoechoic nodules have been shown to represent abscesses or foci of xanthogranulomatous inflammation. Other sonographic findings include disruption of the mucosal line, pericholecystic fluid, stones, and intrahepatic biliary dilatation.

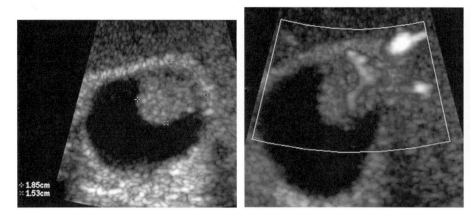

FIGURE 13. Transverse images demonstrate a 1.8-cm gallbladder mass with flow. This lesion contained carcinomatous foci at pathologic evaluation.

37. What are the normal anatomic landmarks of the porta hepatis and where should one measure the common duct?

Search for the "Mickey Mouse." The portal vein forms the head, the hepatic artery forms one ear, and the common duct forms the other ear. The common duct should be imaged in long axis and the lumen measured at the level where the hepatic artery crosses the duct.

38. What is the normal diameter of the intrahepatic bile ducts?

The diameter of a normal bile duct should not be more than 40% of the adjacent portal vein (Fig. 14). Dilated intrahepatic bile ducts can be distinguished from their adjacent portal veins by several features (Fig. 15):

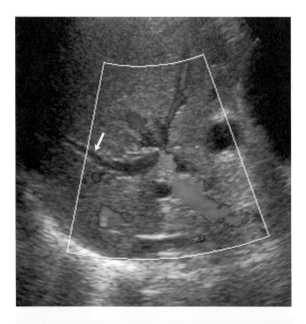

FIGURE 14. Longitudinal ultrasound through the porta shows tubular structures (*arrow*) without flow, indicating ductal diliation.

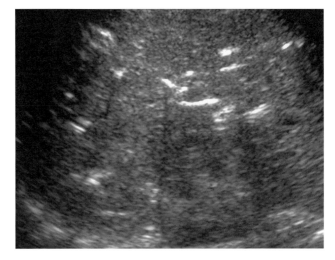

FIGURE 15. Transverse ultrasound shows scattered linear echogenic foci throughout the liver compatible with pneumobilia. Some have posterior acoustic shadows (*arrows*).

- Bile ducts have tortuous walls.
- Bile ducts have increased through transmission.
- Bile ducts have a central stellate configuration.
- Doppler analysis should demonstrate flow in the portal system and the hepatic arteries (if dilated enough to see). The bile ducts lack flow.

39. Can one see normal intrahepatic ducts?

Yes, especially in slender patients and with higher frequency transducers and harmonics. Normal ducts are often seen centrally in the porta hepatis as well as in the left lobe.

40. What measurement is accepted as indicating extrahepatic bile duct dilatation?

Extrahepatic bile duct dilatation is present when the maximum diameter of the common duct is 7 mm or greater. Duct diameter (inner measurements are obtained and the wall should not be included) is measured at the level of the porta hepatis. The common duct diameter increases with increasing age and is wider in patients with a history of cholecystectomy.

41. What is the best scanning approach for evaluation of the common bile duct?

The distal common bile duct should be examined first in the erect right posterior oblique or right lateral decubitus position in the transverse plane to minimize gas in the antrum and duodenum, which would obscure the obtained images. The proximal common bile duct can be evaluated in the same position; however, it is advantageous to scan in the parasagittal plane with the patient in a supine left posterior oblique position.

42. What are the major etiologies and types of biliary obstruction?

Extrinsic ductal obstruction occurs from a pancreatic mass, from enlarged lymph nodes, or from duodenal or ampullary masses. Intrinsic obstruction may be due to stones, strictures, or tumors.

43. Where does choledocholithiasis usually obstruct the common bile duct?

The distal intrapancreatic portion of the duct is the most narrow portion of the duct and is therefore the most common site of obstruction (Figs. 16 and 17).

44. Why is choledocholithiasis difficult to diagnose?

Like gallbladder stones, ductal stones are hyperechoic and shadowing. However, in 20% of cases, a lack of bile surrounding the stone results in lack of posterior acoustic shadowing. Additionally, visualization of the distal duct is often obscured by bowel gas.

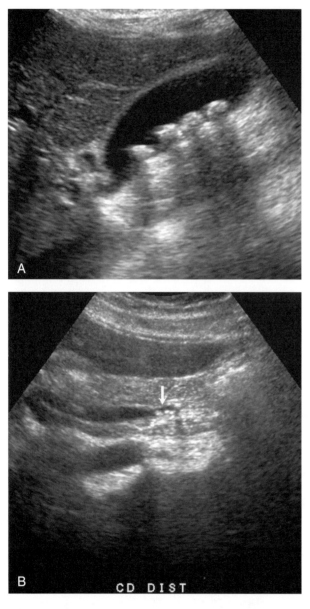

FIGURE 16. Cholelithiasis and choledocholithiasis. Longitudinal image (*A*) shows a distended gallbladder containing multiple stones. Image of the common bile duct (*B*) distally shows an echogenic stone (*arrow*) within it.

45. What can be done to improve visualization of the distal duct?

Place the patient semierect, right side down, to move gas out of the duodenum. Give the patient a few sips of water, if needed. Scan transversely, starting at the porta and moving caudally.

46. What is a Klatskin tumor and what is the classic appearance?

This is a cholangiocarcinoma occurring at the bifurcation of the common hepatic duct. Sonographically this typically appears as dilated intrahepatic ducts with no communication between the left and right ducts. Rarely, a polypoid intraluminal mass can be identified.

47. What radiographic features are suspicious for cholangiocarcinoma?

Abrupt termination of a dilated duct with little or no visible mass is a suspicious feature.

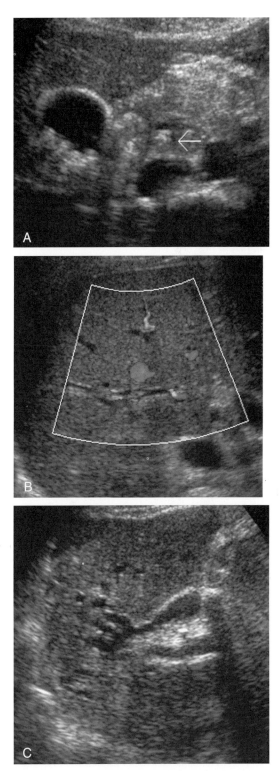

FIGURE 17. Transverse images demonstrate intrahepatic bile duct dilation (*A*) as a result of a stone (*arrow*) in the common bile duct (*B*). *C*, An example of the beaded irregular appearance of the bile ducts with worsening dilation.

48. What is the differential diagnosis of cholangiocarcinoma?

The differential diagnosis of cholangiocarcinoma depends largely on its location. Diagnoses of an abnormality at the ductal confluence that should be considered include cholangiocarcinoma (Klatskin tumor), gallbladder carcinoma, hepatocellular carcinoma, or metastases. Ampullary carcinoma and pancreatic carcinoma should also be considered if obstruction is detected in the distal duct.

49. What are the sonographic findings of sclerosing cholangitis?

Sclerosing cholangitis, most frequently affecting young men and highly associated with inflammatory bowel disease, manifests as a common duct wall thickening that is either smooth or irregular. Multifocal strictures with resultant beading occurs in the intrahepatic ducts and can produce associated intrahepatic bile duct dilatation.

50. What sonographic finding in a patient with sclerosing cholangitis should alert the radiologist to the possibility of cancerous transformation?

A hepatic parenchymal lesion in a patient with sclerosing cholangitis should raise the suspicion for cholangiocarcinoma. Other suspicious findings include duct wall thickening greater than 5 mm and disproportionately dilated intrahepatic bile ducts.

51. What is the differential diagnosis of bile duct wall thickening?

- Choledocholithiasis
- AIDS cholangiopathy (due to infection with cytomegalovirus or *Cryptosporidium*)
- Sclerosing cholangitis
- Pancreatitis
- Oriental cholangiohepatitis (recurrent pyogenic cholangitis caused by biliary flukes)
- *Clonorchis sinensis* or *Ascaris lumbricoides*
- Ascending cholangitis

52. Describe the classification of choledochal cysts.

Type I choledochal cysts are most common and represent 80–90% of the lesions. Type I cysts are dilatations of the entire common hepatic and common bile ducts or segments of each. They can be saccular or fusiform in configuration. These represent 80–90% of all choledochal cysts.

Type II choledochal cysts are relatively isolated protrusions or diverticula that project from the common bile duct wall. They may be sessile or may be connected to the common bile duct by a narrow stalk.

Type III choledochal cysts are found in the intraduodenal portion of the common bile duct. Another term used for these cysts is *choledochocele*.

Type IVA cysts are characterized by multiple dilatations of the intrahepatic and extrahepatic biliary tree. Most frequently, a large solitary cyst of the extrahepatic duct is accompanied by multiple cysts of the intrahepatic ducts. **Type IVB** choledochal cysts consist of multiple dilatations that involve only the extrahepatic bile duct.

Type V (Caroli's disease) choledochal cysts are defined by dilatation of the intrahepatic biliary radicles. Often, numerous cysts are present with interposed strictures that predispose the patient to intrahepatic stone formation, obstruction, and cholangitis. The cysts are typically found in both hepatic lobes. Occasionally, unilobar disease is found and most frequently involves the left lobe.

53. What three factors make up the classic clinical triad of a choledochocele?

1. Jaundice (80%)
2. Palpable mass (50%)
3. Abdominal pain (50%)

54. What is Caroli's disease?

Caroli's disease is segmental cystic dilatation of the intrahepatic biliary system. Its etiology is unknown, it is autosomal recessive, and it is the fifth subset in the clinical spectrum of the choledochal cyst classification. It has an 80% association with medullary sponge kidney (tubular ectasia). Biliary stasis in cystic structures predisposes to stone formation, pyogenic cholangitis, and intrahepatic abscess.

55. What are the sonographic features of Caroli's disease?
Multiple intrahepatic cystic structures are the hallmark. The "central dot" sign is a specific sonographic finding caused by a dilated biliary segment surrounding the adjacent hepatic artery and portal vein, causing these vascular structures to produce a small echogenic focus in the middle of the anechoic dilated duct. Secondary findings of renal disease and portal hypertension aid the diagnosis.

56. What is the differential diagnosis of a choledochal cyst?
- Duplication cyst of the duodenum
- Omental or mesenteric cyst
- Pancreatic pseudocyst
- Hepatic artery aneurysm
- Right renal cyst

57. What is Mirizzi's syndrome?
This is a common duct obstruction caused by mass effect or inflammatory reaction from a stone in the cystic duct or gallbladder neck. This is commonly seen in patients with low insertion of the cystic duct.

BIBLIOGRAPHY

1. Brant WE, Helms CA: Fundamentals of Diagnostic Radiology, 2nd ed. Lippincott, Williams and Wilkins, pp. 836–841.
2. Kurtz AB, Middleton WD: Ultrasound: The Requisites. Philadelphia, Hanley & Belfus, 1996, pp 35–71.
3. Rumack CM, Wilson SR, Charboneau JW (eds): Diagnostic Ultrasound, 2nd ed. St. Louis, Mosby, 1998, 1997, pp 172–195.
4. Parulekar SG: Transabdominal sonography of bile ducts. Ultrasound Q (18)3:187–202, 2002.

16. THE LIVER

Hamad Ghazle, M.S., RDMS, and Deborah J. Rubens, M.D.

1. What are the indications for a liver ultrasound examination?
- Elevated liver function tests (LFTs)
- Jaundice
- Evaluation of blood flow (i.e., portal hypertension [HTN])
- Abdominal or right upper quadrant (RUQ) pain
- Evaluation of liver size, shape, and parenchyma
- Suspicion of primary or metastatic tumors
- Evaluation and follow-up of adult polycystic disease

2. What are the liver lobes?
The right lobe consists of all the tissue lateral to the middle hepatic vein and the gallbladder, and the left lobe is medial to these structures. The caudate lobe is separate from both right and left, and is the tissue anterior to the inferior vena cava (IVC) and posterior to the left portal vein and the ligamentum venosum.

3. Which structure suspends the liver from the diaphragm and the anterior abdominal wall?
The liver is suspended from the abdominal wall by a broad, thin anteroposterior fold of the peritoneal membrane called the **falciform ligament.** It appears as a linear echogenic structure on ultrasound. It is usually better seen when ascites surround it.

4. What is the quadrate lobe?
The medial segment of the left lobe of the liver is also known as the quadrate lobe. It is anterior to the porta hepatis, between the gallbladder fossa (right) and the fissure of the ligamentum teres (left).

5. What is the umbilical vein remnant called?
The umbilical vein remnant is called the **ligamentum teres.** It is usually seen as an echogenic triangular structure in the left lobe of the liver on transverse scans. It may occasionally be round on transverse images and mimic an intrahepatic lesion (Fig. 1).

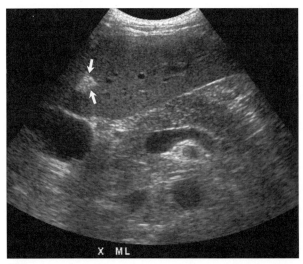

FIGURE 1. Normal liver echotexture. Transverse scan of the left lobe of the liver showing a triangular echogenic area (*arrows*), which is the ligamentum teres.

6. Where is the bare area of the liver located?

A normal liver is almost entirely covered by the peritoneal membrane. Hence, the liver is considered an intraperitoneal structure. At the posterosuperior aspect of the liver, there is a region not covered by the peritoneum called the bare area. This area attaches the liver to the diaphragm and is immediately anterior to the IVC.

7. What is a portal triad?

The portal triad consists of a portal vein, hepatic artery (usually anterior and medial to the main portal vein), and common hepatic duct (anterior and lateral to the main portal vein). Portal triads are surrounded by Glisson's capsule, which contributes to their echogenic walls.

8. What is Morison's pouch and what is its significance?

The earliest accumulation of free fluid within the abdominal cavity occurs in a potential space known as Morison's pouch or the hepatorenal space. It is situated between the right kidney and the right lobe of the liver.

9. What is the significance of the hepatic veins?

In addition to their function of blood drainage , the hepatic veins can be helpful in identifying segmental liver anatomy. The right hepatic vein (which follows the right intersegmental fissure) divides the right lobe into anterior and posterior segments. The left hepatic vein (which follows the left intersegmental fissure) divides the left lobe into lateral and medial segments. The middle hepatic vein (located in the main lobar fissure) divides the liver into right and left lobes.

10. What are two common imaging configurations of the hepatic veins?

- "Bunny." The left and middle hepatic veins form the ears and the IVC is the head of the rabbit.
- "Antlers" or "reindeer." The left and middle veins make the left antler and the right hepatic vein makes the right one. The IVC is the head. This configuration can be obtained by placing the transducer transversely beneath the rib cage (subcostally) and angling superiorly or cephalad, with the transducer face parallel to the right costal margin.

11. What is the papillary process of the caudate lobe?

The papillary process is a normal variant of the caudate lobe that may be confused with an enlarged lymph node or an extrahepatic liver mass. It is usually seen in the anterior and inferior aspect of the caudate lobe. It may present as a round projection of the caudate lobe or as a separate structure on longitudinal or transverse ultrasound images. A key factor in avoiding a misdiagnosis is to demonstrate that the mass or projection has the same echogenicity as the liver.

12. What is Couinaud's system and what is its significance?

This is a segmental liver nomenclature system that is widely used in Europe and French Canada and is becoming universal. Couinaud's system is the anatomic basis for surgical hepatic resections and is based on the portal and hepatic venous segments. There are eight segments.

The three hepatic veins are the longitudinal boundaries and divide the liver into four sections. Each of these sections is divided transversely by an invisible plane through the right and left portal veins. The following table is a summary of the liver segmental anatomy:

SEGMENT	DESCRIPTION/LOCATION
I	Caudate lobe
II and III	Left superior and inferior lateral segments
IV	Medial segment of left lobe
V and VI	Anterior and posterior segments of right lobe (inferior to invisible transverse plane)
VII and VIII	Posterior and anterior segments of right lobe (superior to invisible transverse plane)

13. How can portal veins be differentiated from hepatic veins?

PORTAL VEINS	HEPATIC VEINS
Have echogenic walls due to the fibrous capsule of Glisson	Do not have echogenic walls unless the ultrasound beam is perpendicular to the vessel walls (specular reflector)
Enlarge at the level of the porta hepatis	Enlarge as they approach the diaphragm or the inferior vena cava
Are intralobar and central in the liver	Are interlobar and located posteriorly and at the cranial aspect of the liver
Do not demonstrate through transmission	Demonstrate through transmission or acoustic enhancement

14. What is the significance of the main lobar fissure?

The main lobar fissure is determined by an imaginary line drawn from the gallbladder fossa to the groove of the IVC. This line divides the liver into right and left lobes and is the line of surgical resection of the right lobe.

15. What comprises the hepatic blood supply?

The liver receives its oxygen and nutrients via a dual blood supply. The portal vein supplies approximately 70–75% of the total blood volume to the liver, whereas the hepatic artery supplies the remaining 25–30%. The hepatic artery has a much higher oxygen content than the portal vein and supplies the biliary ducts.

16. What is the normal sonographic appearance of the liver?

The liver parenchyma (often used as a standard to set up the overall scan parameters for the abdomen) has a moderately echogenic (medium gray echoes) and a homogeneous echotexture, which is interrupted only by blood vessels (hepatic and portal veins). When compared with other structures in the abdomen, the liver is either isoechoic or slightly more echogenic than the renal cortex and is isoechoic or slightly less echogenic than the pancreas. The portal triads and hepatic vein walls have thin, bright, echogenic margins, especially when the vessel is perpendicular to the axis of the transducer. The lumen of the vessels are normally anechoic (Fig. 2).

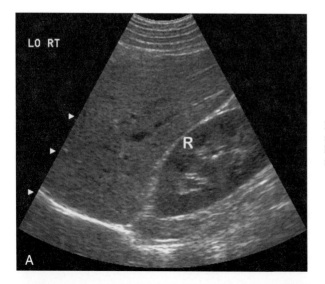

FIGURE 2. *A*, A sagittal scan showing a normal liver slightly hyperechoic compared to the renal cortex (*R*). (*continued*)

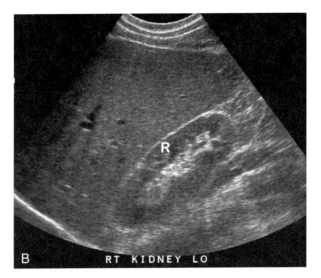

FIGURE 2. (*continued*) *B, A sagittal image showing a normal liver isoechoic to the renal cortex (R).*

17. What is the size of a normal liver on ultrasound?

Several techniques have been used to determine the size of the liver. The longitudinal measurement at the midclavicular (craniocaudal) line is widely used. This approach indicates that the normal liver should measure ≤ 16 cm in length.

18. Is there a specific patient preparation for a liver ultrasound examination?

No special preparation is required to scan the liver, but because a liver examination usually includes a comprehensive study of other upper abdominal organs (e.g., gallbladder, biliary system), fasting for 6–8 hours or overnight fasting before the study is highly recommended.

19. What positions are used for scanning the liver?

Supine and left lateral decubitus positions are used. The latter frequently improves visualization of the right lobe, bringing it down into the abdomen from under the ribs. Semiupright scanning can also be attempted, as can scanning from posteriorly (useful in patients with ascites). Placing the patient's right arm at or above his or her head expands the intercostal spaces for better transducer contact.

20. What transducer is used for imaging the liver?

A transducer with a frequency of 3–7 MHz is used. Depending on patient size, use the highest frequency that penetrates. To penetrate the right lobe, 3–5 MHz is usually needed. A higher frequency can be used on the left, because it is smaller.

Curved linear arrays give good resolution for the left lobe (near field) and a subcostal approach should be used on the right. A sector probe is often needed for intercostal scanning.

21. How is the gain adjusted?

The time-gain compensation and the overall gain should be adjusted to provide adequate penetration of the right lobe of the liver and a smooth homogeneous liver parenchyma, which is the same brightness at all levels.

22. What imaging planes should be used for scanning the liver?

The goal of the ultrasound examination is to survey the entire liver and its margins including the dome. This is accomplished by using multiple orientations including sagittal, transverse, coronal, and oblique planes. A midclavicular sagittal scan provides liver length. Sagittal scans at midline or slightly to the left should include the aorta and the IVC, those slightly to the right should include the IVC in long axis. Additional sagittal or parasagittal images should demonstrate the common hepatic duct, the main portal vein, and the liver parenchyma as compared with the right kidney. Transverse images should include the IVC and hepatic veins, the left lobe including the portal vein, and the right lobe with the right portal vein.

23. What is fatty infiltration of the liver?

Fatty infiltration of the liver occurs when the fat content of the hepatocytes increases. It can be associated with obesity, diabetes mellitus, alcohol abuse, oral contraceptives, pregnancy, starvation, glycogen storage disease, severe hepatitis, and, in the majority of cases, is idiopathic.

24. How is fatty infiltration manifested?

Fatty infiltration may be focal or diffuse (more common). Diffuse disease is classified as:

- **Mild.** Slight increase in liver echogenicity with loss of the normal small intrahepatic vessel borders but normal visualization of the diaphragm.
- **Moderate.** Moderate increase in liver echogenicity with impaired visualization of the distal hepatic parenchyma and slight loss of echogenicity of the diaphragm.
- **Severe.** Marked increase in liver echogenicity with no visualization of the diaphragm or the posterior segment of the right hepatic lobe (Fig. 3).

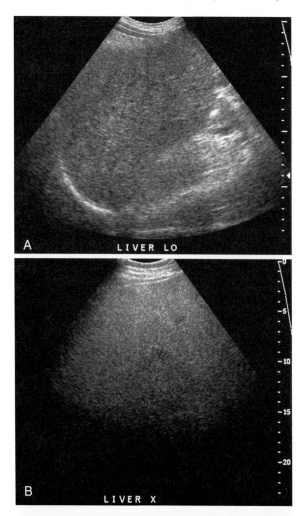

FIGURE 3. Fatty liver. *A,* Diffuse enlargement of the liver with increased echogenicity and loss of peripheral vessels seen in mild fatty infiltration. *B,* Diffuse enlargement of the liver with posterior sound beam attenuation. No diaphragm echo is seen in severe fatty infiltration. (*continued*)

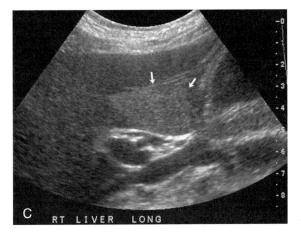

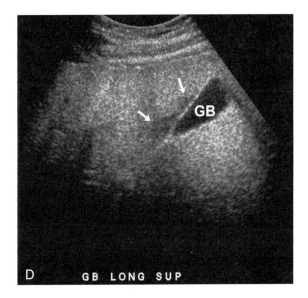

FIGURE 3. (*continued*) *C*, A well-defined echogenic mass (*arrows*) anterior to the portal vein represents focal fatty infiltration. *D*, Hypoechoic masses adjacent to the gallbladder (*GB*), representing focal fatty sparing (*arrows*).

25. What is focal fatty infiltration (FFI)? How can it be distinguished from a true liver mass?

FFI is a discrete area of increased echogenicity, often with geographic (distinct and sharp) margins. Typically, it is seen in the anterior medial segment of the left lobe of the liver adjacent to the falciform ligament. Another common location is adjacent to the gallbladder fossa, although FFI may occur anywhere in the liver. As opposed to a true liver mass, FFI should not distort or displace any adjacent or regional hepatic vessels (*see* Fig. 3).

26. What is focal fatty sparing?

Focal fatty sparing is an area of "normal liver echogenicity" with sharp and well-defined margins in the midst of diffuse fatty infiltration that has caused increased hepatic echogenicity. Typical regions include the posteromedial segment of the left lobe of the liver adjacent to the portal vein and often in nodular areas adjacent to the gallbladder (*see* Fig. 3).

27. How else can fatty infiltration be confirmed?

Magnetic resonance imaging (MRI) can elegantly confirm the presence of fat. Most often, computed tomography (CT) scanning can confirm the diagnosis. A normal sulfur colloid nuclear scan also confirms fatty infiltration, especially for focal lesions greater than 2 cm.

28. What is the liver tumor associated with type I glycogen disease?

Type 1 glycogen (von Gierke's) disease is an autosomal recessive disorder that results from impairment of the enzyme glucose-6-phosphatase. This allows excessive deposition of glycogen in the liver, intestinal tract, and kidneys. Forty percent of patients may have associated liver adenomas.

29. What is hepatitis?

Hepatitis refers to inflammation of the liver (hepatocytes) caused by viruses, parasites, bacteria, or toxins such as alcohol and drugs. If the cause is a virus, it is called viral hepatitis. Presently, there are six distinct viruses that have been detected. These viruses are denoted by the letters A through G.

Type A has only an acute phase with 99% recovery in 4–6 months. Type B is the greatest threat to health care providers. Types B–G progress to chronic infection with potential sequelae of cirrhosis or hepatocellular carcinoma. LFT results are elevated. The severity of elevation depends on the severity and stage of the infection.

Hepatitis A
- Transmitted by oral-fecal route
- Most commonly transmitted by food preparation with unwashed hands
- Patients may present with flulike symptoms (nausea, vomiting, headache)

Hepatitis B
- Transmitted through blood contact including transfusions, unclean needle sharing, and sexual contact
- Has a carrier state (an estimated 300 million people are infected worldwide, especially in Asia, China, Africa, and Greenland)
- Patients may present with malaise, fatigue, anorexia, or changes in taste

Hepatitis C
- Also called non-A/non-B hepatitis
- Usually transmitted through blood contact (90% of hepatitis C patients have had a transfusion)
- 85% of patients infected develop chronic liver disease, which leads to hepatic failure
- Patients may present with vomiting, headache, cough, and low-grade fever

30. What is the ultrasound appearance of hepatitis?

The liver most often is normal with respect to size and echogenicity. Occasionally it is hypoechoic with pronounced increased echogenicity of the portal triads and portal vein walls, the "starry sky" pattern. The liver becomes hypoechoic with respect to the kidney. This should be confirmed by checking that the left kidney remains hypoechoic to the spleen. Otherwise, the relatively increased right renal echogenicity may reflect renal disease. The increased echogenicity of portal vein walls is due to infiltrative changes around the vessels. The decreased liver echogenicity is thought to be due to the edema and swelling of the liver cells due to inflammation (Fig. 4).

31. What other signs of hepatitis may be encountered?

There may be hepatomegaly, a nontender thickened gallbladder wall (> 3 mm), or a contracted gallbladder. These are more common than the starry sky pattern, but less specific. In chronic hepatitis, the liver appears more echogenic due to the spread of fibrosis (becomes coarse) and a decrease in echogenicity of the walls of the portal veins (*see* Fig. 4).

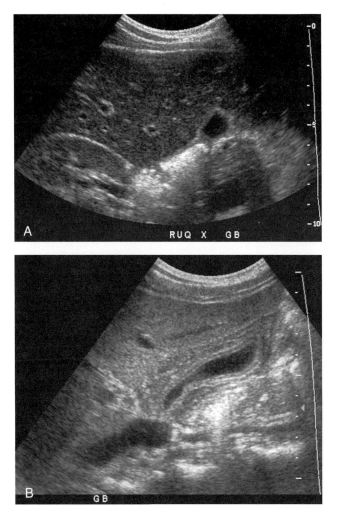

FIGURE 4. Hepatitis. *A,* A transverse image of the inferior segment of the right lobe of the liver shows prominent portal triads and decreased liver echotexture as compared to the adjacent kidney. This is the starry sky appearance. *B,* A sagittal scan of the gallbladder shows increased wall thickness and edema. This patient did not have a sonographic Murphy's sign or acute cholecystitis and tested positive for hepatitis A. The liver echotexture is normal.

32. What is cirrhosis?

Cirrhosis is a diffuse process characterized by fibrosis and the conversion of normal liver tissue into abnormal nodules. It usually results from prolonged and continued insults to the hepatocytes. It is often irreversible and progressive.

33. What are some of the causes of cirrhosis?

Some of the most common causes are alcoholism (70%), viral hepatitis (B, C, D), cholangitis, congestive heart failure, hemochromatosis, Wilson's disease, and hepatic veno-occlusive disease (Budd-Chiari syndrome).

34. What are the clinical manifestations of cirrhosis?

Patients may develop symptoms dependent on the stage of the cirrhosis. Such symptoms include fatigue, weight loss, jaundice, abnormal LFTs, portal hypertension (late stage), hepatic cell failure (late stage), and ascites (late stage). There may be coagulopathy and dilated superficial veins on the abdominal wall as well.

35. What is the typical ultrasound appearance of cirrhosis?

The ultrasound appearance is dependent on the stage of the disease:

- **Early stage.** The liver may appear normal or enlarged due to edema and swelling. In addition, there may be an increase in caudate lobe size compared to the right lobe (CL/RL ratio is > 0.65). The liver may be coarse and heterogeneous (similar to fatty infiltration). The gain controls must be set appropriately, or else the wrong diagnosis is made.
- **Late stage.** The liver capsule surface may be irregular and nodular. This can be appreciated when ascites is present or a high-frequency transducer is used. The liver may become small, atrophied, or shrunken. Regenerating hypoechoic nodules may be seen. Ascites, splenomegaly, varices, and the development of collaterals may also be seen. In addition, portal hypertension (recanalization of the umbilical vein and hepatofugal flow in portal veins) and enlargement of the hepatic arteries (with decrease in blood flow resistance) may develop (Fig. 5).

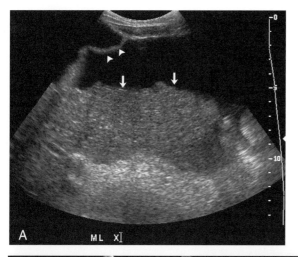

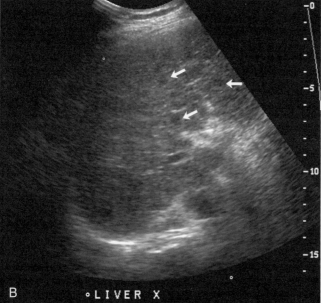

FIGURE 5. Cirrhosis. *A,* The liver is small with diffuse coarse parenchyma. Surface irregularity (*arrows*) can be appreciated in the presence of ascites. The falciform liagment (*arrowheads*) is nicely seen. *B,* This liver is enlarged with diffusely nodular parenchyma (*arrows*). (*continued*)

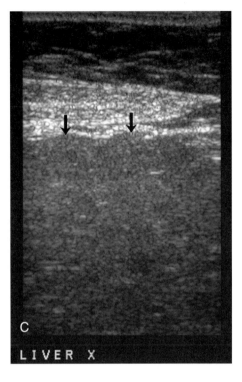

FIGURE 5. (*continued*) *C,* Irregular liver surface (*arrows*) of the left lobe was appreciated by using a high frequency linear transducer.

36. What tumor is associated with cirrhosis?

The tumor associated with cirrhosis is hepatoma or hepatocellular carcinoma. Its incidence is around 5% in the United States.

37. Does seeing lymph nodes imply tumor is present in a patient with cirrhosis?

No. Many patients with cirrhosis have hepatitis or primary biliary cirrhosis (an autoimmune disorder) as causes. These are commonly associated with moderately increased, reactive nodes in the porta hepatis and the gastrohepatic ligament.

38. What are the common sequelae of cirrhosis?

The following are ultrasound findings associated with cirrhosis:

- Portal hypertension. This results from the increased resistance in the scarred, fibrous liver. It causes portal vein (> 13 mm) and splenic vein (> 10 mm) enlargement. Slow to bidirectional and eventually reversed portal venous flow is also seen. Collaterals may also be seen, especially adjacent to the hilum of the spleen. Recanalization of the umbilical vein is diagnostic but not common (present in 20% of cases). (See Chapter 46, Doppler Evaluation of Liver and Transjugular Intrahepatic Portosystemic Shunts).
- Portal vein thrombosis
- Splenomegaly or ascites
- Enlargement of the hepatic arteries with a tortuous corkscrew appearance
- Compression of the hepatic veins: frequent and difficult to see without color Doppler.

39. What is Budd-Chiari syndrome?

The Budd-Chiari syndrome is most common in India, South Africa, and Asia. This disease is characterized by obstruction of the hepatic venous flow. The obstruction can be due to thrombus, congenital fibrous tissue or web (primary), or tumor (secondary). IVC involvement may also be seen. The causes of Budd-Chiari syndrome may include pregnancy, hypercoagulopathy, leukemia, oral contraceptives, trauma, hepatocellular carcinoma, chemotherapy, and renal and adrenal carcinoma. It can also be idiopathic (50–70% of cases).

40. What are the sonographic findings in Budd-Chiari syndrome?
The patient develops ascites. The caudate lobe becomes enlarged (due to increased blood flow) and is more hypoechoic than the liver. The intrahepatic IVC is narrowed or obstructed, and the hepatic veins terminate or increase in size. Blood flow may be absent, turbulent, or reversed in the IVC and hepatic veins. Portal venous flow may reverse. Less common findings may include thickening and increased echogenicity of the hepatic vein walls and the development of intrahepatic and extrahepatic collaterals. (See Chapter 46, Figure 18.)

41. What is the classification of hepatic cysts?
Hepatic cysts are categorized as congenital or acquired.
- **Acquired.** Secondary to exposure to infectious process or trauma (parasitic, traumatic, or inflammatory).
- **Congenital** (hereditary or innate). Can be divided into simple cysts or polycystic liver disease that can be associated with polycystic kidney disease). They are more common in females and can occur anywhere in the liver, but the right lobe is more often affected.

Hepatic cysts are rarely palpable and may not cause liver enlargement. Patients are usually asymptomatic but cysts may cause epigastric pain depending on cyst size or hemorrhage within the cyst.

42. What are the sonographic criteria for a simple liver cyst?
A simple liver cyst should be anechoic or sonolucent and have sharp and well-defined walls with increased through transmission. Cysts may be single or multiple and are usually asymptomatic unless they become very large. If the lesion does not satisfy these criteria, metastasis (carcinoid, breast carcinoma, or lymphoma), infection bacteria abscess, or echinococcal infection should be suspected. A simple cyst may contain internal echoes or debris and septations caused by hemorrhaging or infection.

43. When does adult polycystic liver disease present? What is its sonographic appearance?
In general, adult polycystic disease is an autosomal dominant disease that becomes symptomatic in the fifth to the seventh decade of life (possibly earlier). It affects more females than males (4:1). The number of cysts varies depending on the stage of the disease. Cysts are usually multiple, of variable size, and affect the whole liver. Cysts disrupt the normal liver echotexture but the LFTs may remain normal.

Patients are usually asymptomatic; however, intracyst hemorrhage causes pain.

Sonographically, these cysts have the same characteristics as simple cysts (anechoic with well-defined walls and posterior acoustic enhancement) (Fig. 6).

44. If a patient presents with multiple liver cysts, what organs should be scanned?
If multiple liver cysts are seen in the liver, polycystic disease should be suspected. Polycystic disease usually affects several organs such as the liver, kidneys, pancreas, and spleen. Twenty-five percent to 50% of patients with polycystic renal disease have liver cysts, whereas 60% of patients with polycystic liver disease have renal cysts. Therefore, the kidneys should be evaluated.

45. How does a liver hematoma look on ultrasound?
On ultrasound, a hematoma may have several appearances based on its age. Initially, it appears hypoechoic, then echogenic, and eventually it becomes complex to cystic. Some through transmission may be seen.

46. What is hydatid disease?
Hydatid disease is also known as an echinococcal disease. It is common in third world countries where sheep and cattle are raised. It is induced by the parasite *Echinococcus granulosus* (a

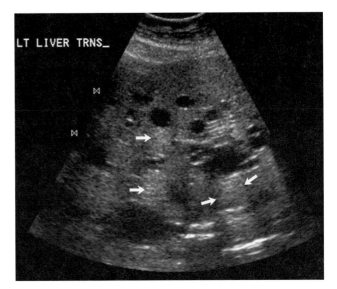

FIGURE 6. Polycystic liver disease. Multiple small cystic lesions are seen throughout the liver. Note the through transmission (*arrows*) seen posterior to the cysts.

tape worm). It has two layers: an inner layer (germinal epithelium), in which daughter cells develop, and an outer (inflammatory) layer. It has a tendency to rupture, and when fluid escapes, anaphylactic shock may occur. Consequently, aspiration is not recommended. It may cause extrinsic compression on blood vessels, causing thrombosis or infarction.

47. What is the ultrasound appearance of echinococcal cysts?
Several ultrasound appearances have been seen:
• Simple cysts with or without calcification
• Multilocular cystic mass
• "Honeycomb" or "cartwheel," which are fluid collection with septations
• "Waterlily," which results from detachment of the germinal layer and appears as a linear collection of echoes floating in the dependent portion of the cyst.
• Mother/daughter: cyst within a cyst
• Complex mass

48. What are common sources of liver abscesses?
• Portal vein: bowel diverticulitis, Crohn's disease, appendicitis (*E. coli,* enteric organisms)
• Hepatic artery: endocarditis, teeth cleaning, bacteremia
• Biliary sources: cholangitis (ascending), biliary obstruction (tumor, nodes in porta) with sepsis, biliary necrosis and stasis (liver transplant)

49. What are the symptoms (presentation) of pyogenic or bacterial abscesses?
The symptoms include fever, right upper quadrant pain, nausea, vomiting, diarrhea, anemia, pleurisy, chills, sepsis, shock, increase in LFTs, and leukocytosis. Jaundice may be present in 25% of the cases. Pyogenic abscesses can be seen anywhere in the liver but are mostly found in the right lobe (80%). They are usually solitary but can be multiple. In adults, it is usually caused by *Escherichia* and in children by *Staphylococcus*. It usually enters the liver through the biliary system (most common), the portal vein, the hepatic artery, or directly through a contagious infection.

50. Is there a typical ultrasound appearance of pyogenic liver abscesses?
There is no typical ultrasound appearance. Some are anechoic to hypoechoic and may have increased through transmission (50% of cases). If they contain gas, they may be predominately echogenic with dirty shadowing and poor margination (Fig. 7):

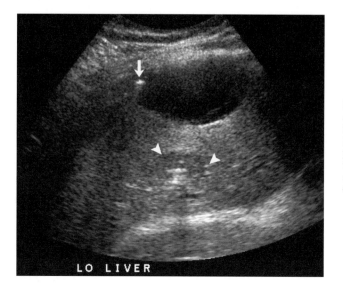

FIGURE 7. Liver abscess. A cystic mass with echogenic foci representing gas bubbles (*arrow*) was proved to be a pyogenic abscess. Note subtler, more solid appearing abscess (*arrowheads*) posteriorly.

- 90% are irregular with poorly defined walls.
- 60% are round and oval.
- Size is variable (1 cm and up).
- Walls may be thickened with some vascularity (depends on age of abscess).

Tip: Turn on Doppler to assess for flow. Abscesses may have peripheral vascularity but should not have central vessels as tumors do.

Pitfall: Ultrasound frequently underestimates the number and size of abscesses. CT or MRI can be used to evaluate blind spots, including the dome and areas under the rib.

51. What is the ultrasound presentation of an amebic abscess?

The appearance may mimic a pyogenic abscess and can be diagnosed by hemoglutination titers (no need for aspiration). It is mostly located peripherally or close to the liver capsule and can be oval or round. It is well defined but has no significant wall echoes. It is mostly hypoechoic with internal echoes (debris) at high gain and shows through transmission. It responds well to antibiotics (metronidazole) but may take up to 2 years to heal. A cyst may persist and become indistinguishable from a simple cyst.

52. What is *Pneumocystis carinii*?

This infection is most commonly seen in acquired immunodeficiency syndrome (AIDS) and immunocompromised (organ and bone marrow transplant, chemotherapy, or corticosteroid therapy) patients. It usually affects the lungs but can spread to liver, spleen, pancreas, lymph nodes, and thyroid.

53. How is *Pneumocystis carinii* infection diagnosed on ultrasound?

It is usually seen as multiple, tiny, nonshadowing echogenic foci dispersed throughout the liver. It has also been referred to as the "starry sky." Caution must be used because infections by cytomegalovirus and *Mycobacterium avium-intracellulare* can have the same ultrasound patterns.

54. What is candidiasis?

It is also known as a fungal abscess. It is uncommon but if it occurs it is the most common type of fungal hepatic infection. It is caused by the *Candida albicans*. It usually travels through the bloodstream in immunocompromised patients (transplant recipient, cancer patients on chemotherapy, or HIV-infected patients). It can also occur during pregnancy and long-term hospital care requiring hyperalimentation.

55. How does candidiasis look on ultrasound?

It appears as a small, uniformly hypoechoic focus (most common) or a small, uniformly hyperechoic focus (late stage of disease). It has also shown a "wheel-within-a-wheel" configuration (outer hypoechoic rim corresponding to fibrosis; inner hyperechoic ring corresponding to inflammatory changes; a small, uniformly hyperechoic focus corresponding to necrosis). It has also been described to have a "bull's eye" appearance that mimics liver metastases. In other occasions, candidiasis may lead to several microabscesses in the liver.

56. What are hemangiomas and how are they imaged?

Liver hemangiomas are the most common benign liver tumors of vascular origin. They are composed of endothelial lined spaces (cavernous sinuses) filled with blood. They are more common in females than males (5:1). They may be solitary or multiple and are usually located in the posterior segment of the right lobe (73%) and the left lobe (27%). They may enlarge during pregnancy and estrogen administration. Therefore, they are hormonal dependent. Very little or no flow is seen on color Doppler (Fig. 8).

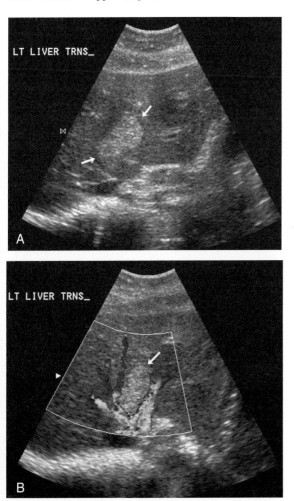

FIGURE 8. Hemangiomas. *A* and *B,* Typical appearance. A hyperechoic mass is seen adjacent to the hepatic veins (*arrow*). No flow was detected on color Doppler due to the nature of the very slow blood flow in these tumors (see also Color Plates, Figure 5). (*continued*)

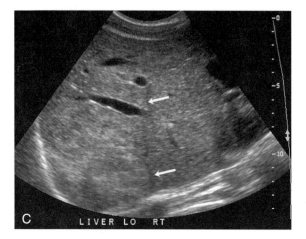

FIGURE 8. (*continued*) *C,* A typical appearance of a hemangioma mimicking hepatocellular carcinoma (*arrows*). A large heterogeneous mass is seen in the posterior segment of the right lobe of the liver. Computed tomography confirmed the diagnosis of giant hemangioma.

Sonographically, hemangiomas appear as well-defined oval or round hyperechoic lesions (may be attributed to the interfaces between the walls of the sinuses). Through transmission may also be seen. As they enlarge in size, they may present as complex masses with hypoechoic areas of necrosis, hemorrhaging, fibrosis, or thrombosis. They can mimic metastatic disease from the gastrointestinal tract, hepatocellular carcinoma, adenoma, and focal nodular hyperplasia.

Tip: If no risk for metastatic disease or primary hepatocellular carcinoma is present, a follow-up examination is recommended in 6 months. Otherwise, CT, MRI, or ^{99m}Tc nuclear medicine examination should be performed.

Pitfall: Variants may be hypoechoic in fatty liver and have a thin halo with peripheral vascularity.

57. What is focal nodular hyperplasia (FNH)?

FNH is a rare benign liver tumor, usually discovered incidentally, consisting of hepatocytes, Kupffer cells, bile ducts, and fibrous connective tissue. It can be solitary or multiple. It is more common in women between the ages of 20 and 40, with increased incidence with the use of oral contraceptives. FNH is frequently located in the lateral aspect of the liver (subcapsular), mostly in the right lobe. Patients are usually asymptomatic.

58. What is the sonographic appearance of FNH?

FNH is usually a nonencapsulated and well-circumscribed tumor ranging from 0.5–20 cm, but is usually < 8 cm. It may have several ultrasound appearances. It can be hypoechoic, hyperechoic, or isoechoic to normal liver. It can be confused with liver adenoma. It is important to keep in mind the constituents of the tumor. FNH contains Kupffer cells, whereas adenoma does not. Kupffer cells have a tendency to absorb the ^{99m}Tc colloid. Consequently, a nuclear medicine examination (^{99m}Tc) can be very helpful in distinguishing between the two tumors. Briefly, the FNH is "hot" due to the absorption of the radionuclide by the Kupffer cells. In addition, FNH may show high arterial flow within the central region radiating out in a linear fashion.

59. What is a liver adenoma?

A liver adenoma is a benign epithelial tumor composed of hepatocytes and lacks Kupffer cells and bile ducts. On ultrasound, it may be hypoechoic in glycogen storage disease type I (liver is usually abnormally echogenic), or it may be a well-defined hyperechoic mass with central hypoechoic areas due to necrosis and hemorrhage. Birth control pills and androgens increase its incidence. Patients are usually asymptomatic, but they may present with severe right upper quadrant pain due to hemorrhage.

60. What are the symptoms associated with hepatocellular carcinomas (HCC)?

Patients may present with right upper quadrant pain, abdominal mass, elevation of serum alpha fetoprotein (two thirds of cases), signs of cirrhosis, weight loss or loss of appetite, unexplained fever, or hepatomegaly.

61. Describe the ultrasound patterns in HCC?

HCC can be solitary, multiple, or diffuse. It can be hyperechoic (50%), hypoechoic, isoechoic, or mixed. It is vascular and has a tendency to invade the portal venous system (tumor or thrombus, 30–68%), hepatic veins (producing Budd-Chiari syndrome), and the IVC (less frequent) (Fig. 9).

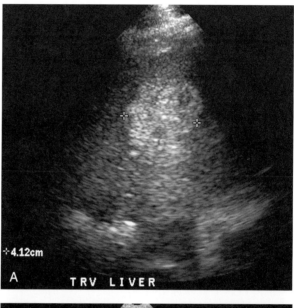

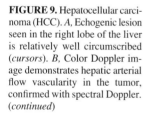

FIGURE 9. Hepatocellular carcinoma (HCC). *A,* Echogenic lesion seen in the right lobe of the liver is relatively well circumscribed (*cursors*). *B,* Color Doppler image demonstrates hepatic arterial flow vascularity in the tumor, confirmed with spectral Doppler. (*continued*)

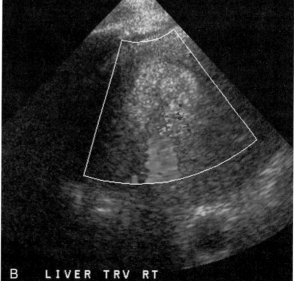

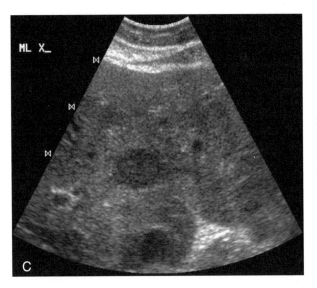

FIGURE 9. (*continued*) *C,* Hypoechoic lesions seen in the right and left lobes of another patient demonstrate the variable ultrasound appearance of HCC.

62. What are the primary sites that cause metastatic disease to spread to the liver?

In adults, the primary sites are the gastrointestinal tract (colon, pancreas, rectum), breasts, and lungs. In children, they are neuroblastoma, Wilm's tumor, and leukemia. Metastases can spread to the liver through the portal vein (gastrointestinal tract), the hepatic artery, or the lymphatic system or direct from gallbladder and stomach tumors (less common).

63. What are the sonographic patterns of liver metastatic disease?

Metastatic disease is more frequent than HCCs in the United States (approximately 20% higher). It can be solitary or multiple. It can present in several ways (Fig. 10):

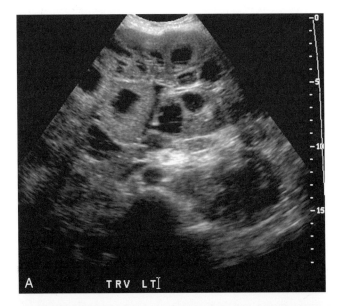

FIGURE 10. Metastases—spectrum of appearances. *A,* Cystic lesions with echogenic rims seen dispersed throughout the liver. This primary tumor was carcinoid. (*continued*)

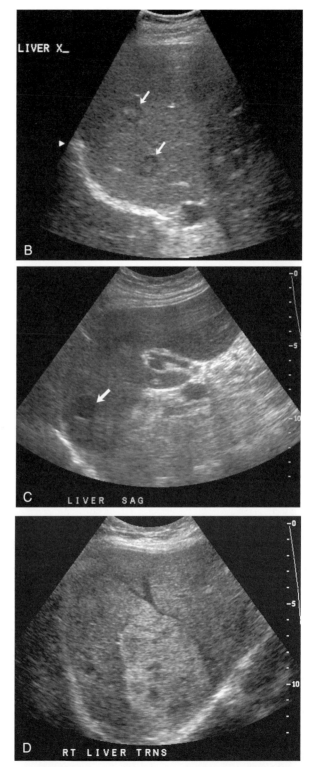

FIGURE 10. (*continued*) *B,* Multiple hypoechoic lesions that can be seen with breast and lung cancer and melanoma. These have a target or "bulls eye" appearance, with an echogenic center and a hypoechoic rim (*arrows*). These were metastatic lung carcinoma. *C,* Hypoechoic lesion in the right lobe consistent with lymphoma (*arrows*). *D, E,* Hyperchoic lesions that are well circumscribed and mimic hemangioma, except for increased central hepatic arterial vascularity. Typical primaries include colon, breast, and neuroendocrine lesions. (*continued*)

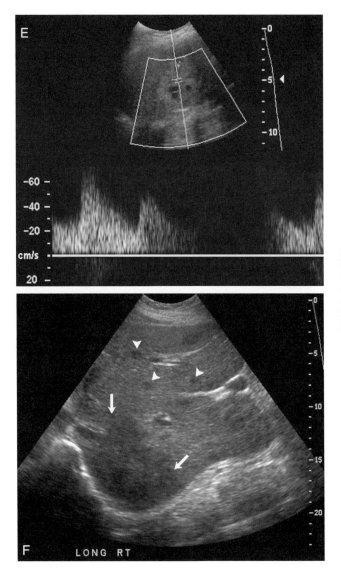

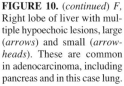

FIGURE 10. (*continued*) *F,* Right lobe of liver with multiple hypoechoic lesions, large (*arrows*) and small (*arrowheads*). These are common in adenocarcinoma, including pancreas and in this case lung.

- **Hypoechoic.** It is usually hypovascular and may have a halo around the mass due to necrosis or hemorrhage, which gives it the bull's eye or target sign appearance. It is usually associated with breast and bronchial carcinomas, or with lymphoma.
- **Echogenic.** It is usually hypervascular and may have calcifications (especially with colon and rectal cancer). This appearance is usually seen in cancers of the colon, pancreas (islet cell tumors), rectum, or urogenital tract (ovary, kidney [renal cell carcinoma]).
- **Cystic or anechoic.** It is due to necrosis or hemorrhage as seen in leiomyosarcoma.
- **Diffuse or infiltrative.** It can be seen with lung and breast carcinomas as well as melanoma.

BIBLIOGRAPHY

1. Chafetz N, Filly RA: Portal and hepatic veins: Accuracy of marginal echoes for distinguishing intrahepatic vessels. Radiology 130:725–728, 1979.
2. Donoso L, Martinez-Noguera A, Zidan A, Lora F: Papillary process of the caudate lobe of the liver: Sonographic appearance. Radiology 173:631–633, 1989.
3. Freeman MP, Vick CW, Taylor KJW, et al: Regenerating nodules in cirrhosis: Sonographic appearance with anatomic correlation. Am J Roentgenol 146:533–536, 1986.
4. Gibney RG, Hendin AP, Cooperberg PL, et al: Sonographically detected hepatic hemangiomas: Absence of change over time. Am J Roentgenol 149:953–957, 1987.
5. Grant EG, Perrella R, Tessler FN, et al: Budd-Chiari syndrome: The results of duplex and color Doppler imaging. Am J Roentgenol 152:377–381, 1989.
6. Hussain S: Diagnostic criteria of hydatid disease on hepatic sonography. J Ultrasound Med 4:603–607, 1985.
7. Kuhman JE: Pneumocystic infections: The radiologist's perspective. Radiology 198:623–635, 1996.
8. LaBreque DR: Acute and chronic hepatitis. In Stein JH (ed): Internal Medicine, 4th ed. St. Louis, Mosby, 1994.
9. Levine E, Cook LT, Granthem JJ: Liver cysts in autosomal-dominant polycystic kidney disease: Clinical and computed tomographic study. Am J Roentgenol 145:229–233, 1985.
10. Low V, Khangure MS: Hepatic adenoma and focal nodular hyperplasia: A diagnostic dilemma. Aust Radiol 44:124–130, 1990.
11. Marks WM, Filly RA, Callen PW: Ultrasonic anatomy of the liver: A review with new applications. J Clin Ultrasound 7:137–146, 1979.
12. Mittelstaedt CA. Liver. In Mittelstaedt CA (ed): Abdominal Ultrasound. New York, Churchill Livingstone, 1992, pp 173–248.
13. Moody AR, Wilson SR: Atypical hemangioma: A suggestive sonographic morphology. Radiology 188:413–417, 1993.
14. Needleman L, Kurtz AB, Rifkin MD, et al: Sonography of diffuse benign liver disease. Am J Roentgenol 146:1011–1015, 1986.
15. Newlin N, Silver TM, Stuck KJ, et al: Ultrasonic features of pyogenic liver abscesses. Radiology 139:155–159, 1981.
16. Quinn SF, Gosink, BB: Characteristic sonographic signs of hepatic fatty infilteration. Am J Roentgenol 145:753–755, 1985.
17. Smith D, Downey D, Spouge A, Soney S: Sonographic demonstration of Couinaud's liver segments. J Ultrasound Med 17:375–381, 1998.
18. Spouge AR, Wilson SR, Gopinath N, et al: Extrapulmonary *Pneumocystis carinii* in a patient with AIDS: Sonographic findings. Am J Roentgenol 155:76–78, 1990.
19. Wernecke K, Vassallo P, Bick U, et al: The distinction between benign and malignant liver tumors on sonography: Value of a hypoechoic halo. Am J Roentgenol 159:1005–1009, 1992.
20. Yoshida T, Matsue H, Okazaki N, et al: Ultrasonographic differentiation of hepatocelluar carcinoma from metastatic liver cancer. J Clin Ultrasound 15:431–437, 1987.

17. THE KIDNEYS

Ryan K. Lee, M.D.

1. When is a renal scan indicated?
The most common indication is suspected obstruction in a patient with renal failure. Renal ultrasound is also requested to screen for stones or renal masses and sometimes to confirm indeterminate masses seen on computed tomography (CT), such as renal cysts.

2. What is the function of the kidney?
The major function of the kidney is to excrete metabolic waste, filtering over 1700 L of blood per day into approximately 1 L of urine. The kidney is also an endocrine organ and secretes hormones, such as renin, erythropoietin, and prostaglandins.

3. What is the embryology of the kidney?
Actually, three sets of kidneys develop in the human body. The **pronephros** is rudimentary and does not function. The **mesonephros** develops next and functions as an interim kidney. The **metanephros** is the permanent kidney; it develops in the fifth week of gestation and consists of the ureteric bud and metanephrogenic blastema.

4. How should a kidney be scanned?
The upper poles of the kidneys are often best seen with a high intercostal posterior approach using the liver or spleen as a window. The lower poles can be seen subcostally during a deep inspiration. Having the patient lie in a decubitus position and scanning anterolaterally is also useful for obese patients. Depending on the body habitus, a 2.5–5-MHz transducer is generally appropriate.

5. What are the normal dimensions of the kidney?
The adult kidney is 11 cm long, 5 cm wide, and 2.5 cm thick and weighs between 120 and 170 gm. Normal length is considered to be between 10 and 12 cm.

6. What is the accepted size discrepancy between the two kidneys?
Kidney length should be within 2 cm of each other. A > 2 cm discrepancy suggests that one of the kidneys is either too large or too small.

7. What is the normal echogenicity of the kidney?
The cortical echogenicity is normally equal or somewhat less than the echogenicity of the liver (Fig. 1) and is less echogenic compared to the spleen. The pyramids are hypoechoic structures, being less echogenic than the cortex (Fig. 2).

8. What is a junctional parenchymal defect?
The junctional parenchymal defect is a wedge-shaped echogenic defect usually along the anterior aspect of the upper kidney. It is a normal variant caused by incomplete embryologic fusion of the upper and lower poles (Fig. 3).

9. What is a dromedary hump?
This bulge along the lateral border of the left kidney results from molding of the adjacent spleen and is a normal variant (Fig. 4).

10. What is a column of Bertin?
The column of Bertin is a normal cortical tissue projected toward the hilum of a normal kidney. The column of Bertin forms the lateral boundaries of each pyramid defined by inward ex-

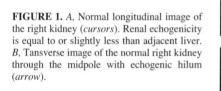

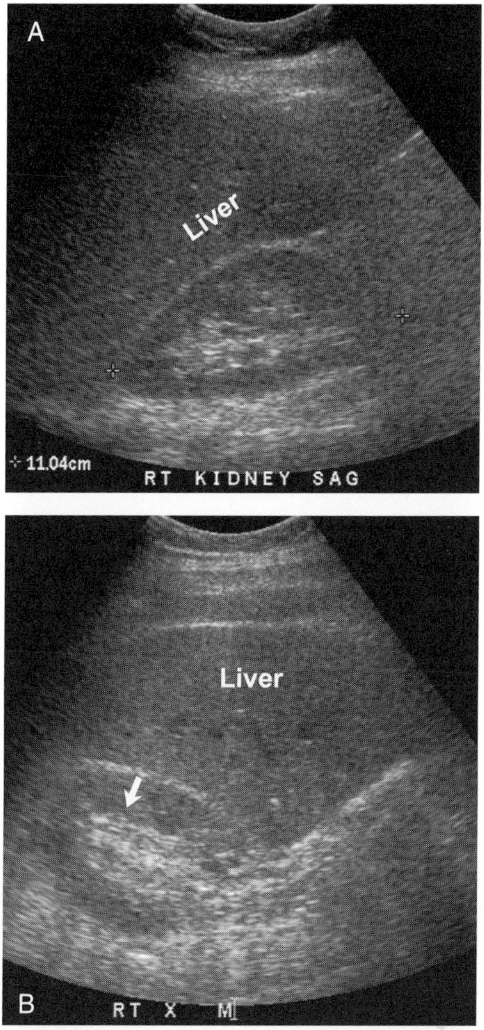

FIGURE 1. *A,* Normal longitudinal image of the right kidney (*cursors*). Renal echogenicity is equal to or slightly less than adjacent liver. *B,* Tansverse image of the normal right kidney through the midpole with echogenic hilum (*arrow*).

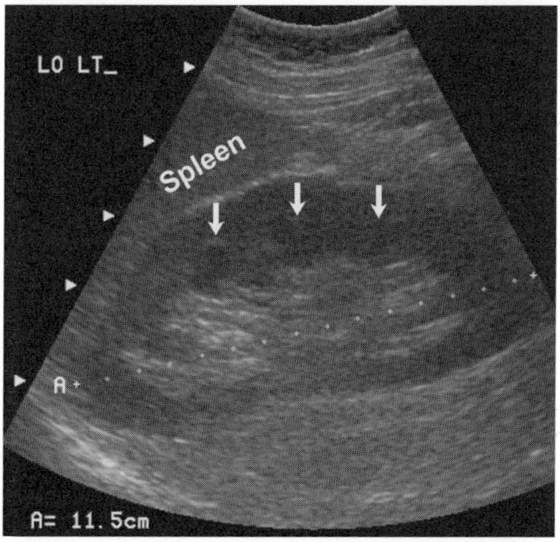

FIGURE 2. Normal left kidney. The kidney echotexture is slightly less than the adjacent spleen. Normal hypoechoic renal pyramids are present (*arrows*).

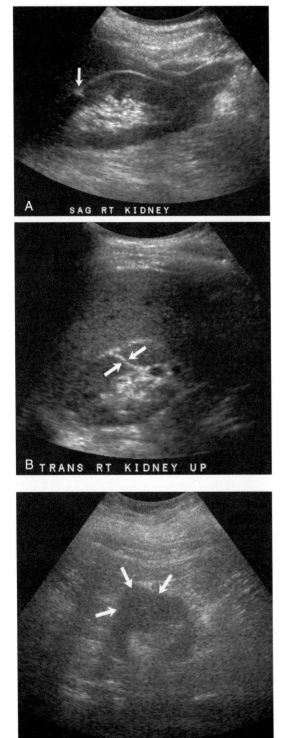

FIGURE 3. Junctional parenchymal defect. Longitudinal (*A*) and transverse (*B*) images of the right kidney demonstrate a normal junctional defect (*arrows*) not to be mistaken for a scar.

FIGURE 4. Dromedary hump. Transverse and longitudinal images of this normal variant (*arrows*) configuration of renal parenchyma, more common in the left kidney.(*continued*)

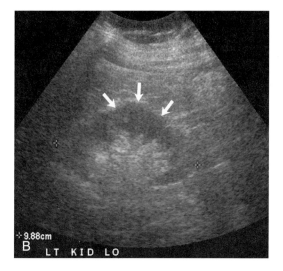

FIGURE 4. (*continued*)

tensions of the cortical tissue. Sometimes this normal column of Bertin hypertrophies and protrudes into the renal sinus giving the appearance of a pseudotumor. This usually occurs at the junction of the mid and upper one third of the kidney. It is not pathologic but is an incidental finding (Fig. 5).

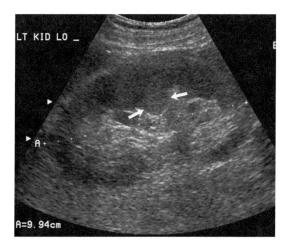

FIGURE 5. Column of Bertin. Abnormal column of parenchymal tissue (*arrows*) indents the renal sinus. It does not represent a renal mass.

11. What are fetal lobulations?

Normal and commonly seen cortical indentations secondary to incomplete fusion of the embryologic renal lobules.

12. What is a horseshoe kidney?

Horseshoe kidney results when there is embryologic fusion of the lower poles. The tissue connecting the lower poles can be either functioning renal parenchyma or fibrous tissue.

13. What is the significance of a horseshoe kidney?

It is associated with an increased risk of reflux, infection, obstruction, calculi, duplicated collecting systems, and cardiovascular and skeletal abnormalities. There is also an increased risk of injury to the renal parenchyma after trauma.

14. What is ureteropelvic junction (UPJ) obstruction?

UPJ obstruction is a congenital idiopathic obstruction at the level of the UPJ. Some believe that excessive collagen deposition within the muscle causes the obstruction; other theories include intrinsic valves, true luminal stenosis, and aberrant arteries. The obstruction results in a dilated renal pelvis and calyces, and a "beaking" pattern at the level of the obstruction often can be noted, which is also known as the *UPJ configuration*.

15. What is hydronephrosis?

Hydronephrosis is the dilatation of the pelvis and calyces (pelvicaliectesis) secondary to an accumulation of urine within the kidney. This can be caused by an anatomic obstruction, such as a renal calculus, or may be nonobstructive in nature.

16. How is hydronephrosis graded?

Mild hydronephrosis refers to visualization of the collecting system with blunting of the fornices, still with visible sinus echoes.

Moderate hydronephrosis is dilatation of the collecting system that fills the sinus without evidence for cortical thinning.

Severe hydronephrosis refers to severely dilated, clubbed calyces with associated thinning of the cortical parenchyma (Fig. 6).

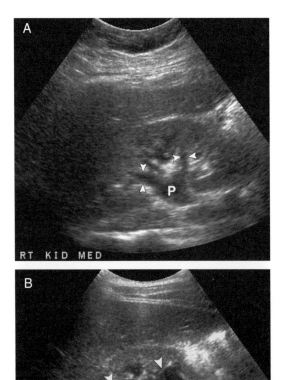

FIGURE 6. Hydronephrosis. Mild (*A*), moderate (*B*), (*continued*)

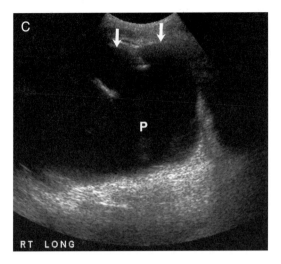

FIGURE 6. (*continued*) and severe (*C*) hydronephrosis show progressive calyceal (*arrows*) and pelvis (*P*) dilatation. Note parenchymal loss with severe hydronephrosis.

17. What are the false positives for obstructive hydronephrosis?
- Overly distended bladder with transmitted backpressure
- Overhydration or diuresis
- Prominent renal pelvis, UPJ
- Congenital megacalyces
- Postobstructive dilatation
- Vesicoureteral reflux (Fig. 7)
- Parapelvic cysts
- Hydronephrosis of pregnancy (physiologic decreased ureteral peristalsis (2nd trimester) accompanied by uterine pressure (3rd trimester)

18. What are false negatives in patients who are obstructed?
- Insufficient hydration. Many patients who are acutely obstructed are dehydrated, so the collecting system is not distended.
- Decompression caused by forniceal rupture. Look for perinephric fluid.
- Retroperitoneal fibrosis. The collecting system cannot dilate.

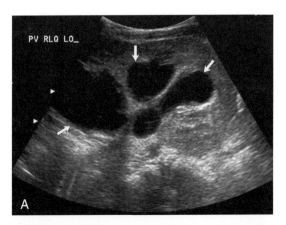

FIGURE 7. False positives for hydronephrosis. Longitudinal postvoid (*A*) (*continued*)

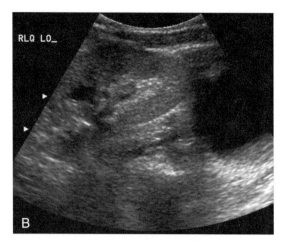

FIGURE 7. (*continued*) and prevoid (*B*) images through a transplant show moderate hydronephrosis (*arrows*). Postvoid hydronephrosis is caused by reflux. Prevoid image is normal.

19. What is acute pyelonephritis and what does it look like?

Acute pyelonephritis is tubulointerstitial inflammation of the kidney. It most commonly arises from a lower urinary tract infection secondary to *Escherichia coli* (ascending infection). Sonographic findings include renal enlargement, loss of corticomedullary differentiation, abnormal echogenicity, poorly marginated masses, and compression of the renal sinus. Focal areas of infection may be of increased or decreased echogenicity and may present as mass lesions (Fig. 8).

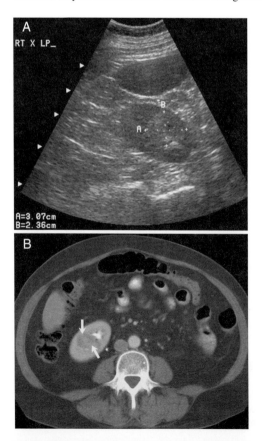

FIGURE 8. Pyelonephritis. Transverse right lower pole has a 3-cm hyperechoic mass corresponding to the low attenuation lesion (*arrows*) on enhanced CT. This represents focal pyelonephritis.

20. How does chronic pyelonephritis appear on ultrasound?

Chronic pyelonephritis presents as a dilated blunted calyx with a thinned, scarred adjacent cortex and may affect multiple calyices. It is often associated with vesicoureteral reflux.

21. What is the difference between a renal abscess and pyonephrosis?

Renal abscesses are abscesses within the renal parenchyma. These appear on sonography as round, thick-walled echogenic or hypoechoic complex masses that may have septations. They may or may not demonstrate through transmission (Fig. 9).

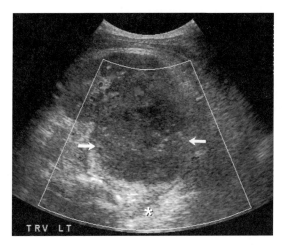

FIGURE 9. Renal and perirenal abscess. Transverse color Doppler image through the left kidney shows a solid-appearing mass (*arrows*) with internal echoes. However, it lacks any vascularity and has enhanced through transmission (*), suggesting its complex fluid nature. This abscess originated in the kidney and extended into the perirenal space.

Pyonephrosis is purulent material within an obstructed collecting system. It is often seen in young adults who have UPJ obstruction or renal calculi. Ultrasound is neither sensitive nor specific in identifying pyonephrosis. The nonspecific finding of hydronephrosis with or without hydroureter is usually the only finding. Sometimes echogenic pus can be noted to fill or layer within the collecting system.

22. What is XGP?

Xanthogranulomatous pyelonephritis (XPG) is a chronic inflammatory renal process that causes replacement of normal renal parenchyma with lipid-laden macrophages; it is usually associated with longstanding obstruction. Ultrasound classically demonstrates posterior acoustic shadowing from a central staghorn calculus, enlarged kidney, and multiple dilated calyces.

23. Hoes does papillary necrosis appear on ultrasound?

Sonography does not detect the early stages of papillary necrosis very well. In the later stages in which the papilla sloughs, echogenic nonshadowing material can be seen within a dilated collecting system. Passage of this sloughed debris into the ureters can then cause obstruction and hydronephrosis.

24. How do renal calculi appear sonographically?

Renal calculi appear as echogenic foci, which are markedly hyperechoic to renal parenchyma. The most important characterizing feature of calculi is the posterior acoustic shadow. This occurs because calculi prevent sound waves from propagating through them, causing an anechoic streak opposite the position of the transducer (Fig. 10).

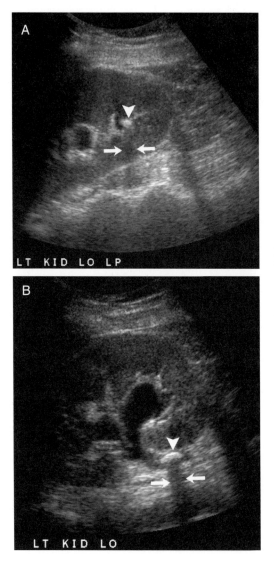

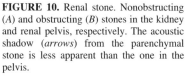

FIGURE 10. Renal stone. Nonobstructing (*A*) and obstructing (*B*) stones in the kidney and renal pelvis, respectively. The acoustic shadow (*arrows*) from the parenchymal stone is less apparent than the one in the pelvis.

25. What are the limitations to detecting calculi?

Vascular calcifications in the renal arteries may be mistaken for calculi. Calculi may be difficult to detect in an echogenic renal sinus background. Small stones (< 5 mm) may not shadow, especially if not located in the focal zone of the transducer. Detection can be aided by using color or power Doppler to generate a twinkle artifact at the stone (Fig. 11).

26. What is nephrocalcinosis? Can it be seen by ultrasound?

Nephrocalcinosis is the term used to describe calcifications within the renal parenchyma. **Medullary nephrocalcinosis** refers to calcification within the medullary pyramids. Common causes for medullary nephrocalcinosis include medullary sponge kidney, hyperparathyroidism, and renal tubular acidosis type I (type I affects distal tubules). A less common form of nephrocalcinosis is **cortical nephrocalcinosis,** or calcification in the cortical parenchyma. Causes for cortical nephrocalcinosis include chronic glomerulonephritis, renal transplant rejection, and acute cortical necrosis.

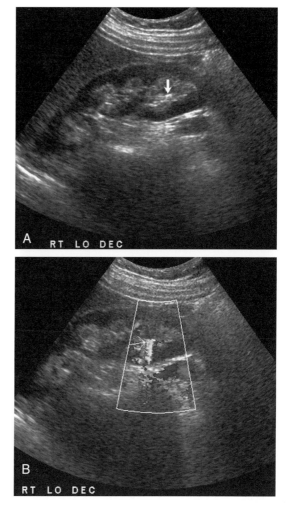

FIGURE 11. Stones without shadowing. *A,* Grayscale image shows a faint echo (arrow) in the lower pole renal sinus with no shadow. *B,* Color Doppler image shows a marked "twinkle" artifact (arrow) behind the stone, confirming its presence.

Nephrocalcinosis can be seen by ultrasound as echogenic foci in either the medullary pyramids (**medullary nephrocalcinosis**) or the cortex (**cortical nephrocalcinosis**). If the calcifications are very small, shadowing may not be appreciated (Fig. 12).

27. What is Alport syndrome?
This X-linked hereditary nephritis is accompanied by sensorineural hearing loss. Patients with Alport syndrome may develop cortical calcifications as their kidneys fail.

28. What is medullary sponge kidney?
Also known as **benign tubular ectasia,** medullary sponge kidney is the dilatation, or ectasia, of the distal collecting ducts. The dilatation causes stasis in the collecting ducts, encouraging stone formation. It is not surprising then, that it is often associated with medullary nephrocalcinosis. The cause of medullary sponge kidney is not known. Medullary sponge kidney is difficult to identify by ultrasound, but, when complicated by nephrocalcinosis, multiple, echogenic foci can be seen in the medullary pyramids.

29. What are the characteristics of simple cysts?
The major characteristics of **simple cysts** include an anechoic lumen, sharply defined thin smooth walls, and posterior acoustic enhancement. Posterior acoustic enhancement occurs be-

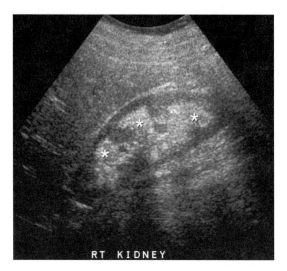

FIGURE 12. Medulary nephrocalcinosis. Longitudinal ultrasound shows the pyramids (*) to be as bright as the renal sinus. Normally, they should be iso- or hypoechoic to the parenchyma.

cause sound traveling through fluid is not as attenuated as sound traveling through soft tissue, thus higher amplitude echoes are produced posterior to the fluid-filled cyst (Fig. 13).

30. What are the characteristics of complex cysts?

The major characteristics of **complex cysts** include septations, calcifications, thickened walls, and internal echos. The lack of posterior acoustic enhancement is another feature of complex cysts.

31. What are parapelvic cysts?

Parapelvic cysts are cysts that are found in the renal sinus. They are thought to be lymphatic in origin and have characteristics of simple cysts. They are usually asymptomatic, but if large enough, they can cause hydronephrosis and hypertension. Parapelvic cysts may at times be difficult to distinguish from hydronephrosis, but in the latter case, calyces can usually be seen to connect with the collecting system (Fig. 14).

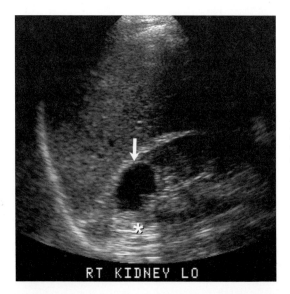

FIGURE 13. Renal cyst. Simple renal cyst (*arrow*) is anechoic with a sharp back wall and enhanced through transmission (*).

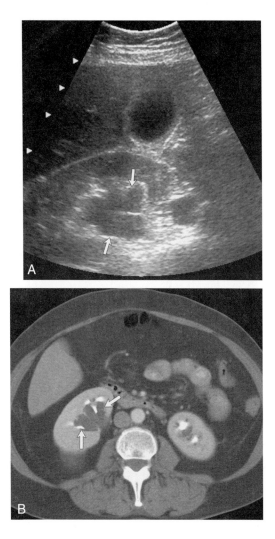

FIGURE 14. *A*, Parapelvic cyst. Longitudinal ultrasound image shows hypoechoic cystic lesions in the renal sinus which are not necessarily interconnected, not connecting with the pelvis. *B*, CT image of the same patient shows fluid attenuation cysts (*arrows*) interspersed with the brightly enhanced renal collecting system (*white*).

32. What is a milk of calcium cyst?

Crystalline material composed of calcium can develop in cysts and create echogenic material, which layers dependently and causes posterior acoustic shadowing. These cysts have no clinical significance other than to be differentiated from a more malignant process.

33. How are cystic lesions classified?

The Bosniak Classification

CLASSIFICATION	DESCRIPTION
Bosniak I	Simple cysts
Bosniak II	Septated, minimal calcium, nonenhancing high-density cysts, infected cysts (Fig. 15)
Bosniak II F	When a cyst does not meet the criteria of Bosniak II or Bosniak III cyst, it is placed in the II F category. *F* stands for follow-up. The main difference from category II is that II F cysts are > 3 cm in size.
Bosniak III	Multiloculated, hemorrhagic, with dense calcification, or a nonenhancing solid component
Bosniak IV	Contains an enhancing component with marginal irregularity

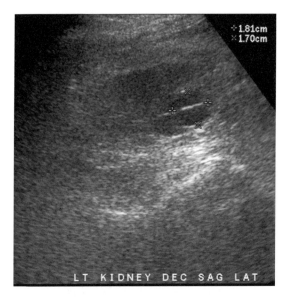

FIGURE 15. Complex cyst. This lower pole cyst (*cursors*) has a central echogenic line or septation and therefore is classified as a Bosniak II lesion.

The significance of this classification scheme is that Bosniak III and IV cysts usually require operative management.

34. What is a multicystic dysplastic kidney?

Multicystic dysplastic kidney is a developmental anomaly in which normal renal parenchyma has been primarily replaced by multiple noncommunicating cystic structures with little to no renal function. It is usually a unilateral process; a bilateral process is not compatible with life. Ultrasound demonstrates a small kidney with multiple noncommunicating cystic structures and absence of normal renal parenchyma. The renal artery and ureter are absent or atretic. There is high association of contralateral abnormalities such as UPJ obstruction.

35. What is multilocular cystic nephroma?

This rare, benign cystic neoplasm demonstrates multiple cysts of various sizes contained in a thick pseudocapsule. Age distribution is bimodal; half of patients are boys younger than 10 years, and the other half are women aged 30–40 years. Sonographic findings are nonspecific, and differentiation from a cystic renal cell carcinoma can be difficult. The septa may show blood flow. A classic description of a cystic mass herniating into the renal pelvis can be suggestive but is not diagnostic.

36. What is the most common malignant primary renal tumor, and what does it look like on ultrasound?

Renal cell carcinoma (RCC) is the most common primary adult renal malignancy, accounting for over 80% of primary renal tumors. The classic triad of flank pain, palpable mass, and hematuria is, in fact, seen in only a minority of patients. RCCs are more common in men than women, with peak incidence between 50 and 70 years. RCC can have a variety of appearances, many of which are nonspecific. Most RCCs present as solid tumors that can be hyper-, iso-, or hypoechoic (Fig. 16). About 7% of all RCCs will have cystic components that may be difficult to differentiate from benign complex cysts.

37. Which disease processes have an increased risk of RCC?

- Chronic renal failure requiring long-term dialysis with acquired cystic kidney disease
- Von Hippel–Lindau disease
- Tuberous sclerosis

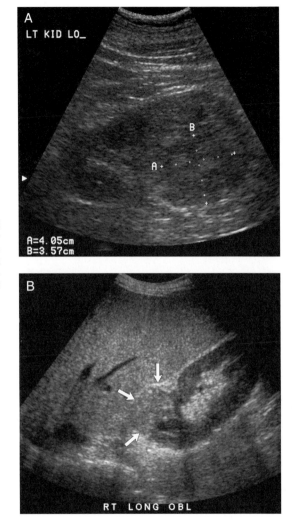

FIGURE 16. *A,* Longitudinal ultrasound shows a 4-cm hypoechoic mass, nearly isoechoic with the kidney. *B,* Longitudinal ultrasound of a different patient shows a hyperechoic mass *(arrows)* arising from the upper pole. Both were renal cell carcinoma.

38. How is renal carcinoma staged?

STAGE	DESCRIPTION
I	Confined within renal capsule
II	Penetrates beyond renal capsule but stays within Gerota's fascia; may involve ipsilateral adrenal gland
IIIA	Involves renal vein
IIIB	Involves regional lymph nodes
IIIC	Both renal vein and regional nodes are involved
IV	Invasion of adjacent organs or distant metastases

39. What complications of renal cancer can be identified by ultrasound?

Thrombosis of the renal vein and inferior vena cava (IVC) are two of the most important complications of renal cell cancer that are well evaluated with ultrasound. Ultrasound demonstrates echogenic material in these vessels, with a lack of flow on color Doppler interrogation. Detecting these thrombi are important in the staging of RCC. Overall staging, however, is still better performed with CT or magnetic resonance imaging (MRI).

40. How does RCC differ from oncocytoma?

Oncocytomas represent 3–6% of all renal tumors and may be benign or malignant. They mimic RCC on imaging, although occasionally they can be suspected due to a central scar, but this is not specific. They tend to be multicentric and bilateral in up to 10%, as are RCCs.

41. What is medullary carcinoma?

Renal medullary carcinoma is a rare tumor of the kidney. This tumor occurs exclusively in young black patients with sickle cell trait (hemoglobin SA or hemoglobin SC) but not sickle cell anemia. The radiographic appearance of renal medullary carcinoma is that of a prototypical infiltrative lesion. The tumors are heterogeneous at ultrasound. The constellation of renal medullary mass, black race, sickle cell trait, and hemoglobin SC disease suggest the diagnosis. The mean survival is approximately 15 weeks from diagnosis.

42. Name the common renal metastases.

The most common malignancies to metastasize to the kidney are lung, breast, and RCC of the opposite kidney. They can be single or multiple masses or a diffusely infiltrative process. Lesions are most often discrete and hypoechoic.

43. What is renal lymphoma?

Renal lymphoma (most commonly non-Hodgkin's) arises either from hematogenous dissemination or direct extension because the kidney has no lymphoid tissue. Usually there is disseminated involvement throughout the body when disease is detected in the kidney. Sonographic findings suggestive of renal lymphoma include focal parenchymal involvement, diffuse infiltration, perirenal involvement, and invasion from a retroperitoneal mass. Usually, lesions are hypoechoic and may or may not be vascular.

44. What is the appearance of transitional cell carcinoma (TCC)?

TCC accounts for 7% of all primary renal tumors, but it is difficult to detect with ultrasound. This is a solid hypoechoic mass, located within the collecting system. It may be mimicked by hypoechoic fat and may be difficult to distinguish from thrombus if it lacks flow on Doppler interrogation. Screening for TCC is still done best by urography or retrograde ureterography.

45. What is the difference between autosomal dominant and autosomal recessive polycystic kidney disease?

Autosomal recessive polycystic kidney disease results from pathologically dilated collecting tubules and hepatic cysts. There is an inverse relationship between the severity of the renal and liver disease. The more severe the renal disease, the less severe the liver disease is, and the higher the mortality. These cysts are small and usually not seen by ultrasound. Instead, the kidneys are echogenic, due to the multiple interfaces created by the walls of the cysts.

Autosomal dominant polycystic kidney disease results in a large number of renal cysts bilaterally. Signs often do not present until the mid 40s and include hypertension, palpable masses, pain, and hematuria. Cysts also can appear in other organs including the spleen, pancreas, and liver. Infection, stone formation, and cyst rupture are all potential complications in addition to renal failure.

46. What is von Hippel–Lindau disease (VHLD)?

VHLD disease is autosomal dominant with high penetrance and is caused by a genetic defect in the short arm of chromosome 3. Manifestations of VHLD include retinal angiomas, central nervous system hemangioblastomas, pancreatic cysts, islet cell tumors, pheochromocytomas, endolymphatic sac tumors, cystadenomas of the epididymis, and broad ligament and renal cysts and tumors. RCCs, which are often multifocal and bilateral, are reported to develop in 24–45% of VHLD patients. Predominantly cystic lesions with solid components are characteristic of VHLD. The solid component usually represents RCC. VHLD not associated with pheochromocytoma is subclassified as VHLD-1 and with pheochromocytoma as VHLD-2.

47. What is tuberous sclerosis?

Tuberous sclerosis complex (TSC) may be inherited as an autosomal dominant trait or may occur sporadically. Tuberous sclerosis is an autosomal dominant disorder often associated with a chromosome 9 (*TSC1*) and chromosome 16 (*TSC2*) abnormality, although up to 60% of cases occur spontaneously. The classic presentation includes mental retardation, seizures, and adenoma sebaceum. Renal lesions are seen in 50% of TSC patients and include multiple cysts, angiomyolipomas (AMLs), tumors and perirenal cystic collections, and lymphangiomas. Other associations include subependymal nodules, giant cell astrocytoma, peripheral tubers, retinal hamartomas, cardiac rhabdomyoma, lymphangioleiomyomatosis, shagreen patches, subungual fibromas, and bone cysts. This is another autosomal dominant disorder associated with renal cysts, and it, too, is inherited in an autosomal dominant manner. Associations include cortical hamartomas and, in 80% of patients, bilateral angiomyolipomas.

48. What is an angiomyolipoma (AML)?

This benign renal tumor is composed of blood vessels, muscle cells, and adipose tissue. These tumors typically are unilateral (except in TSC patients) and occur in middle-aged women. Angiomyolipomas in patients with TSC are usually bilateral in 80% of cases. Sporadic angiomyolipomas are more common. The sonographic appearance is a hyperechoic mass, but RCC can also have similar appearance. AMLs are usually asymptomatic but do have the propensity to hemorrhage, especially those larger than 4 cm. They can also invade the inferior vena cava. The presence of fat within an AML on CT or MRI is diagnostic (Fig. 17).

49. How effective is ultrasound in diagnosing renal artery stenosis?

The detection of **renal artery stenosis** requires a two-part approach, with both parts using Doppler interrogation. The first approach for determining renal artery stenosis involves establishing peak main renal artery velocities (> 180 cm/sec) and the ratio of peak renal artery velocity to peak aortic velocity (> 3.5).

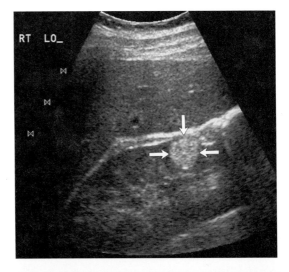

FIGURE 17. Angiomyolipoma. Longitudinal ultrasound shows a very echogenic and well-circumscribed mass (*arrows*) in the lower pole. This was confirmed to contain fat on CT. By ultrasound, it cannot definitely be distinguished from renal cell carcinoma.

The second approach involves measuring the intrarenal vasculature waveforms. Renal artery stenosis results in a characteristic waveform consisting of a slowed systolic upstroke and a low-amplitude systolic peak, which is known as a parvus-tardus waveform. Additionally, measuring the resistive index ([peak systolic velocity — peak diastolic velocity]/peak systolic velocity) has also been advocated, with a resistive index < 0.5 suggestive of proximal stenosis.

The effectiveness of these techniques is controversial. It is often difficult to image the entire main renal artery, which makes the first approach difficult to implement. Studies evaluating the second technique have yielded mixed results.

50. What is the differential diagnosis for a unilateral small kidney?

Reflux nephropathy	Chronic pyelonephritis
Previous renal surgery	Renal hypoplasia
Unilateral renal artery stenosis	Radiation therapy

51. What is the differential diagnosis for bilateral small kidneys?

Chronic renal insufficiency	Chronic glomerulonephritis
Reflux nephropathy	Nephrosclerosis from hypertension
Analgesic nephropathy	Remote acute tubular necrosis

52. What is the differential diagnosis for a unilateral large kidney?

- Ureteral obstruction
- Duplicated collecting system
- Compensatory hypertrophy from a poorly functioning contralateral kidney
- Acute pyelonephritis
- Xanthogranulomatous pyelonephritis
- Infiltrating tumor
- Contusion
- Acute renal vein occlusion

53. What is the differential diagnosis for bilateral large kidneys?

- Diabetic nephropathy
- Lymphoma
- Amyloid
- Autosomal dominant polycystic kidney disease
- Autosomal recessive polycystic kidney disease
- Metastatic disease
- Myeloma
- Collagen vascular disease

54. What is the purpose of determining bladder jets?

Doppler examination of the bladder to evaluate for bladder jets can help increase the sensitivity for determining renal obstruction. Absence of an identifiable urine jet from the ureter into the bladder has been advocated as a means of identifying obstruction on the ipsilateral side.

BIBLIOGRAPHY

1. Dunnick NR, Sandler CM, Amis ES, et al (eds): Textbook of Uroradiology, 3rd ed. Philadelphia, Lippincott Williams & Wilkins, 2001.
2. Kurtz AB, Middleton WD: Ultrasound: The Requisites. Philadelphia, Hanley & Belfus, 1996.
3. Rumack CM, Wilson SR, Charboneau JW (eds): Diagnostic Ultrasound, 2nd ed. St. Louis, Mosby, 1998.
4. Zagoria RJ, Tung GA: Genitourinary Radiology: The Requisites. St. Louis, Mosby, 1997.

18. THE URINARY BLADDER

Osbert Adjei, M.D.

1. What are the standard ultrasound imaging planes used for the urinary bladder?
Longitudinal and transverse planes are used, with the patient supine. The lateral decubitus position may be used for patients who cannot be positioned supine.

2. What are the indications for imaging patients in both the supine and lateral decubitus positions?
To evaluate suspected bladder masses for motion, both supine and lateral decubitus positions are used. Lesions that are not anatomically related to the bladder wall such as stones or blood clots move to the dependent position under gravity, whereas bladder wall–related lesions such as polyps or tumors do not.

3. What are the frequencies of the probes used for urinary bladder ultrasound?
For urinary bladder ultrasound, 3–5 MHz probes are used. Lower frequency probes are used for larger patients, whereas the higher frequency probes are used for smaller patients.

4. Is breath-holding required for urinary bladder ultrasound?
No. The bladder is a retroperitoneal pelvic organ, far removed from respiratory motion, which is primarily a thoracoabdominal process.

5. What are the landmarks used to localize the urinary bladder?
The full bladder itself is its own best landmark. In males, one can look for the prostate gland below the bladder neck. In nonhysterectomized females, the anteverted uterus can be seen in the midline, posterosuperior to the bladder. The bladder is anterior in the pelvis and should extend beneath the pubic symphysis.

6. What are the routine preparations for a urinary bladder ultrasound examination?
A moderately full bladder is the standard requirement. An overdistended bladder causes pain and distracts from the examination as well as distorting the bladder anatomy and adjacent organs. If the patient is unable to drink or fill the bladder, it can be filled retrograde by a catheter.

7. What are the clinical indications for a full bladder in ultrasound?
- *Ultrasound diagnosis:* both as an acoustic window (pelvic approach) and as a landmark for evaluation of the uterus and adnexae, prostate, seminal vesicles, and intravesical lesions
- *Pathologic diagnosis:* transrectal biopsy of the prostate, seminal vesicles, and other retroperitoneal and intraperitoneal lesions such as lymph nodes and metastases. The bladder needs to be partly full (hence visible) to avoid injury during the procedure, and to serve as a landmark.

8. What are the indications for postvoid ultrasound evaluation?
- To evaluate for change (resolution) in hydronephrosis or determine the degree of postvoid hydronephrosis
- To measure postvoid residual volume in patients with suspected outlet obstruction, neurogenic bladder, and urinary incontinence
- To identify cystic pelvic lesions that persist postvoid such as lymphoceles, loculated ascites, or cystic pelvic tumors (Fig. 1).

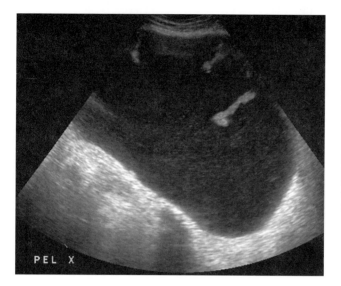

FIGURE 1. Large cystic mass in the pelvis with a polypoid internal component. The mass persisted postvoid. The differential diagnoses included distended bladder with a polypoid lesion. Surgery revealed a right ovarian mass, which on histology turned out to be adenocarcinoma.

9. **What are the differential diagnoses for a cystic structure adjacent to the urinary bladder?**
   - Urinary bladder diverticulum (Fig. 2)
   - Lymphocele (especially after radical pelvic surgery)
   - Cysts of the prostate or seminal vesicle, including müllerian duct cysts
   - Urinoma
   - Incontinence device
   - Neobladder
   - Patent urachus
   - Aneurysm of the internal or external iliac artery
   - Ovarian cysts

10. **What is the cystic abnormality most commonly misdiagnosed as urinary bladder diverticula in male patients and how can the two be differentiated?**
    Müllerian duct cysts are midline embryologic remnants located within the cranial portion of the prostate. They range in size from 1–3 cm, although they can occasionally be larger.

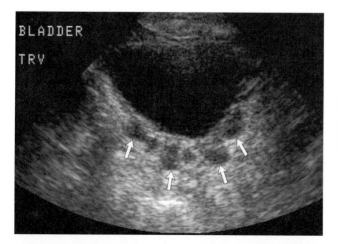

FIGURE 2. Bladder diverticuli. Ultrasound shows multiple hypoechoic structures projecting outward through the bladder wall (*arrows*).

Unlike bladder diverticula, müllerian duct cysts do not empty postvoid and do not fill with contrast on intravenous urography (IVU).

11. What are the two forms of neurogenic bladder and their ultrasound characteristics?
- Neurogenic bladder due to lower motor neuron disease is typically a thin-walled, large capacity bladder, without upper urinary tract dilatation.
- Neurogenic bladder due to upper motor neuron disease is typically a thick-walled bladder with trabeculation, often associated with upper urinary tract dilatation (Fig. 3).

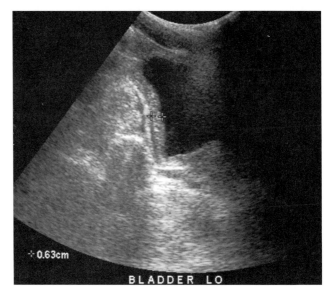

FIGURE 3. Thick-walled bladder (*cursors*) in a patient with a history of spina bifida. Findings are consistent with neurogenic bladder due to upper motor neuron disease.

12. How does a thick-walled neurogenic bladder differ from cystitis?
A thick-walled neurogenic bladder appears moderately to markedly distended with a markedly thickened wall with trabeculations. Cystitis is also characterized by diffuse wall thickening but without trabeculae or diverticula. The latter are a result of muscle hypertrophy, whereas the wall thickening in cystitis is due to edema.

13. What are the potential complications in patients with neurogenic bladders?
These include recurrent infections, stone formation, diverticula (which further predispose to both stones and infections caused by urine stasis), and hydronephrosis caused by ureteral obstruction or reflux.

14. What further imaging examinations should be recommended to evaluate focal lesions and why?
Cystoscopy and, if negative, computed tomography (CT) or magnetic resonance imaging (MRI) could be used to evaluate the soft tissue characteristics. MRI is diagnostic for endometriosis with high signal intensity on fat-suppressed T_2-weighted imaging.

15. A 60-year-old man was found to have a soft tissue mass projecting into the bladder on ultrasound. What are the possible differential diagnoses?
- Prostate mass. Epicenter of mass should be in the prostate (Fig. 4).
- Bladder wall tumor. Check for vascularity to differentiate from hematoma or abscess.
- Hematoma. The lesion should be avascular buy may be hypoechoic to hyperechoic in echogenicity.

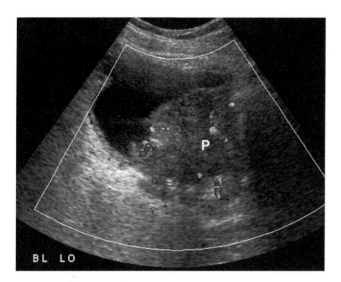

FIGURE 4. Prostate cancer (*P*). The mass has a hypoechoic appearance, projects into the bladder, and simulates denovo bladder tumor.

- Focal cystitis. This is rare. When it occurs it is often due to infections. Other causes include:
  - Malakoplakia (a chronic granulomatous disease characterized by Michaelis-Gutmann bodies) seen more commonly in immunosuppressed patients
  - Cyclophosphamide cystitis, usually presents as an nonglomerular hemorrhage, which may be complicated by transitional cell carcinoma in the long term
  - Cytitis glandularis (glandular transformation of Brunn's nests from chronic inflammation)
  - Schistosomiasis

16. What are the common bladder tumors and what are their typical appearances on ultrasound?
- Transitional cell carcinoma (3:1 male-to-female ratio) may be polypoid, fungating, sessile, or, less likely, diffuse. Tissue is hypoechoic and may demonstrate flow on color or power Doppler (Fig. 5).

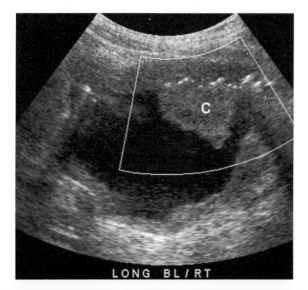

FIGURE 5. Bladder carcinoma (*C*). Ultrasound shows an antidependent hypoechoic mass that demonstrates flow on color Doppler. The presence of flow differentiates tumors from clot.

- Squamous cell carcinoma tends to be hypoechoic, large, solid, and infiltrative.
- Adenocarcinoma is rare ($< 1\%$) but should be suspected if there is a mass at the dome adjacent to a patent urachus or within an urachal diverticulum.
- Metastases to the bladder are not common.

17. What are the common metastases to the bladder?
In order of decreasing likelihood these are:
- Malignant melanoma
- Lung carcinoma
- Gastric carcinoma
- Breast carcinoma

18. What is the most common etiology of extravesical tumor invasion into the bladder?
- Uterine cancer in women
- Prostate cancer in men

19. A 20-year-old patient with human immunodeficiency virus (HIV) infection is found to have a rounded soft tissue mass, non-shadowing, with intermediate echogenicity in his urinary bladder. What is the likely diagnosis and which other organs should be evaluated?
Fungal ball is the most likely cause. In this patient, the kidneys should also be evaluated because the renal pelvis is a more common site for fungal balls.
Fungal balls may also occur in diabetic patients.

20. A well-defined mass of intermediate echogenicity is found within the bladder wall of a (middle aged) 50-year-old woman. What is the most likely diagnosis?
Leiomyoma.

21. What are the causes of focal bladder wall thickening?
Common causes include cystitis (including those caused by indwelling catheter), Crohn's disease (may lead to fistula formation), and endometriosis. Pelvic malignancies (metastasis or local tumors) also may invade the bladder locally. Benign tumors such as leiomyomas may occur in the bladder wall. A focal mass could also be caused by a tumor of the urachus (if at bladder dome).

22. What is considered a normal postvoid residual volume for adult patients on ultrasound and what factors may influence the postvoid volume?
A volume of 100 ml is considered normal if the period between voiding and postvoid ultrasound is not more than 5 minutes. Postvoid residual volume is influenced by a number of factors:
- The time interval between voiding and imaging
- Underlying illnesses such as diabetes
- Medications such as diuretics
- Whether the patient strained on voiding
- The setting of the examination

23. What are some of the factors that predispose to elevated postvoid residual volumes?
- Bladder outlet obstruction. Causes include benign prostatic hypertrophy, urethral strictures, urethral stone, and chronic fecal impaction.
- Neurogenic bladder. Causes include diabetes mellitus and spinal cord injury.
- Medications including anticholinergics and diuretics.

24. How is postvoid residual volume (PVR) calculated and what is the significance of a PVR of 200 ml in an elderly patient?
The "prolate ellipsoid method: **(length × width × height × 0.52)** gives an estimate of prevoid or postvoid volume.

A large postvoid residual volume (as above) is associated with an increased risk of:
- Stone formation
- Infections
- Hydronephrosis
- Overflow incontinence

25. What is the most common cause of a small volume bladder with associated wall thickening?

Tuberculosis is most common. In middle-aged women, a possible cause is interstitial cystitis, a disease of unknown etiology but which has been found to be associated with systemic diseases including rheumatoid arthritis and systemic lupus erythematosus. Patients typically present with symptoms of irritation during voiding.

26. What is the appearance of intravesical air on ultrasound and what are the causes of intravesical air?

Antidependent hyperechoic foci with ring down is the appearance of intravesical air, which is caused by:
- Instrumentation: Foley catheter and stent placement, cystoscopy, and ureteroscopy
- Fistulas: vesicovaginal, vesicouterine, vesicoenteric, and vesicocutaneous
- Emphysematous cystitis due to gram-negative organisms (usually *Escherichia coli*) seen in diabetics

27. What is the most likely cause of diffuse bladder wall calcification in a patient with hematuria and what are the possible long-term complications of the underlying disease?

The most likely cause worldwide is schistosomiasis. The long-term complications include transitional cell carcinoma and ureteral obstruction with subsequent hydronephrosis. In the United States, chronic calcific cystitis is a result of chronic infection.

28. What is the utility of Doppler ultrasound in the evaluation of urinary bladder?

Doppler is most commonly used to assess ureteral jets. Because Doppler is based on the principle of fluid motion, the presence of a strong Doppler jet excludes total ureteric obstruction; however, it does not exclude partial obstruction. Asymmetry may be useful to confirm obstruction, that is, an absent jet on the symptomatic side is strong evidence for obstruction (Fig. 6).

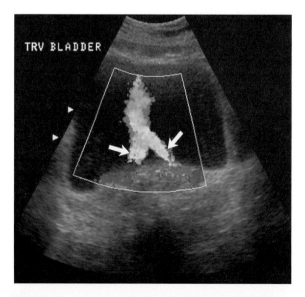

FIGURE 6. Transverse image of the normal bladder shows simultaneous right and left bladder jets (*arrows*) at the trigone (see also Color Plates, Figure 6).

29. What are other indications for Doppler ultrasound in the bladder?

Doppler may also be used to differentiate between tumors and clots. Tumors may exhibit flow while clots do not (except when there is active bleeding). The absence of flow in a bladder mass, however, does not exclude tumor. Remember that tumors may bleed and form clots that may then obscure the tumors, especially if the tumors are small.

30. What is the utility of ultrasound in the assessment of bladder injury?

The utility of ultrasound in this case is very low and may detract from time and effort. CT is the modality of choice or, if unavailable, cystogram is used to assess for bladder rupture.

31. How does one look for bladder jets?

To look for bladder jets, first image the bladder in a transverse plane, making sure the base of the bladder is included in the image. In real time, turn on the color Doppler so the color box is over the entire base of the bladder and make sure the setting is set for slow flow (low wall filter, low scale, and color gain just below the point of seeing noise.) The jets appear as bursts of color across the base of the bladder. Keep watching until jets are seen from both the right and left sides of the bladder (*see* Fig. 6).

32. How long should one persist in looking for bladder jets?

If 5–8 minutes have elapsed and jets from only one side have appeared, chances are the other side is obstructed. Usually 10 minutes is long enough.

33. What is the typical ultrasound appearance of an ureterocele?

A ureterocele appears as a well-defined, thin-walled hypoechoic mass. It may be confused with a diverticulum. Ureteroceles are invariably located inferolaterally where the ureters enter the bladder (Fig. 7).

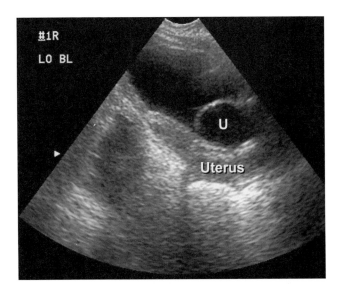

FIGURE 7. Ureterocele. Bladder ultrasound shows an inferolateral extravesical cystic lesion (*U*) bulging into the bladder.

34. What is the typical ultrasound appearance of a bladder stone?

A bladder stone appears as a well defined (sometimes mobile) mass. It may demonstrate posterior acoustic shadowing and twinkle artifacts (Fig. 8).

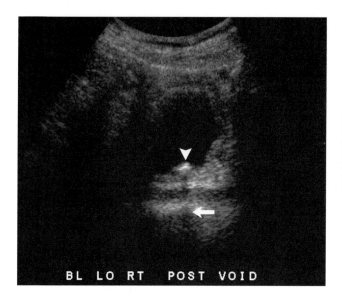

FIGURE 8. Bladder calculus. Image of the bladder shows an echogenic intraluminal mass (*arrowhead*). The mass demonstrates posterior acoustic shadowing (*arrow*) and was mobile.

35. What is the significance of bladder calculi?

Bladder calculi predispose patients to infection, which in turn promotes the formation of more calculi. Bladder calculi may cause bladder outlet obstruction or urethral obstruction. The presence of calculi may signify the presence of other diseases including inflammatory bowel disease, primary gout, and myeloproliferative diseases.

BIBLIOGRAPHY

1. Cooperberg MR, Chambers SK, Rutherford TJ, Foster HE Jr: Cystic pelvic pathology presenting as falsely elevated postvoid residual urine measured by portable ultrasound bladder scanning: Report of three cases and review of the literature. Urology 55:590, 2000.
2. Heiken JP, Forman HP, Brown JJ: Neoplasm of the bladder, prostate, and testis. Radiol Clin N Am 32:81–98, 1994.
3. Matsuda T, Saitoh M: Detection of ureteric jet phenomenon using Doppler color flow mapping. Int J Urol 2:232–234, 1995.
4. Singer AJ, Durinzi KL. Importance of a filled bladder for the detection of intravesical pathology. Urology 56:506–507, 2000.
5. Sulman A, Goldman H: Malakoplakia presenting as a large bladder mass. Urology 60:163, 2002.

19. THE SPLEEN

Dean A. Nakamoto, M.D.

1. What are the indications for splenic ultrasound?
The spleen is usually scanned as part of the left upper quadrant examination as a window to the pancreatic tail and the left kidney. Specific indications for splenic ultrasound include left upper quadrant pain, enlarged spleen at physical examination, or suspected splenic infection (usually in immunocompromised hosts).

2. When is the spleen used as an acoustic window?
Splenic scanning is useful as a window to the left upper quadrant for visualization of the pancreatic tail, the left adrenal, the fundus of the stomach, and the upper pole of the left kidney.

3. What transducer is used to examine the spleen?
A transducer with the same frequency as that used for the liver (3–5 MHz). Intercostals sector scanner is preferred.

4. How is the patient scanned?
The spleen is posterior, so the right lateral decubitus position works best, with the patient's arms overhead and the transducer placed posterior to the mid axillary line, intercostally, in breath-hold on inspiration.
Tip: If lung obscures the spleen, try scanning in expiration instead of inspiration.

5. What images should be acquired?
• Transverse through the upper pole, hilum, and lower pole
• Longitudinal (coronal) through the hilum, with real-time examination scanning anteriorly and posteriorly
Tip: Scanning is best with the patient in the left lateral decubitus (LLD) position. The anterosuperior (AP) window is usually obscured by stomach gas unless the spleen is enlarged enough to displace the stomach medially.

6. What is normal echogenicity?
The spleen normally appears medium gray (fine echoes), slightly smaller than the liver, and more echogenic than the kidney. If kidney echogenicity is greater than that of the spleen, then kidney is abnormal.

7. What are the causes of splenomegaly?
• Causes of mild to moderate splenomegaly: portal hypertension, infection, acquired immunodeficiency syndrome (AIDS)
• Causes of marked splenomegaly: leukemia, lymphoma, myelofibrosis

8. How does one determine splenomegaly?
Typically, the spleen is less than 13 cm in maximum length. For borderline cases, measurements of 12 cm in length, 7 cm in AP diameter, and 5 cm in transverse diameter can be used.

9. What are the primary neoplasms of the spleen?
The benign neoplasms are hemangioma, hamartoma, and lymphangioma. The malignant neoplasms are lymphoma and angiosarcoma. Metastases, although rare, do occur as well.

10. What is the most common benign neoplasm of the spleen?

Although rare, hemangioma is considered the most common primary neoplasm of the spleen. The incidence ranges from 0.3% to 14%. Typically the patient is asymptomatic; however, 25% of splenic hemangiomas may rupture or cause symptoms of hypersplenism.

11. What is the sonographic appearance of hemangioma?

Splenic hemangiomas can have variable appearances. They may be well-defined, echogenic lesions. However, they may also have small anechoic foci and can appear as complex mixed solid and cystic lesions. The lesions are usually small, but can be as large as 17 cm (Fig. 1).

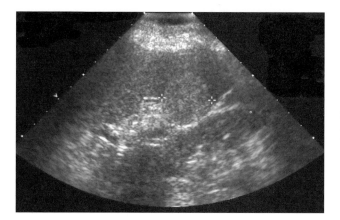

FIGURE 1. Splenic hemangioma. This is the typical appearance of a splenic hemangioma (*cursors*). It is well defined and hyperechoic.

12. Are there any syndromes associated with splenic hemangioma?

Kasabach-Merritt syndrome (anemia, thrombocytopenia, and coagulopathy) has been reported with large hemangiomas. When splenic hemangiomas are multiple, the patient may have generalized angiomatosis (Klippel-Trénaunay-Weber syndrome). If the entire organ is replaced by hemangiomas, it is called hemangiomatosis.

13. How does one confirm the diagnosis of splenic hemangioma?

Splenic hemangiomas appear similar to liver hemangiomas. On computed tomography (CT) they are low in attenuation and demonstrate peripheral enhancement. On magnetic resonance imaging (MRI), they are typically low in signal on T_1-weighted images and increased in signal relative to normal spleen on T_2-weighted images. They demonstrate progressive enhancement following intravenous gadolinium and retain contrast on the delayed images. On technetium-99m tagged red cell study, they usually take up pharmaceutical.

14. What are the non-neoplastic cystic lesions of the spleen.

There are three main types of non-neoplastic cystic lesions of the spleen: congenital epithelial cysts, post-traumatic pseudocysts, and hydatid cysts. Splenic abscesses and infarcts may appear cystic. Pancreatic pseudocysts may also extend into the spleen.

15. What are epithelial cysts?

The epithelial (also called epidermoid, mesothelial, or primary) cysts are congenital in origin and are true cysts with an epithelial lining. They are usually unilocular and solitary, but they may be multiple.

16. What are post-traumatic pseudocysts?

Post-traumatic pseudocysts are thought to represent the end stage of splenic hematomas. They do not have an epithelial lining and are therefore called pseudocysts (Fig. 2). Although they

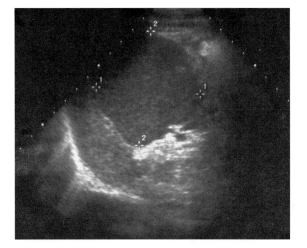

FIGURE 2. Hemorrhagic cyst of the spleen. This well-defined lesion with echogenic debris (*within calipers*) was a hemorrhagic splenic cyst and presumably represents a post-traumatic pseudocyst.

are presumed to be post-traumatic, a history of previous trauma is present in one fourth to one half of the cases; however, the trauma may have been in the distant past and not recalled. Post-traumatic pseudocysts are more likely to have peripheral curvilinear calcification than epithelial cysts. Post-traumatic pseudocysts are the most common splenic cystic lesions in the United States.

17. What are hydatid cysts?

Hydatid disease of the spleen is uncommon and occurs in less than 2% of all patients with *Echinococcus* infection. On ultrasound, the lesions have a variable appearance. They may be anechoic with daughter lesions and calcifications; however, they can also appear solid with fine internal echoes from hydatid sand.

18. What is the most common malignant neoplasm of the spleen?

Lymphoma is the most common malignancy of the spleen. Splenic lymphoma can be primary, which accounts for up to 2% of all lymphomas, or secondary as part of diffuse systemic involvement. The spleen is involved in 25–33% of patients with Hodgkin's or non-Hodgkin's lymphoma.

19. How does splenic lymphoma appear on imaging?

The imaging appearance of the splenic lymphoma is determined by the four gross pathologic patterns of splenic lymphoma:
1. Homogeneous enlargement without discrete mass
2. Miliary nodules < 5 mm in size
3. Multifocal masses of various sizes from 1 to 10 cm
4. Solitary mass

The most common imaging finding is splenomegaly, although splenomegaly may be absent in one third of the patients. When focal lesions are visualized by ultrasound, they can appear similar to cysts and be hypoechoic and almost anechoic. There may even be through transmission, but the amount of through transmission is less than what would be expected for a cyst. Even if hypoechoic, they often are perfused on color or power Doppler imaging.

20. Does splenomegaly in a patient with lymphoma always indicate splenic lymphoma?

No. Up to 30% of enlarged spleens in lymphoma patients are benign in origin.

21. What is an angiosarcoma of the spleen?

Angiosarcoma of the spleen as a primary tumor is rare. Hepatic angiosarcomas may be associated with toxic exposure (vinyl chloride, arsenic); primary splenic angiosarcoma may not have this association.

22. Which primary neoplasms metastasize to the spleen?

Splenic metastases are relatively rare and occur in approximately 7% of patients with malignancy at autopsy. The common sites of primary tumor are breast, lung, ovary, stomach, melanoma, and prostate. Most of these are likely due to hematogenous spread. Although melanoma is not the most common source of splenic metastases, it has the highest frequency of metastasis to the spleen. Up to 36% of melanomas metastasize to the spleen. The most common metastasis to spleen is from lung carcinoma.

23. Which primary neoplasms can cause cystic splenic metastasis?

Cystic metastasis can be seen with melanoma, ovary, breast, and endometrial carcinoma.

24. Which primary neoplasms can cause hyperechoic splenic metastasis?

Hyperechoic metastases are rare, but can be seen with plasmacytoma, hepatocellular carcinoma, melanoma, and prostate and ovarian carcinoma.

25. What are the different mechanisms of infection of the spleen?

- Metastatic or embolic infection (e.g., subacute bacterial endocarditis, sepsis)
- Contiguous infection (e.g., perinephric abscess, infected pancreas)
- Immunodeficiency states
- Trauma
- Embolic noninfectious events causing ischemia and subsequent infection

The abscesses may be bacterial, fungal or mycobacterial in origin. Although splenic abscesses are considered uncommon, they have become more frequent due to an increasing number of immunosuppressed patients, such as those patients with leukemia who receive aggressive chemotherapy and bone marrow transplants, and those patients with human immunodeficiency and AIDS.

26. Describe the sonographic appearances of bacterial splenic abscesses.

Splenic abscesses are usually solitary but may be multiple. Initially, they may appear as an ill-defined low echogenicity mass. They may subsequently form septations, debris, and thick walls. Most splenic abscesses do not contain air. Although ultrasound is useful for screening, contrast-enhanced CT is the imaging modality of choice.

27. What are the features of fungal abscesses?

Fungal microabscesses are usually 5–10 mm in size, although they can be up to 2 cm. The liver and spleen are usually both involved. They can be difficult to visualize by ultrasound. When visualized, fungal microabscesses may have a central echogenic nidus surrounded by hypoechoic circles, causing "bull's-eye lesions" (Fig. 3). If there is necrosis within the central echogenic

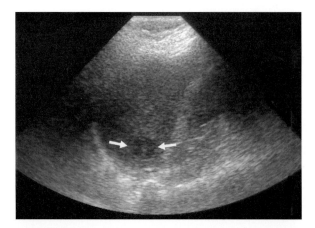

FIGURE 3. Fungal abscess with bull's-eye appearance. This bull's-eye lesion occurred in a neutropenic patient with acute lymphocytic leukemia (*arrows*). Note the central echogenicity. Lesions were also noted in the liver.

nidus, a hypoechoic focus can develop causing a "wheel-within-a-wheel" appearance. MRI is probably the best way to detect and characterize fungal microabscesses.

28. What types of splenic abnormalities can be seen in AIDS patients?

The most common finding is splenomegaly, which is usually moderate. Focal lesions may be due to opportunistic infections such as with *Candida, Pneumocystis,* or mycobacteria. These can present as foci of low echogenicity, target lesions, or small calcifications. Peliosis due to bacillary angiomatosis can occur. Neoplastic lesions such as Kaposi's sarcoma and lymphoma can also be seen.

29. What is the appearance of splenic infarcts?

Splenic infarcts are a common cause of focal splenic lesion. The typical sonographic appearance is a peripheral, wedge-shaped, hypoechoic lesion. In the later stages, they can be hyperechoic due to fibrosis. Contrast-enhanced CT best delineates the areas of splenic infarct (Fig. 4). The lack of mass effect can help differentiate an infarct from a splenic abscess or neoplasm such as lymphoma. In leukemia and lymphoma, splenic infarcts are often round and central, and may mimic neoplasm or abscess. Atypical infarcts can have cystic appearance on ultrasound (Fig. 5)

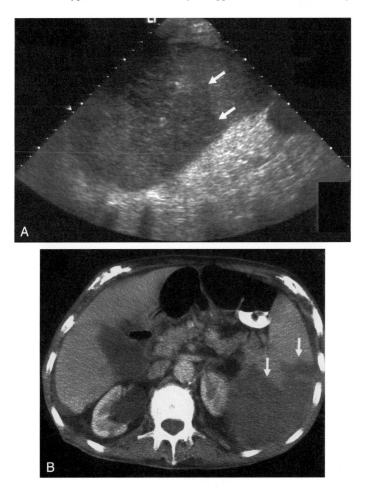

FIGURE 4. Splenic infarct. *A,* This is the typical appearance of a splenic infarct (*arrows*) involving the upper pole. It is hypoechoic relative to the noninfarcted spleen. Note the geographic margins. *B,* Corresponding computed tomography scan.

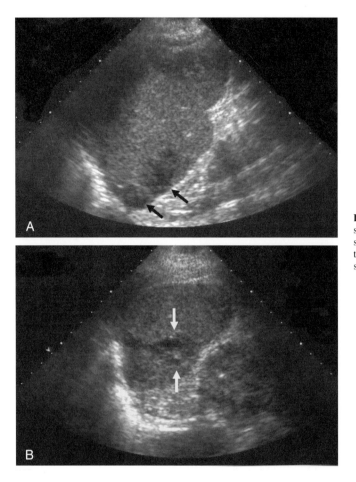

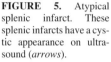

FIGURE 5. Atypical splenic infarct. These splenic infarcts have a cystic appearance on ultrasound (*arrows*).

30. What are the common causes of splenic infarct?

In younger patients, splenic infarcts may occur from local thrombosis due to hematologic diseases, such as the various sickle hemoglobinopathies. In elderly patients, splenic infarcts are most commonly due to embolic events from cardiovascular diseases. Other causes include myeloproliferative disorders, splenic artery aneurysm, pancreatitis, splenic torsion, and portal hypertension.

31. What are the potential complications of splenic infarct?

Complications may be seen in up to 20% of splenic infarcts. These include abscess, pseudocyst formation, and hemorrhage.

32. What is the role of ultrasound in blunt splenic trauma?

The spleen is the most frequently injured solid abdominal organ. In general, contrast-enhanced CT is the modality of choice to image patients with trauma. However, in many trauma centers, there is a role for ultrasound in the acute care of the unstable post-trauma patient. Such patients are evaluated with the Focused Assessment with Sonography for Trauma (FAST) technique. This technique is used in the resuscitation area and evaluates for intraperitoneal fluid or tamponade.

Perisplenic, subcapsular hematomas and parenchymal lacerations can be seen sonographically. Hematomas appear hyperechoic immediately after trauma. However, once the blood clots and for the subsequent 24–48 hours, the hematomas may be similar in echogenicity with the normal parenchyma. Patients with known splenic injury can be followed up with ultrasound.

Tip: A transverse left lobe of the liver in the left upper quadrant may overlap the spleen and mimic a perisplenic hematoma. Turn on Doppler to see normal hepatic vasculature.

33. What important sequelae of trauma can be identified by ultrasound?

Post-traumatic pseudoaneurysms of the spleen may result from non-operative management of splenic lacerations or with spleen salvaging surgery.

34. How are pseudoaneurysms identified?

On grayscale imaging, a cystic space is observed. On color Doppler, color fills the space and spectral Doppler shows the characteristic to and from flow through the aneurysm neck.

35. What is the significance of a splenic pseudoaneurysm?

These may expand and cause delayed splenic rupture with a risk of 6–10%.

36. How are splenic pseudoaneurysms treated?

Rarely, these resolve spontaneously. Usually, catheter embolization is performed, with a reported 77% success rate. If embolization fails, open repair is an option.

37. What are some unusual locations of accessory spleens?

Accessory spleens are typically located at the splenic hilum. They can occur almost anywhere in the abdomen. They are usually on the left and above the renal pedicle. They have been described in paratesticular, diaphragmatic, gastric, and pararenal sites. Confirmation of splenic tissue can be obtained with technetium-labeled, heat-damaged red blood cells. They are usually solitary, although they can be multiple. When multiple, they tend to be clustered in a single location.

38. What is the differential diagnosis of multiple spleens?

The main differential considerations are polysplenia, post-traumatic splenosis, and multiple accessory spleens.

39. What is the difference between polysplenia and asplenia?

Polysplenia and asplenia are two of the major congenital splenic anomalies. These conditions are part of the spectrum of visceral heterotaxy. Patients with polysplenia may have bilateral left-sidedness, or a dominance of left-sided over right-sided body structures. Polysplenia patients may have two morphologic left lungs, left-sided azygous continuation of an interrupted inferior vena cava, biliary atresia, absence of the gallbladder, gastrointestinal malrotation, and cardiovascular abnormalities.

Asplenia patients may have bilateral right-sidedness. They may have two morphologic right lungs, reversed position of the abdominal aorta and inferior vena cava, anomalous pulmonary venous return, and horseshoe kidneys.

40. What are the indications for splenic biopsy?

- Diagnosis of infections, especially in the immunocompromised population, including tuberculosis and infection with *Candida* and *Pneumocystis carinii*
- Biopsy of a focal solid mass, usually lymphoma or metastasis
- Aspiration of a fluid collection for diagnosis of infection

41. What complications are encountered?

The major complication risk is bleeding, which occurs in up to 10% of patients. As many as 8% of patients have major bleeding requiring splenectomy. Bleeding may be a delayed complication, occurring hours to days after the biopsy. Risk factors for bleeding include coagulopathy, low platelet count, and peripherally located lesions. When investigating metastatic disease, it is still deemed safer to biopsy sites other than the spleen, because the splenic risk of bleeding complications exceeds that of most other sites.

42. Does the needle size relate to biopsy success or bleeding risk?

No. Commonly used needles include 20–23 gauge for fine needle aspiration and 18–20 gauge core needles, with biopsy accuracy of 85–90% for most series, independent of needle size. Similarly, the bleeding risk seems to be equivalent, independent of needle size.

BIBLIOGRAPHY

1. Civardi G, Vallisa D, Berte R, et al: Ultrasound-guided fine needle biopsy of the spleen: High clinical efficiency and low risk in a multicenter Italian study. Am J Hematol 67:93–99, 2001.
2. Dachman AH, Friedman AC: Radiology of the spleen. St. Louis, Mosby, 1993.
3. Fitoz S, Atasoy C, Dusunceli E, et al: Post-traumatic intrasplenic pseudoaneurysms with delayed rupture: Color Doppler sonographic and CT findings. J Clin Ultrasound 29:102–104, 2001.
4. Franquet T, Montes M, Lecumberri FJ, et al: Hydatid disease of the spleen: Imaging findings in nine patients. Am J Roentgenol 154:525–528, 1990.
5. Mathieson JR, Cooperberg PL: The spleen. In Rumack CM, Wilson SR, Charboneau JW (eds): Diagnostic Ultrasound, 2nd ed. St. Louis, Mosby, 1998.
6. Nakamoto DA, Onders RP: The spleen. In Haaga JR, Lanzieri CF (eds): Computed Tomography and Magnetic Resonance Imaging of the Whole Body, 4th ed. St. Louis, Mosby, 2003.

20. THE PANCREAS

Deborah J. Rubens, M.D.

1. What are the indications for pancreatic ultrasound?

Pancreatic ultrasound is used to identify tumors or masses within the pancreas, usually for biopsy or to identify the complications of pancreatitis (peripancreatic fluid collections or pseudocysts for follow-up or for drainage) and to stage pancreatic carcinoma.

2. What transducer is used to examine the pancreas?

Examination is done with a transducer with the highest frequency possible with a curved linear array or sector probe with a 3.5–7 MHz center frequency. Harmonics are used to detect cysts and calcifications.

3. What planes are scanned?

- Transverse: Head (including uncinate), body, and tail. This may require several sweeps to accommodate the length of the pancreas and the common location of the head caudal to the body and tail.
- Longitudinal: Sagittal images of the head should include the common duct and superior mesenteric artery (SMA) and superior mesenteric vein (SMV).

4. What is optimal positioning for scanning the pancreas?

- Start supine and then use other positions as needed. *Tip:* Start at beginning of ultrasound examination, before patient swallows too much air with breathholding
- Left lateral decubitus (LLD): For tail (gas rises to stomach antrum), scan transverse in left upper quadrant (LUQ) with compression.
- Right lateral decubitus (RLD): Use spleen as window for tail. Fluid in stomach enters antrum and duodenum, and the head is better visualized.
- Semierect: Left lobe of liver displaces bowel and is useful as window to head and body.

5. What preparation is needed for examination of the pancreas?

- Patient should have nothing by mouth (NPO) to diminish bowel gas.
- To displace stomach and duodenal gas, patient should drink 1–2 glasses of water through a straw. (A straw is used so gas is not swallowed.)
- The patient is positioned semierect and in the right posterior oblique (RPO) position to have water filling the antrum and duodenum, displacing gas.

6. Are there any oral contrast agents available to help visualize the pancreas better?

Sonorex, a cimethacone compound, has been approved by the Food and Drug Administration (FDA) as an oral contrast agent. It works by decreasing gas bubble size and diminishes the reflectivity of the air bubbles. The head and tail are frequently better visualized. However, displace enough gas to image the head, and the splenic window may be adequate to image the tail.

7. What are the normal anatomic components of the pancreas and their size?

- Head: 2–3 cm anteroposterior (the most caudal and to the patient's right).
- Body: 2 cm anteroposterior
- Tail: 3 cm anteroposterior
- Duct: Mean dimensions are 3 mm in head, 2 mm in body, and 1.6 mm in tail, with 2.5 mm considered the upper limit of normal.

8. What vascular landmarks are used to find the pancreas?

The normal pancreas (Fig. 1) is bounded by the following vessels:

- SMA is posterior to the body.
- SMV is posterior to the neck.
- Inferior vena cava is posterior to the head.
- Aorta identifies the midline. The left of the aorta is the beginning of the tail.
- Gastroduodenal artery is anterior to the pancreas and identifies the neck.
- Splenic vein is posterior to the body and tail.

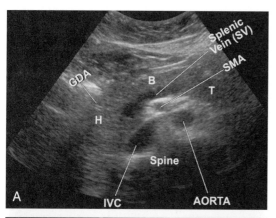

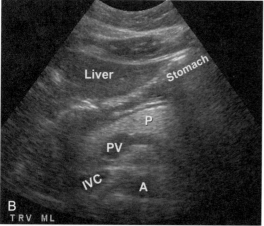

FIGURE 1. Normal pancreas. *A,* Transverse image through the body and head with normal vascular landmarks. Note the low level of homogenous echoes. *B,* Fluid in the stomach improves visualization of the pancreatic body and head. A, aorta; B, body; GDA, gastroduodenal artery; H, head; IVC, inferior vena cava; P, pancreas, PV, portal vein; SMA, superior mesenteric artery.

9. What anatomic structures identify the pancreatic neck?

The neck is directly anterior to the portal venous confluence. The gastroduodenal artery is anterior to the neck on the surface of the pancreas and divides the head and neck.

10. What separates the body from the tail?

The body and tail junction is defined as the left lateral border of the vertebral column.

11. What is the normal echogenicity of the pancreas?

The echogenicity of a normal pancreas should be uniform and slightly higher than the liver. Focal contour abnormality or altered echogenicity are suspicious for mass or tumor.

12. What is the significance of decreased echogenicity of the uncinate?

Decreased echogenicity of the uncinate is a normal variant. This is due to a lower number of interfaces, often with decreased fat because the uncinate (ventral anlage) and the rest of the pancreas have a different composition. This area of decreased echogenicity should have a geographic boundary, and no vascular displacement or mass effect. Diagnosis can be confirmed with computed tomography (CT) or magnetic resonance imaging (MRI). CT may show higher attenuation of this region, because it contains less fat (Fig. 2).

FIGURE 2. Hypoechoic uncinate. Transverse image of the head shows the uncinate (*arrows*) to be hypoechoic compared with the rest of the pancreas. This is a normal variant with no mass effect and should not be mistaken for a tumor or pancreatitis.

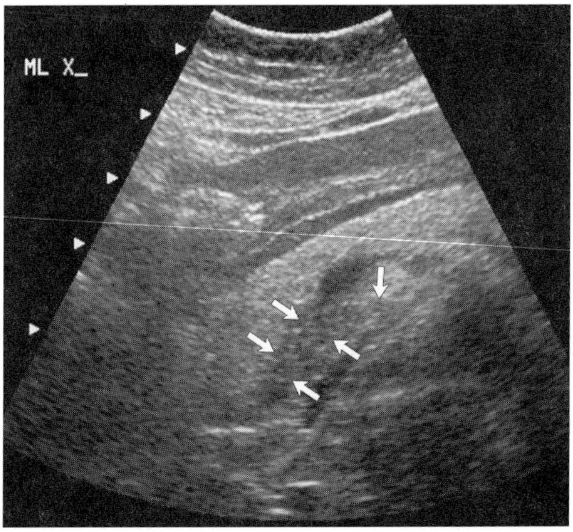

13. What diseases involve the pancreas?

Pancreatitis and tumors (malignant or benign) are most common. Pancreatic cysts are often associated with other disease processes.

14. What are the clinical features of pancreatitis?

Pancreatitis is an inflammatory condition characterized by edema inside and around the pancreas, sometimes accompanied by hemorrhage or necrosis. Pancreatitis can be complicated by pseudocyst formation, peripancreatic fluid collections, and splenic artery or vein thrombosis.

15. Can ultrasound diagnose acute pancreatitis?

Frequently the ultrasound is normal, even when pancreas is abnormal by CT or laboratory values. Ultrasound does not readily detect the edema in the peripancreatic fat. Only discrete fluid collections are seen (i.e., lesser sac, anterior pararenal space, pseudocysts). Signs suggestive of pancreatitis include swelling of the gland and obstruction of the common duct or pancreatic duct. The gallbladder should be evaluated as a potential cause (gallstone pancreatis) (Fig. 3).

16. Does echogenicity help diagnose acute pancreatitis?

No. Pancreatitis may be hypoechoic or echogenic due to edema or even hemorrhage in the tissue. The pancreas with pancreatitis may have normal echogenicity as well.

17. What are pseudocysts and where do they occur?

A pseudocyst is a fluid collection with a nonepithelial wall containing pancreatic enzymes. They occur in 10–20% of patients with pancreatitis, may resolve spontaneously, and occasionally require drainage when infected. Common locations include the pancreas, the lesser sac, and the anterior pararenal space. They also may occur in the spleen, stomach wall, liver, and even the chest (Fig. 4).

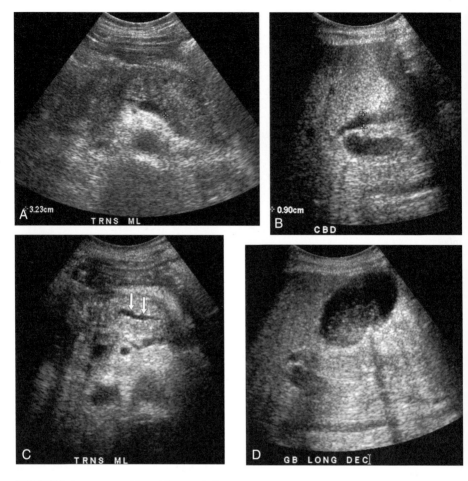

FIGURE 3. Acute pancreatitis. *A,* Ultrasound of acute pancreatitis shows an enlarged body (*cursors*). *B,* The common bile duct is dilated. *C,* The pancreatic duct (*arrows*) is dilated. *D,* The gallbladder is filled with sludge and stones, the potential cause of the pancreatitis.

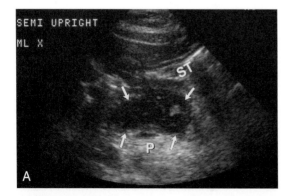

FIGURE 4. Pancreatic pseudocyst in the lesser sac. Transverse (A) (*continued*)

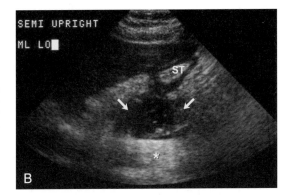

FIGURE 4. (*continued*) and longitudinal (B) images of a typical lesser sac pseudocyst (*arrows*) posterior to the stomach (*ST*). Note the echogenic debris within the collection and posterior acoustic enhancement, which makes the pancreas (*P*) more echogenic.

18. What vascular complications of pancreatitis may be identified with ultrasound?

These include splenic or portal vein thrombosis, splenic artery pseudoaneurysm, and splenic infarcts.

19. What are the diagnostic features of chronic pancreatitis?

Pancreatic calcifications occur in intraductal or periductal locations, often in association with pancreatic duct obstruction and dilation (Fig. 5). A focal hypoechoic mass is found in about 40% of patients (Fig. 6). Pseudocysts are common (25–40% of patients) and tend to persist. Common bile duct dilatation is associated in 5–10% of cases. Pancreas echogenicity is variable, often a mix of hyperechoic and hypoechoic regions due to fibrosis and edema (Fig. 7). Acute exacerbation results in focal enlargement but, overall, chronic pancreatitis results in tissue atrophy.

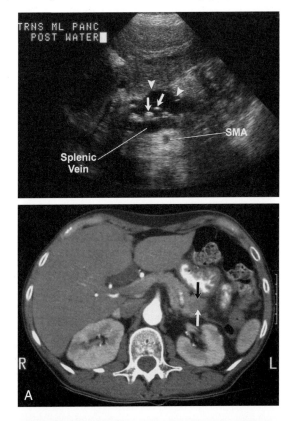

FIGURE 5. Chronic pancreatitis. Note dilated duct (*arrowheads*) with periductal calcifications (*arrows*).

FIGURE 6. Chronic pancreatitis. *A*, Transverse CT shows a hypoechoic mass (*arrows*) in the pancreatic tail. (*continued*)

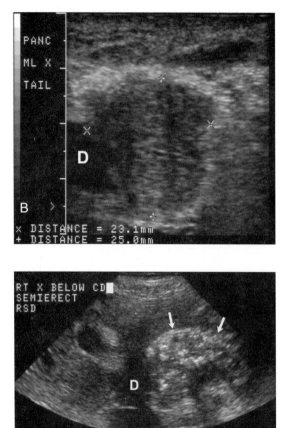

FIGURE 6. (*continued*) *B*, Transverse intraoperative ultrasound shows a hypoechoic mass corresponding to the CT lesion in (*A*). The adjacent pancreatic duct (*D*) terminates abruptly.

FIGURE 7. Chronic pancreatitis. Transverse image through the body and pancreatic head (*arrows*) shows diffuse and heterogeneous increased echoes resulting from calcifications. D, duodenum.

20. What is the goal of ultrasound in pancreatitis?
- To find the etiology of the disease, including gallstones or tumor
- To identify complications: pseudocysts, fluid collections, abscess, splenic arterial, or venous thrombosis.

21. How is a dilated pancreatic duct distinguished from a pancreatic vessel?
Color Doppler or power Doppler can be used if the transducer is perpendicular to the direction of the duct. The duct travels in the center of the pancreas. The splenic vein is on the dorsal border.

22. What is the appearance of a pancreatic tumor on ultrasound?
This is typically a hypoechoic mass that may or may not deform the contour (Fig. 8). It may be in the head (70%), body (15–20%), or tail (5%). Adenocarcinoma is most common, followed by islet cell tumors and cystic pancreatic neoplasms. Secondary signs of pancreatic tumors include an obstructed (dilated) pancreatic duct, adjacent lymphadenopathy, encasement of adjacent vessels, and liver metastases.

23. What is a double duct sign?
This refers to obstruction of the common bile duct and the pancreatic duct. It is caused most commonly by a mass in the head of the pancreas (tumor, chronic pancreatitis) but may also be secondary to ampullary or duodenal tumors.

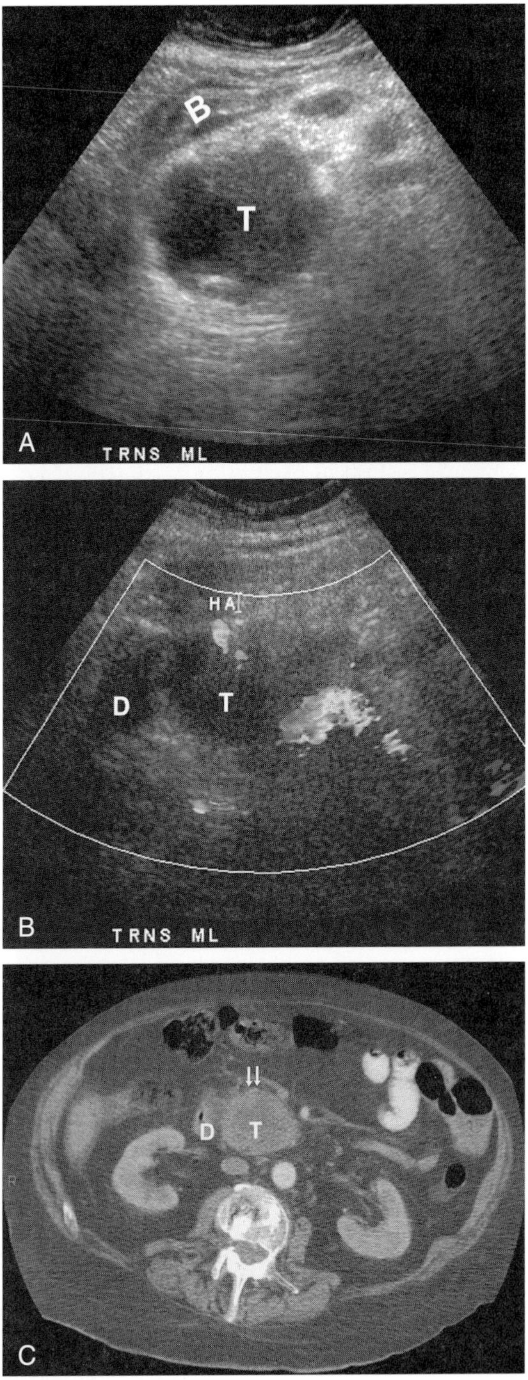

FIGURE 8. Pancreatic cancer. *A*, Transverse midline image of hypoechoic pancreatic cancer (*T*) with bowel (*B*) anteriorly. *B*, Color Doppler image shows encasement of the hepatic artery (*HA*) by the tumor (*T*) (see also Color Plates, Figure 7). D, duodenum. *C*, Corresponding CT image shows HA (*arrows*) at the margin of the tumor (*T*) but not definite encasement. D, duodenum. (*continued*)

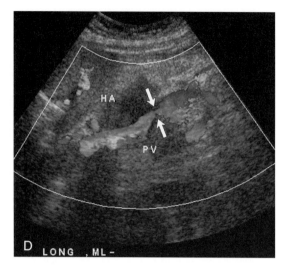

FIGURE 8. (*continued*) *D,* Tumor. Note encasement of portal vein (*arrows*) by tumor (see also Color Plates, Figure 8).

24. What are the islet cell tumors of the pancreas?
These are solid tumors arising from multipotential stem cells in ductal epithelium, the so-called APUD (amine precursor uptake and decarboxylation) system. These tumors produce hormones that may result in clinical symptoms. Tumor types include insulinoma, gastrinoma, glucagonoma, somatostatinoma, vipoma, and adrenocorticotropic hormone (ACTH)-producing tumors. They are often small (< 2 cm) and hypervascular.

25. Which is the most common functioning islet cell tumor?
Insulinoma is most common. It is unusually benign, solitary, and intrapancreatic.

26. What is the significance of nonfunctioning islet cell tumors?
These comprise up to one third of all islet cell tumors and have a high likelihood of malignancy. They often manifest with liver metastases and a large pancreatic mass.

27. What is the typical ultrasound appearance of islet cell tumors?
They may be cystic, solid, or heterogeneous and may contain calcifications. On endoscopic or intraoperative ultrasound, lesions are usually hypoechoic and well circumscribed (Fig. 9).

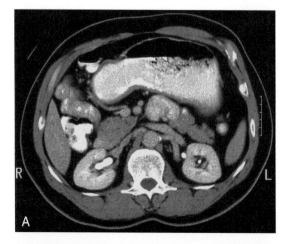

FIGURE 9. Insulinoma in the head of the pancreas. CT (*A*) is normal while intraoperative ultrasound (*continued*)

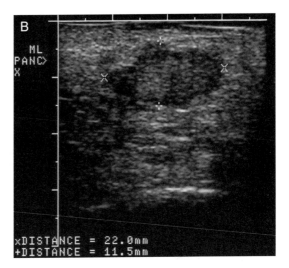

FIGURE 9. (*continued*) (*B*) shows a typical small hypoechoic mass. This mass was nonpalpable and was localized by ultrasound.

28. What is the sensitivity of ultrasound to detect islet cell tumors?

Ultrasound is 20–75% sensitive for insulinoma and only 20–30% sensitive for gastrinoma, because the latter tends to be extrapancreatic and multiple.

29. Which islet cell tumor is associated with the multiple endocrine neoplasia (MEN) type I syndrome?

Gastrinoma is most commonly associated with MEN I (also known as Werner's syndrome), which also includes pituitary hyperplasia and parathyroid adenoma. Insulinomas are less commonly associated. Islet cell tumors in MEN I tend to be multiple and have an increased risk of malignancy.

30. What is the best screening modality for islet cell tumors?

These should be identified chemically and then localized with MRI or with biphasic (arterial phase) thin section multislice CT, looking for enhancing lesions.

31. What is the role of intraoperative or endoscopic ultrasound in detecting islet cell tumors?

Endoscopic ultrasound identifies as many as 80% of lesions, and intraoperative ultrasound has a similar sensitivity. The detection rate of ultrasound combined with palpation approaches 100%. All modalities are limited when lesions are multiple and small.

32. What is Zollinger-Ellison syndrome?

This is classically severe peptic ulcers in multiple locations caused by gastrinoma. However, many patients with gastrinoma present with a solitary ulcer or with diarrhea caused by gastric hypersecretion. The clinical diagnosis is made by a serum gastric level > 1000 ng/ml or a positive secretin test.

33. What masses mimic pancreatic cancers and how can they be distinguished?

Lymph nodes adjacent to the pancreatic head may simulate a pancreatic head mass. Harmonies are used to check texture. Lymph nodes often lack internal echoes, whereas adjacent pancreatic tissue is subtly nodular and displaced. Focal pancreatitis may be a hypoechoic mass and may cause dilatation of the pancreatic duct and common duct when acute. By ultrasound, it cannot be distinguished from a tumor. However, pancreatic cancer often invades the adjacent mesentery, encasing vessels or occluding them. A hypoechoic uncinate process can mimic a tumor. However, it has geographic margins and no mass effect.

34. What cystic pancreatic tumors occur?

Cystic neoplasms are 1% of all pancreatic cancers and are microcystic (serous) adenomas which are benign, or macrocystic (mucinous) cystadenomas or cystadenocarcinomas. Mucinous lesions may be benign or low-grade malignancies, which are difficult to distinguish pathologically. Therefore surgical excision is recommended. Both serous and mucinous types occur in middle-aged patients with a female predominance.

35. What is a solid and papillary epithelial neoplasm?

These are large, well-defined, encapsulated tumors with cystic areas resulting from necrosis and hemorrhage. They typically occur in young women, involve the pancreatic tail, and are locally invasive. Patients have a better prognosis than those with adenocarcinoma because the lesions are less likely to metastasize.

36. How is the pancreas involved in cystic fibrosis?

The pancreas echogenicity increases as the glands atrophy and are replaced by fibrosis or fat. With advanced disease, the pancreas atrophies and is replaced by fat, fibrosis, and small cysts as a result of duct obstruction.

37. How is the pancreas involved in adult polycystic kidney disease (APCKD)?

Pancreatic cysts occur in 10% of patients with APCKD and are usually asymptomatic. The pancreas function is normal.

38. What are the pancreatic manifestations of von Hippel-Lindau syndrome (VHL)?

These include true pancreatic cysts, seen in up to 25% of patients with VHL on ultrasound. They are present in 72% of autopsy results. Other tumors include islet cell tumors, microcystic adenomas, ductal adenocarcinomas, ampullary cell carcinomas, and hemangioblastomas.

BIBLIOGRAPHY

1. Atri M, Finnegan PW: The pancreas. In Rumack CM, Wilson SR, Charboneau JW (eds): Diagnostic Ultrasound, vol 1, 2nd ed. St. Louis, Mosby, 1998, pp 225–277.
2. Buetow PC, Miller DL, Parrino TV, et al: From the archives of the AFIP. Islet cell tumors of the pancreas: Clinical, radiologic, and pathologic correlation in diagnosis and localization. RSNA Radiographics 17(2):453–472, 1997.
3. Fried AM: Retroperitoneum, pancreas, spleen, and lymph nodes. In McGahan JP, Goldberg BB (eds): Diagnostic Ultrasound: A Logical Approach. Philadelphia, Lippincott-Raven, 1998, pp 761–785.

21. THE PROSTATE GLAND

Deborah J. Rubens, M.D., David Schmanke, RDMS, and Mark A. Hall, B.S., RDMS

1. What are common indications for a prostate ultrasound?
- Elevated prostate-specific antigen (PSA)/prostate cancer detection
- Prebrachytherapy volume assessment
- Guidance of brachytherapy
- Tumor, palpable mass, enlarged prostate on physical examination
- To direct prostate biopsy
- Infertility, looking for ejaculatory duct obstruction or cysts
- Hematospermia, looking for calculi
- Abscess, prostatitis, infection
- Urinary hesitancy

2. What are the common imaging methods for prostate ultrasound?
These include transabdominal, transperineal, and transrectal ultrasound. Transabdominal scanning uses a 3–5 MHz transducer through a partially filled urinary bladder with caudal angulation to send the ultrasound beam under the pubic arch. This permits global sizing of the gland. Transperineal prostate ultrasound is performed with similar equipment from the perineum in patients who lack a rectum or who cannot tolerate transrectal ultrasound, usually to provide biopsy guidance. The best prostate ultrasound imaging is via the transrectal approach.

3. What transducer is used for transrectal prostate ultrasound?
An end-firing intracavity probe transducer of ≥ 7.5 MHz or a dedicated side-firing transducer is placed into the rectum. The prostate is imaged in axial and coronal planes. Two side-firing transducers can be combined in one probe (biplane) to image the axial and sagittal planes.

4. Is there an advantage to one transrectal transducer over the other?
- Side-firing linear arrays may limit the field of view in the sagittal plane.
- Axial curved linear arrays or endocavity linear arrays have a small footprint, which may limit the transverse field of view in the near field.
- An endocavity probe can be used for both transrectal and transvaginal scanning.
- Biplane transducers offer electronic switching of scan planes without having to rotate, remove, or insert a probe.

5. Are there disadvantages to these probes?
High resolution is obtained at the expense of limited penetration and field of view. It may be difficult to penetrate large glands. The option to lower the frequency to 5 MHz is useful. A large gland is often cut off by a limited field of view or a small footprint probe. Using a water-filled balloon as a stand-off helps to place the gland within the image.

6. How is the scan oriented on the monitor?
For sagittal and axial images, the rectum appears at the bottom of the screen. At the top of the screen is the anterior aspect of the patient. On sagittal images, the base of the prostate is on the left side of the screen and the apex to the right.

7. What is the normal anatomy of the prostate?
The following are the three main zones of the prostate:
- The peripheral zone, which is located posterior and lateral and comprises approximately 70–75% of the gland

- The central zone, which comprises 20–25% of the gland
- The transitional zone, which surrounds the urethra anteriorly and comprises about 5% of the gland.

Also included in the prostate anatomy is the capsule, which surrounds the gland, the seminal vesicles, which course laterally and superiorly from the base of the prostate, the prostatic urethra, which extends from the base anteriorly, coursing posteriorly and inferiorly toward and through the apex, and the ejaculatory ducts, which extend from the seminal vesicles through the central zone and join the prostatic urethra near the mid portion of the gland at an area called the *verumontanum* (Fig. 1).

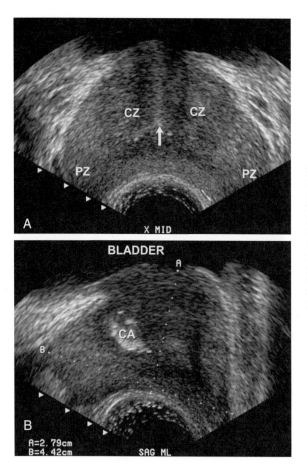

FIGURE 1. *A,* Normal prostate. Normal image of the prostate at the level of the veru montanum (*arrow*). The peripheral zone (*PZ*) is slightly hyperechoic with respect to the central zone (*CZ*). *B,* Normal sagittal image. The prostate anteroposterior dimension (A: 2.8 cm) is measured perpendicular to the long axis of the gland (B: 4.4 cm). Echogenic foci in the central gland represent calcifications (corpora amylacea).

8. **What are the ultrasound features of the prostate zones and the seminal vesicles?**
   - The peripheral zone is isoechoic to the transition zone in young men but becomes relatively hyperechoic in older patients as the transition zone becomes hypoechoic with stromal benign prostatic hyperplasia (BPH).
   - The central zone is echogenic compared to the peripheral zone and is the site of entry for the seminal vesicles, the vas deferens, and the ejaculatory ducts.
   - The transitional zone is of variable echogenicity as it becomes hypoechoic with most cases of BPH. It may contain periurethral calculi.
   - The seminal vesicles are hypoechoic to the gland.
   - The capsule is invisible on ultrasound. It is open at the apex where the urethra exits, at the

base where the seminal vesicles join the prostate, and laterally near the apex where the neurovascular bundles enter. These represent potential avenues for spread of prostatic carcinoma.

9. What are corpora amylacea and where do they occur?
These "white bodies" are calcifications that form in the central zone, presumably due to reflux of urine into the ducts. These may cast acoustic shadows, depending on their density and size (Figs. 1 and 2).

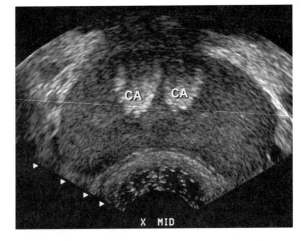

FIGURE 2. Transverse image of a normal prostate with echogenic calcifications in the central gland, the corpora amylacea (CA) or white bodies. In this case, these are dense enough to cause an acoustic shadow anteriorly.

10. What is the function of the seminal vesicles?
These elaborate seminal fluid, which comprises up to 80% of the ejaculate. They also secrete fructose and prostaglandins.

11. What is the normal size of a prostate?
The prostate is about 4 cm wide, 3 cm long, and 2 cm anteroposteriorly. This gives a volume of approximately 12.5 cubic centimeters (cm^3).

12. How is the cubic volume of the prostate calculated?
Cubic volume is determined by taking the height (H) × width (W) × depth (D) × 0.52, which is the formula for a prolate ellipse.

13. How accurate is ultrasound for sizing the prostate volume?
With the ellipse formula of H × W × D × 0.52, there is a ± 20% error rate.
If one uses sequential axial images with the probe fixed in a mechanical stepper and steps through the gland in 0.5-cm sequential slices, and then adds their volumes, the error rate is ± 10%.

14. What is the size of the normal seminal vesicles?
Each seminal vesicle is about 3 cm long and 1.5 cm anteroposteriorly.

15. What steps should be taken to ensure a good scan?
• A good coupling agent inside the cover is essential. Most times gel is sufficient.
• Occasionally using a water-filled standoff permits better assessment of the posterior margin of the gland.

16. What landmarks are used to locate the prostate?
The prostate is an inverted pyramid located behind the inferior arch of the pubic symphysis, anterior to the rectum and posteroinferior to the bladder. The apex, the more caudal portion, lies

on the superior aspect of the urogenital diaphragm. The base is the more cephalad end, is the largest portion, and is adjacent to the bladder. The seminal vesicles are superior to the prostate and posterior to the bladder.

Tip: If it is difficult to visualize the prostate, have the patient fill his bladder and use it as a landmark.

17. Does ultrasound examination of the prostate visualize cancer?

Many cancers are invisible. Visualization ranges from 30–60%. Often, patients with a lesion seen on one side have an invisible tumor on the other.

18. What are the ultrasound features of prostate cancer?

- In the peripheral zone, cancer appears hypoechoic (50% of lesions) (Fig. 3), but often these cancers are isoechoic (20–30%) or even hyperechoic (10–20%). Usually they are found within 0.3 cm of the capsule. Seventy-five to 80% of prostate cancers are in the peripheral zone, 10–20% in the transition zone, and 5–10% in the central zone.

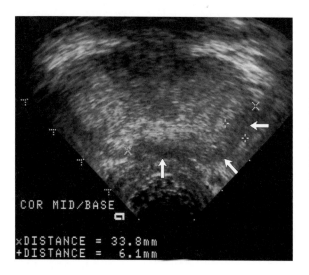

FIGURE 3. Prostate carcinoma. Transverse image of the prostate demonstrates a peripheral hypoechoic lesion (*arrows*) involving the left peripheral zone and extending across the midline. This was prostatic carcinoma on biopsy.

19. What are the Doppler features of prostatic cancer?

In as many as 11% of prostate cancer patients whose grayscale ultrasound results are normal, increased flow is seen on focal color Doppler. However, BPH and prostatitis also have increased vascularity. A negative color Doppler ultrasound should not preclude biopsy, but adding color Doppler ultrasound to prostate biopsy to identify abnormal areas increases biopsy yield.

20. What is the differential diagnosis of hypoechoic prostate lesions?

- Carcinoma
- Benign prostatic hyperplasia (adenomatoid nodule)
- Atrophy
- Prostatitis
- Abscess

21. How is prostate cancer detected?

PSA is produced by the prostate and is detected in the blood. Elevated levels may indicate prostate cancer, but they can also be seen with prostatitis and with benign hyperplasia. Most cancers are detected with a screening serum PSA. Some are still detected on rectal examination.

22. What PSA levels are considered to be abnormal?

Greater than 4 ng/dl is considered abnormal; however, larger glands (e.g., those with BPH) also may result in higher serum PSA levels. Therefore, some clinicians use a ratio known as PSA density. PSA density is determined by dividing the PSA by the volume of the gland. The volume of the gland equals L × W × H × 0.52.

23. How are the results of the PSA density used?

APSA density > 0.12 is considered abnormal and is used as a threshold for prostate biopsy. More aggressive centers use a PSA density of 0.10 as their cutoff.

24. How is prostate biopsy performed?

With the patient in a left lateral decubitus position, a transrectal transducer that supports a biopsy needle is inserted. A minimum of six 18-gauge core biopsies are obtained, one each from the base, midgland, and apex bilaterally, avoiding the urethra. Additional samples are obtained in any focally suspicious lesion (Fig. 4).

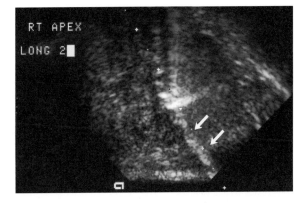

FIGURE 4. Prostate biopsy. Sagittal view shows the echogenic needle following the dotted line guide to a depth of 2 cm within the prostate (*arrows*). At a minimum, biopsies are taken from the base, midgland, and apex bilaterally, with additional samples from any focal suspicious lesions.

25. Is there any preparation needed before a biopsy?

The patient needs antibiotics before and after the biopsy to prevent prostatitis and sepsis. We use ciprofloxacin 500 mg twice a day, two doses before and four doses after the biopsy.

26. What is prostate brachytherapy?

Prostate brachytherapy is surgical implantation of radioactive seeds into the prostate gland using ultrasound guidance. This prostate cancer therapy is designed for patients with nonaggressive cancers that are contained within the prostate.

27. What role does ultrasound play in prostate brachytherapy?

Ultrasound for brachytherapy planning is a controlled sequential scan through the gland to determine the volume and shape of the prostate for the number of seeds and seed distribution. It can also determine whether there is pubic arch interference that limits access to the gland. Similar to planning ultrasound, the transducer is also used intraoperatively in the same controlled, sequential fashion to monitor seed implantation (Fig. 5).

28. What types of cystic lesions occur in the prostate?

- Prostatic utricle cysts: These result from dilatation of the prostate utricle, are small, and extend anteriorly from the veru montanum. They can be associated with unilateral renal agenesis.
- Müllerian duct cysts: These arise from the remnants of the müllerian duct. They may extend lateral to midline and be quite large, frequently extending up to the base of the gland (Fig. 6).

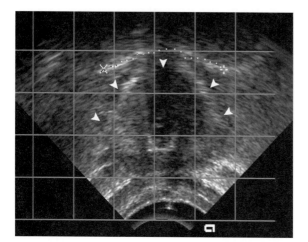

FIGURE 5. Brachytherapy planning. Axial image through the prostate apex. The prostate margins (*arrowheads*) are monitored to ensure there is no overlap with the pubic symphysis, marked with dotted line anteriorly. The lines are used to align the grid through which the needles are passed into the prostate.

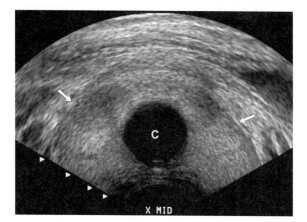

FIGURE 6. Müllerian cyst. Transverse image in the midgland shows a round anechoic midline cyst (*C*). These typically extend to the base of the gland. Arrows demonstrate the prostate margins anteriorly.

- Ejaculatory duct cysts: These are usually small and are due to obstruction of the ejaculatory duct. These cysts are often seen in patients being evaluated for infertility or painful ejaculations. They contain spermatazoa and tend to lateralize more than the other midline cysts.
- Cystic degeneration of adenomas in the transition zone, secondary to prostatic hyperplasia.

29. Do these cysts have the same characteristics as any other type of cyst in the body?

Cysts in the prostate have the same ultrasound characteristics as other cysts (i.e., they are completely anechoic, have good through transmission of the sound beam, and have smooth walls).

30. Does a patient with prostate cysts have any symptoms?

Most patients are asymptomatic. Occasionally a cyst may become infected, resulting in pain and fever.

31. What is the significance of seminal vesicle cysts?

These may be congenital (rare) or acquired and are due to obstruction of the ejaculatory ducts. Congenital cysts are associated with ectopic drainage into the seminal vesicle and unilateral renal agenesis. Acquired cysts are associated with history of infection and often are accompanied by stone formation

32. What is prostatitis?
Prostatitis is the inflammation of the prostate with or without signs of infection. It may be acute or chronic.

33. What are the symptoms of acute prostatitis?
- Urinary frequency
- Dysuria
- Burning or pain while urinating
- Fever and chills
- Lower abdominal, groin, back, and flank pain
- Pain around the anus

34. What is the primary symptom of chronic prostatitis?
Repeated bladder infections.

35. What are the sonographic findings of acute prostatitis?
The prostate is generally hypoechoic with focal areas of increased blood flow.

36. What are the sonographic findings of chronic prostatitis?
- Focal masses of different degrees of echogenicity
- Ejaculatory duct calcifications
- Thickening or irregularity of the capsule
- Periurethral irregularities
- Dilatation of periprostatic veins
- Distended seminal vesicles

37. What does a prostatic abscess look like on ultrasound?
A prostatic abscess appears as an anechoic to hypoechoic mass, which may or may not enlarge the prostate. It is avascular on color Doppler, but may have increased flow at the margins.

38. How do prostatic calcifications appear on ultrasound?
Brightly echogenic with acoustic shadowing.

39. Are calcifications a sign of benign or malignant disease?
Calcifications are a sign of benign disease and are frequently found in patients with BPH.

40. What is BPH?
BPH is hyperplasia of the periurethral glands of the prostate. This process occurs in the transition zone. Ninety percent of men older than age 40 years BPH. The hyperplasia may be stromal (hypoechoic) or glandular. Glandular hyperplasia may respond to medical therapy, with relief of the patient's symptoms (Fig. 7).

41. What are the symptoms of BPH?
Symptoms of benign prostatic hypertrophy include:
- Difficulty initiating voiding
- Nocturia
- Small urine stream
- Urinary frequency due to incomplete bladder emptying

42. Can ultrasound help determine the cause of male infertility?
Ultrasound could be used to determine whether the seminal vesicles or vas deferens are congenitally absent. Ultrasound can determine whether the ejaculatory ducts are dilated or obstructed, and assess for stones.

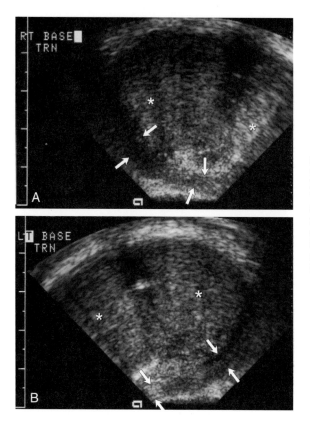

FIGURE 7. Benign prostatic hypertrophy. The prostate is markedly enlarged, measuring > 6 cm transverse. The peripheral zone (*arrows*) is markedly compressed by the periurethral glandular hypertrophy (*asterisks*). The entire prostate cannot be imaged in a single frame, and the right (*A*) and left (*B*) sides must be imaged separately.

BIBLIOGRAPHY

 1. Boulos MTB, Rifkin MD, Ross J: Should prostate-specific antigen or prostate-specific antigen density be used as the determining factor when deciding which prostates should undergo biopsy during prostate ultrasound. Ultrasound Q 17(3):177–180, 2001.
 2. Bree RL: The prostate. In Rumack CM, Wilson SR, Charboneau JW (eds): Diagnostic Ultrasound, 2nd ed. St. Louis, Mosby, 1998, pp 399–429.
 3. Cheng S, Rifkin MD: Color Doppler imaging of the prostate: Important adjunct to endorectal ultrasound of the prostate in the diagnosis of prostate cancer. Ultrasound Q 17(3):185–189, 2001.
 4. Czerwinskyj C, Rifkin MD: Efficacy of including the transition zone in routine biopsies of the prostate in men at high risk. Ultrasound Q 17(3):181–184, 2001.
 5. Fleischer AC: Renal and urological sonography. In Fleischer AC, Kepple DM (eds): Diagnostic Sonography. Principals and Clinical Applications, 2nd ed. Philadelphia, WB Saunders, 1995, pp 521–541.
 6. Hagen-Ansert SL: Introduction to abdominal techniques and protocols. In Hagen-Ansert SL (ed): Textbook of Diagnostic Ultrasound, 4th ed. St. Louis, Mosby, 1995, pp 55.
 7. Newman JS, Bree RL, Rubin JM: Prostate cancer: Diagnosis with color Doppler sonography with histologic correlation of each biopsy site. Radiology 195(1):86–90, 1995.
 8. Rifkin MD (ed): Ultrasound of the prostate. New York, Raven Press, 1988.
 9. Rubens DJ, Gottlieb RH, Maldonado CE, Frank IN: Clinical evaluation of prostate biopsy parameters: Gland volume and elevated PSA. Radiology 199(1):159–163, 1996.
10. Strang JG, Rubens DJ, Brasacchio RA, et al: Real-time US versus CT determination of pubic arch interference for brachytherapy. Radiology 219:387–393, 2001.
11. Vo T, Rifkin MD, Peters TL: Should ultrasound criteria of the prostate be redefined to better evaluate when and where to biopsy. Ultrasound Q 17(3):171–176, 2001.

22. THE RECTUM

Deborah J. Rubens, M.D., David Schmanke, RDMS, and Mark A. Hall, B.S., RDMS

1. What are the indications for performing a rectal ultrasound?
- Rectal and anal tumor staging
- Evaluate for perirectal abscess or fistula
- Evaluation of rectal sphincter

2. What patient preparation is required?
The patient's bladder should be emptied for comfort. An enema is not necessary, but if there is a large amount of stool in the rectum, the patient should be instructed to try to have a bowel movement. Not only does this make the examination more comfortable, but it also helps improve the ultrasound image.

3. What probe is used to perform a transrectal ultrasound?
Dedicated endorectal probes are available from most manufacturers. They are end firing or side firing, usually operating at 6–10 MHz. The probe should be covered with a latex or nonlatex probe cover.
Tip: Make sure there is some scanning gel in the tip of the cover. After the examination, the probe should be soaked in a disinfecting solution such as glutaraldehyde.

4. How is the probe inserted into the rectum?
A digital examination is performed first to identify any obstruction to the probe and to localize the lesion if palpable.
A. Lubricate the probe (K-Y Jelly or Xylocaine Viscous)
B. Have the patient breathe in and out deeply.
C. Make sure the probe is angled toward the umbilicus.
D. Have the patient bear down slightly to relax the sphincter.

5. If a probe cannot be inserted into the rectum, what other ultrasound options exist?
- An endovaginal approach can be used with a female patient. Looking posteriorly may visualize a rectal tumor or abscess, or the anal sphincter.
- A transperineal method may also visualize anal lesions, low perirectal lesions, and the anal sphincter.

6. What is the optimal patient position for performing a transrectal ultrasound?
The optimal position is the left lateral decubitus position with the legs together and knees bent.
Pitfall: Gas rises and may obscure the lesion of interest if it is on the right side.
Tip: Position the patient in the right or left lateral decubitus position to visualize lesions on the right or left walls, respectively. Position the patient with knees to chest facing prone for anterior lesions.

7. What can be done to improve imaging of the rectal wall?
Some probes have an optional water path, which acts as a standoff and permits better visualization of the near field. There is also better contact between the probe and the rectal wall.

8. What is the normal ultrasound appearance of the rectal wall?
- Hyperechoic: Mucosa-probe interface
- Hypoechoic: Mucosa

- Hyperechoic: Submucosa
- Hypoechoic: Muscularis propria
- Hyperechoic: Serosa (adventia) and adjacent connective tissue

9. What is the appearance of a rectal mass on ultrasound?
These masses are usually hypoechoic, and disrupt the normal bowel wall signature. Their depth of invasion can be determined by which layers they disrupt (Fig. 1).

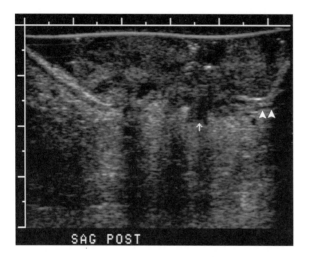

FIGURE 1. Invasive rectal tumor. Normal rectal wall layers (*arrowheads*) are disrupted as the tumor extends through the wall. The irregular hypoechoic tumor projections (*arrow*) are typical.

10. Why is ultrasound used for rectal tumor staging?
Because of the close proximity of the ultrasound probe to the lesion, greater detail is obtained than with pelvic or transperineal scanning. The motion of the tumor can also be assessed to determine whether it is mobile or fixed (more invasive).

11. What normal findings can be encountered that mimic a tumor when transrectal ultrasound is performed for tumor staging?
Collapsed bowel or fluid-filled bowel may mimic a tumor. Look for peristalsis and use color Doppler to help distinguish solid mass from fluid.

12. What imaging modality should be used to help locate the lesion before performing ultrasound?
A computed tomography (CT) or magnetic resonance imaging (MRI) scan is helpful to determine the location of the lesion, anterior, posterior, right, or left. The report of a colonoscopy or physical examination is helpful as well.

13. How is the transducer oriented for rectal wall examination?
All lesions should be imaged in two planes to obtain information about all margins. If the probe is not a biplane probe, an endfire probe or angle phased-array probe should be rotated 90° to visualize all aspects of a lesion.

14. What are the four stages of rectal tumors?
- T1—Tumor confined to mucosa or submucosa
- T2—Invasion of the muscularis propria or serosa
- T3—Tumor invading the perirectal fat
- T4—Tumor involving adjacent organ

15. How accurate is ultrasound in staging rectal tumors?

Overall, ultrasound is about 80–85% accurate in determining the T staging, similar to endo-luminal MRI. Ultrasound performs better in T1 lesions than T2–T4 lesions (Fig. 2).

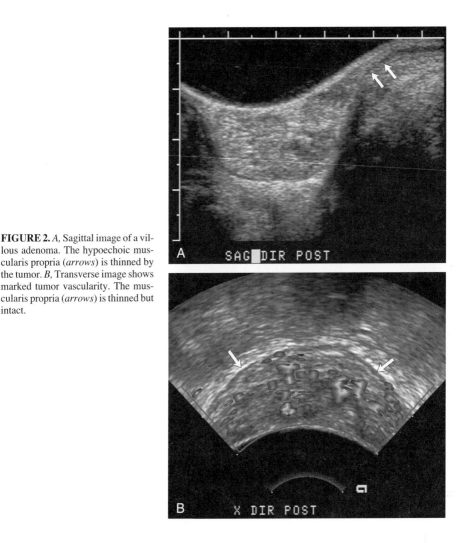

FIGURE 2. *A*, Sagittal image of a villous adenoma. The hypoechoic muscularis propria (*arrows*) is thinned by the tumor. *B*, Transverse image shows marked tumor vascularity. The muscularis propria (*arrows*) is thinned but intact.

16. How large are abnormal perirectal lymph nodes?

Size is less important than appearance. Nodes as small as 5 mm may be metastatic, and 1-cm nodes may be normal. Abnormal nodes are hypoechoic (lacking an echogenic helium) and are round. Ultrasound has an accuracy of about 65–70% for nodal staging.

17. Where are abnormal lymph nodes located?

They are located perirectally and above the rectum, with drainage into the internal iliac chain. This area cannot be reached by standard transrectal ultrasonography (TRUS). If both size greater than 1 cm and abnormal ultrasound features are used to diagnose abnormal lymph nodes, accuracy increases to 85% and specificity improves, but sensitivity decreases to 50%.

18. What is the indication for performing an anal sphincter ultrasound?

An anal sphincter ultrasound is performed to evaluate the sphincter muscle in the assessment of fecal incontinence. This is most common in postpartum women after tearing or trauma to the muscle during delivery.

19. How is the examination performed?

This can be performed with a linear array transducer on the perineum, transvaginally looking posteriorly, or with a dedicated radial endorectal probe. The patient is supine with knees bent.

20. What is the appearance of the anal sphincter on ultrasound?

- The internal anal sphincter appears as a hypoechoic, continuous ring that is 3–4 mm in thickness.
- The anterior muscle thins normally superiorly (Fig. 3).

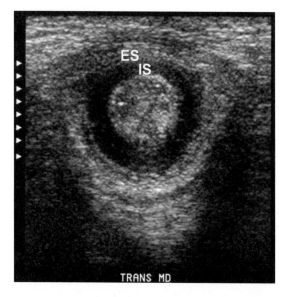

FIGURE 3. Transverse image of a normal intact rectal sphincter. The hypoechoic internal sphincter (*IS*) is slightly thinner anteriorly. The external sphincter (*ES*) is echogenic and tends to blend with adjacent connective tissue.

- When scanning in the transverse plane, there is focal thinning or defects, which usually occur anteriorly in the line with episiotomy (Fig. 4).

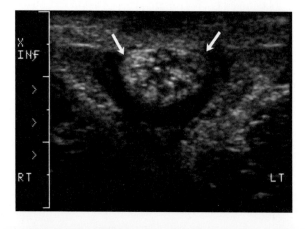

FIGURE 4. Patient with fecal incontinence and disrupted internal sphincter (*arrows*) anteriorly.

- The patient can be asked to tighten the rectum, and the motion of the muscle (or lack of motion) observed in real time.
- The external sphincter is hyperechoic and blends with the perirectal fat and connective tissue. It is difficult to visualize sonographically.

21. How are fistulas or fluid collections identified?

Fistulas appear as hypoechoic, fluid-filled (or echogenic gas-filled) tracts extending from the sphincter toward a skin surface (Fig. 5).

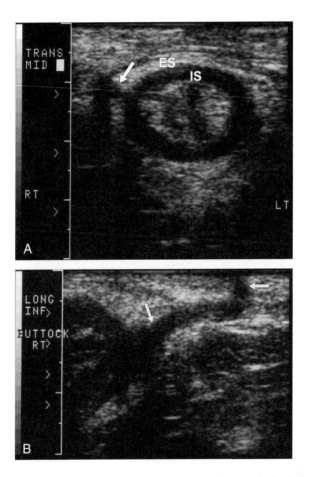

FIGURE 5. Anal fistula extending to the right buttock. Transverse image at the level of the sphincter (*A*) shows tract beginning at the 10-o'clock position on the right (*arrows*). Sagittal image (*B*) following the fluid tract (*arrows*) can follow it to the skin.

BIBLIOGRAPHY

1. Alexander AA, Liu j-B, Merton DA, et al: Fecal incontinence: Transvaginal US evaluation of anatomic causes. Radiology 168:1263–1267, 1996.
2. Beynon J: Rectum. In Dubbins PA, Joseph AEA (eds): Ultrasound in gastroenterology. New York, Churchill Livingstone, 1994, pp 169–183.

3. Campbell DM, Behan M, Donnelly VS, et al: Endosonographic assessment of postpartum anal sphincter injury using a 120 degree sector scanner. Clin Radiol 51:559–561, 1996.
4. Hagen-Ansert SL: Introduction to abdominal techniques and protocols. In Hagen-Ansert SL (ed): Textbook of Diagnostic Ultrasound, 4th ed. St. Louis, Mosby, 1995, p 55.
5. Hussain SM, Stoker J, Schouten WR, et al: Fistula in ano: Endoanal sonography versus endoanal MR imaging in classification. Radiology 200:475–481, 1996.
6. Rubens DJ, Strang JG, Bogineni-Misra S, Wexler IE: Transperineal sonography of the rectum: Anatomy and pathology revealed by sonography compared with CT and MR imaging. Am J Roentgenol 3:637–642, 1998.
7. St. Ville EW, Jafri SZH, Madrazo BL, et al: Endorectal sonography in the evaluation of rectal and perirectal disease. Am J Roentgenol 157:503–508, 1991.
8. Wilson SR: The gastrointestinal tract. In Rumack CM, Wilson SR, Charboneau JW (eds): Diagnostic Ultrasound, 2nd ed. St. Louis, Mosby, 1998, pp 279–327.

23. ULTRASONOGRAPHY OF BOWEL DISORDERS

Raj Mohan Paspulati, M.D.

1. What is the most common cause of right lower quadrant pain?

Acute appendicitis is the most important cause. Other causes include diverticulitis, renal calculi, ectopic pregnancy, and ovarian torsion.

2. Is there a high false-positive rate for diagnosing appendicitis in women?

Yes. The highest incidence of false-positive diagnosis (30–40%) is in women between ages 20 and 40 years. It is secondary to high incidence of pelvic inflammatory disease (PID) and other gynecologic conditions that mimic appendicitis.

3. Describe the ultrasonographic technique used in evaluation of appendicitis.

Graded compression technique with 5–10 MHz linear transducers from the right upper quadrant down to the right lower quadrant is the standard method. Graded compression helps to displace air-filled loops of bowel, enabling the visualization of appendix with ease. Inflamed appendix is not compressible.

4. What are the advantages of ultrasound over computed tomography (CT)?

Ultrasound in women of reproductive age helps exclude the gynecologic causes that can mimic acute appendicitis, such as ovarian torsion and tubo-ovarian abscess. The endovaginal sonogram is helpful in identifying an inflamed appendix that is lying low in the pelvis.

5. What are the sonographic features of a normal appendix?

A normal appendix appears as a blind-ending, tubular, aperistaltic structure attached to the base of the cecum. It has a maximum outer diameter of 6 mm and maximum wall thickness of 2 mm.

6. What is sonographic "gut signature"?

Alternating echogenic and hypoechoic concentric layers of bowel seen on sonography is referred to as *sonographic gut signature*. It is best seen on transverse view. These alternating layers correspond to five distinct layers of the bowel wall: (1) an innermost hyperechoic layer that corresponds to the interface between the mucosa and intraluminal contents, (2) a hypoechoic layer corresponding to muscularis mucosa, (3) a middle hyperechoic layer corresponding to submucosa, (4) an outer hypoechoic layer corresponding to the muscularis propria, and (5) a peripheral hyperechoic layer corresponding to serosa.

7. What are the sonographic features of acute appendicitis?

Features include noncompressible, blind-ending, tubular, aperistaltic structure attached to the base of the cecum, whose outer diameter is > 6 mm. A wall thickness of > 3 mm is also suggestive of acute appendicitis (Fig. 1).

8. What are the other sonographic findings in acute appendicitis?

Sometimes one may see inflamed periappendiceal fat as an echogenic area surrounding the appendix. Circumferential increased flow within the wall of the appendix on color Doppler is strong supportive evidence of acute inflammation.

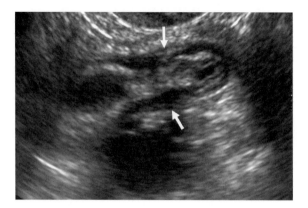

FIGURE 1. Acute appendicitis. Blind ending tubular structure measuring > 6 mm in the right lower quadrant representing an inflamed appendix (*arrows*).

9. What is the significance of an appendicolith?

Demonstration of an appendicolith contributes to the diagnosis of appendicitis. Appendicolith can be seen in the absence of acute appendicitis. Appendicolith appears as a bright echogenic intraluminal focus with a clear distal acoustic shadow. The echogenicity and the acoustic shadow depend on the degree of calcification (Fig. 2).

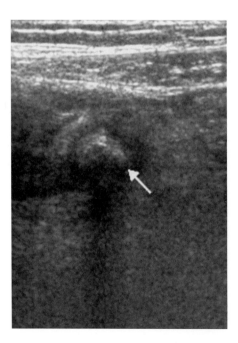

FIGURE 2. Inflamed appendix with an echogenic intraluminal focus causing acoustic shadow consistent with an appendicolith (*arrow*).

10. What factors are responsible for false-negative diagnosis of appendicitis?

- Poor technique and inadequate experience of the operator
- Obese patients with gas-distended bowel in the right lower abdomen
- Inflammation localized to the tip of the appendix, such that the entire appendix cannot be visualized
- Retrocecal appendix or when the appendix is in the true pelvis surrounded by bowel loops

- Perforation of the appendix, leading to decompression of its lumen, which obscures of the characteristic sonographic features of the appendix
- Gas in the lumen of the appendix caused by gas-forming organisms or reflux from the cecum resulting in acoustic shadowing that may mask the sonographic features of appendicitis

11. What are the causes of false-positive diagnosis of appendicitis?

This is most often due to misinterpretation of terminal ileum as the appendix. Following are the differentiating features of terminal ileum from appendix:

- The terminal ileum is a non–blind-ending structure with demonstration of peristalsis.
- It is more often seen as an oval in cross section, compared with the appendix, which is round.

12. What are the sonographic signs of ischemia and gangrene of the appendix?

Signs include focal or generalized interruption of the echogenic submucosal layer of the appendix. Thickened periappendiceal fat due to extension of inflammation is an ancillary sign.

13. What are the sonographic signs of perforated appendix?

- Periappendiceal phlegmon, which appears as ill-defined hypoechoic areas within the echogenic periappendiceal mesenteric fat
- Abscess formation, identified as loculated fluid collections, with or without demonstrable gas (Fig. 3)
- Sympathetic mural thickening of the cecum and terminal ileum

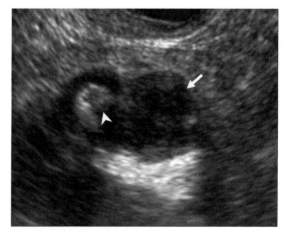

FIGURE 3. Perforated appendix. Inflamed appendix with focal interruption (*arrowhead*) and a well-defined fluid collection representing a periappendiceal abscess (*arrow*).

14. What are the other causes of right lower quadrant pain?

- **Colon:** Typhlitis, segmental colitis, cecal diverticulitis, cecal neoplasm
- **Terminal ileum:** Nonspecific terminal ileitis and Crohn's disease, mesenteric lymphadenitis, omental infarction, epiploic appendagitis
- **Gynecologic causes:** Ovarian cyst with complications such as hemorrhage or torsion, pelvic inflammatory disease, endometriosis, ectopic pregnancy, postpartum ovarian vein thrombosis
- **Urologic causes:** Acute pyelonephritis, ureteric calculi

15. Describe acute terminal ileitis.

It is caused by *Yersinia, Campylobacter,* and *Salmonella* species of bacteria. Clinical symptoms are right-sided abdominal pain, diarrhea, and nausea. Sonographic features include hypoechoic mural thickening of the terminal ileum and cecum with hypoechoic edematous mucosal folds. Color Doppler shows increased vascular flow of the bowel wall. Hypoechoic enlarged mesenteric lymph nodes may be seen.

16. Describe Crohn's disease.

Crohn's disease affects the digestive system from the esophagus to rectum, and its most common manifestation is diffuse bowel wall thickening of the terminal ileum. Submucosa is especially thickened, producing a hyperechoic band caused by lymphedema. Because of transmural involvement, the perienteric fat is inflamed, appearing echogenic and thickened, resulting in separation of adjacent bowel loops. Mesenteric adenopathy is noted in about 20% of patients.

17. Describe sonographic features of colonic diverticulitis.

It is usually left sided. It is characterized by diffuse thickening of the bowel wall along with echogenic pericolonic fat secondary to pericolic inflammation. Focal tenderness can be elicited, and color Doppler ultrasound may show increased flow in the adjacent pericolic fat (Fig. 4).

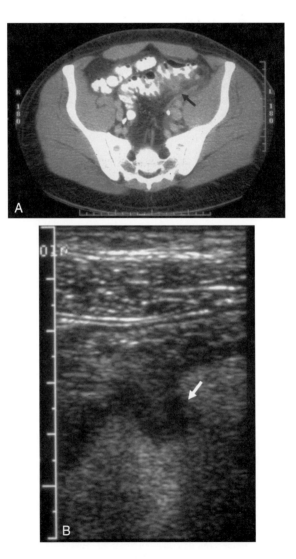

FIGURE 4. Sigmoid diverticulitis. *A,* Axial image through pelvis demonstrates thickening of sigmoid colon with infiltrative changes in the sigmoid mesentery (*arrow*). *B,* Corresponding sonograph shows a sigmoid diverticulum (*arrow*) with surrounding echogenic area secondary to inflamed mesenteric fat.

18. What is right-sided colonic diverticulitis?

It tends to occur in younger patients, is more common in women, and is more common in the Asian population. Right-sided colonic diverticula are usually solitary and congenital in origin.

On ultrasound, right-sided diverticulitis is diagnosed when a diverticulum is identified arising from the cecum or ascending colon with echogenic pericolic fat resulting from pericolic inflammation. Focal tenderness can be elicited, and color Doppler ultrasound may show increased flow in the adjacent pericolic fat. The distinction of right-sided diverticulitis from acute appendicitis is important, because diverticulitis is treated conservatively.

19. Describe epiploic appendagitis.

Epiploic appendages are fatty tags that are attached to the serosal surface of the colon. Torsion or venous thrombosis of an epiploic appendage causes ischemia or infarction, resulting in localized inflammation called epiploic appendagitis. Epiploic appendagitis of the right-sided colon can mimic acute appendicitis. It is important to correctly diagnose epiploic appendagitis, because its treatment is conservative.

20. Describe the sonographic features of epiploic appendagitis.

On ultrasound, an oval, echogenic, finger-like projection extending from the colonic wall is noted. The adjacent pericolic fat is echogenic and forms a mass. The adjacent colonic wall may show thickening.

21. Describe omental infarction.

Omental infarction is typically triangular and involves the inferior aspect of the right side of the omentum. It is characteristically situated between the anterior abdominal wall and the transverse or ascending colon. On sonography, a hyperechoic ovoid shape or a cakelike soft tissue mass is seen between the anterior abdominal wall and the ascending or transverse colon. The various theories about the causes of omental infarction include anomalous arterial supply to omentum, kinking of veins from increased intra-abdominal pressure, and vascular congestion after large meals.

In most patients, omental infarction is a self-limited, benign condition that resolves spontaneously. It resolves with retraction and fibrosis, leading to either complete healing or autoamputation. Reported complications include adhesions with bowel obstruction and abscess formation. Treatment is either conservative or laparoscopic excision to resolve pain and prevent possible complications. Clinically, right-sided omental infarction mimics acute appendicitis.

BIBLIOGRAPHY

1. Balthazar EJ, Birnbaun BA, Yee J, et al: Acute appendicitis: CT and US correlation in 100 patients. Radiology 190:31–35, 1994.
2. Birnbaun BA, Jeffrey RB Jr: CT and sonographic evaluation of right lower quadrant pain. Am J Radiol 170:361–371, 1998.
3. Gronroos JM, Gronroos P: Diagnosis of acute appendicitis. Radiology 219:297–298, 2001.
4. Jeffrey RB Jr, Jain KA, Nghiem HV: Sonographic diagnosis of acute appendicitis: Interpretive pitfalls. Am J Radiol 162:55–59, 1994.
5. Jeffrey RB Jr, Laing FC, Townsend RR: Acute appendicitis: Sonographic criteria based on 250 cases. Radiology 167:327–329, 1988.
6. Lim HK, LeeWJ, Kim TH, et al: Appendicitis: Usefulness of color Doppler US. Radiology 201:221–225, 1996.
7. Ooms HWA, Koumans RKJ, Ho Kang You PJ, Puylart JB: Ultrasonography in the diagnosis of acute appendicitis. Br J Surg 78:315–318, 1991.
8. Rioux M: Sonographic detection of the normal and abnormal appendix. Am J Radiol 158:773–778, 1992.

24. TRAUMA ULTRASOUND

Deborah J. Rubens, M.D., and Jodie Crowley, B.S., RDMS

1. What are the indications for trauma ultrasound?
Trauma ultrasound is indicated in patients with blunt abdominal trauma who are hypotensive and cannot be stabilized for computed tomography (CT) scan, or for triage of stable patients.

2. What is a trauma ultrasound or FAST scan?
FAST is an acronym for *focused abdominal sonography for trauma*. It is performed at the bedside in unstable patients in place of peritoneal lavage.

3. Where does one look for trauma (which quadrants)?
A trauma ultrasound is a limited scan looking for fluid in six major areas (Fig. 1):
1. Heart for pericardial fluid (Fig. 2)
2. Right upper quadrant and Morrison's pouch for peritoneal fluid (Fig. 3)
3. Right lower quadrant for peritoneal fluid (Fig. 4)
4. Left upper quadrant for peritoneal fluid (Fig. 5)
5. Left lower quadrant for peritoneal fluid
6. Midline pelvis for peritoneal fluid (Fig. 6)

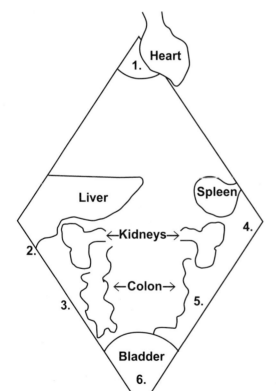

FIGURE 1. Coronal diagram denoting the areas in which one should image during a FAST scan. Results are recorded as positive or negative in each of these areas.

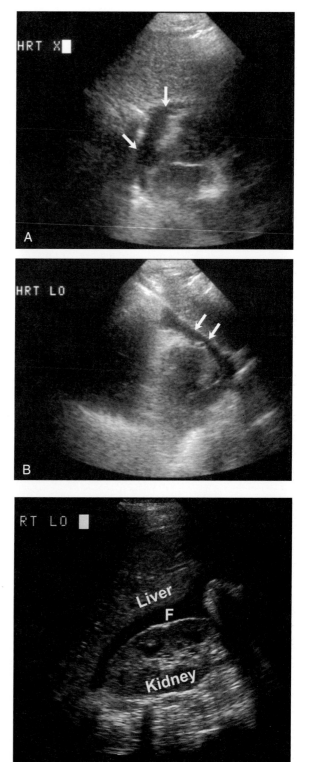

FIGURE 2. Pericardial Fluid. Transverse (*A*) and longitudinal (*B*) images of the heart from a subxiphoid approach. *Arrows* denote pericardial fluid.

FIGURE 3. Right upper quadrant fluid. Longitudinal images shows intraperitoneal fluid (*F*) in Morrison's pouch between the liver and the kidney.

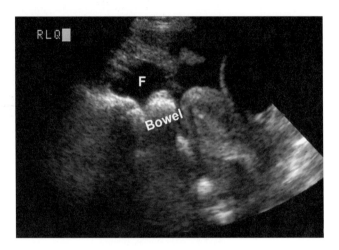

FIGURE 4. Right lower quadrant fluid. Fluid (*F*) displaces bowel from the flanks in the lower quadrants.

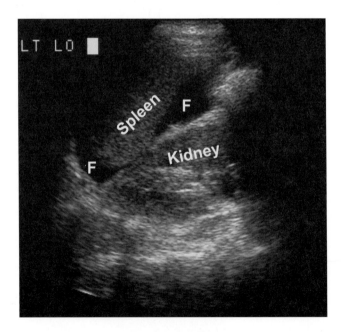

FIGURE 5. Left upper quadrant fluid. Longitudinal ultrasound identifies the spleen and kidney with fluid (*F*) between them and tracking between the spleen and the diaphragm.

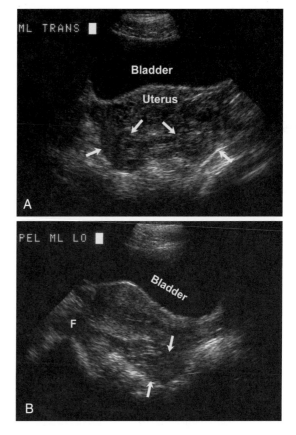

FIGURE 6. Blood and fluid in the pelvis. *A,* Transverse ultrasound shows the uterus surrounded by a heterogeneous solid mass (*arrows*). *B,* Longitudinal ultrasound shows the mass (*arrows*) in the cul-de-sac, posterior to the uterus, with a small amount of fluid (*F*) superiorly. This patient had a ruptured follicular cyst with 2 L blood in the peritoneum at laparotomy.

4. What is considered a positive scan?

The major sign of blood in the abdomen or pelvis appears either as fluid or a solid (*see* Fig. 6). Other things to note are major organ shifts, missing organs, pregnancy, and major organ laceration (liver, spleen, or kidney).

5. What causes false-negative examinations?

- A blood clot may be mistaken for normal tissue (i.e., liver, bowel, spleen). Ultrasound is less sensitive than CT for parenchymal injuries to liver, spleen, and kidneys and does not detect bowel injuries.
- Foley catheter in bladder and bowel obscures free pelvic fluid. This causes false-negative results in up to 20% of cases.
- Subcutaneous emphysema, pneumoperitoneum, bowel gas, or patient body habitus may limit the examination.
- Retroperitoneal hematoma is often undetected by ultrasound (Fig. 7).

6. What causes false-positive examinations?

- Diseases that cause ascites (i.e., liver failure, renal failure, metastatic tumor)
- Peritoneal dialysis
- Ruptured ovarian cyst with physiologic fluid or blood (*see* Fig. 6)
- Ruptured appendicitis, gastroenteritis, or other gastrointestinal source of peritoneal fluid
- Lymphoceles
- Left lobe of liver over spleen mistaken as blood (Fig. 8)
- Stomach mistaken as free fluid in the left upper quadrant (Fig. 9)

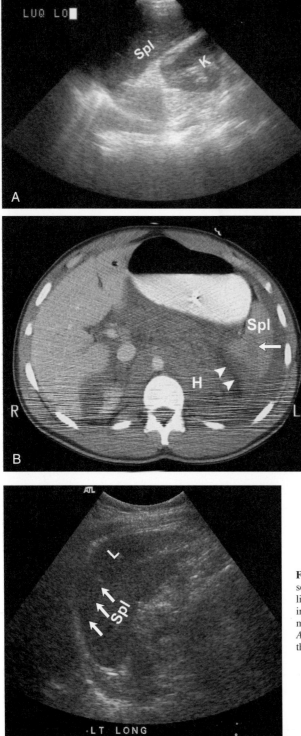

FIGURE 7. False-negative ultrasound. *A,* Longitudinal ultrasound image shows normal kidney (*K*) and spleen (*Spl*) with no free fluid. *B,* performed within 30 minutes shows a splenic laceration (*arrow*) as well as fluid around the spleen (*arrowheads*) and massive retroperitoneal hematoma (*H*). The right kidney is also partially infarcted.

FIGURE 8. False-positive ultrasound. The normal left lobe of the liver (*L*) may cross the midline and be imaged superior to the spleen (*Spl*) mimicking a perisplenic hematoma. *Arrows* denote the margin between the liver and spleen.

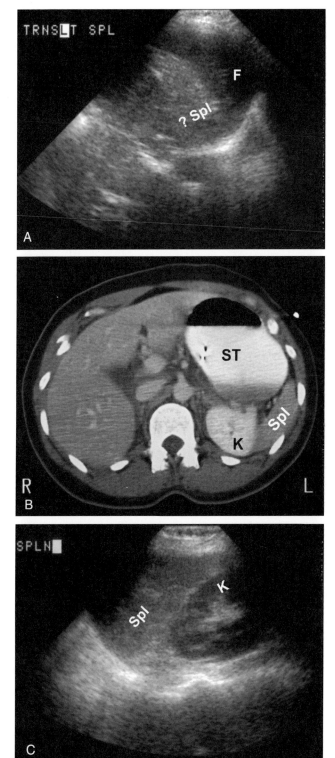

FIGURE 9. Stomach as pseudosplenic hematoma. *A,* Ultrasound image from anteriorly shows a mass with hypoechoic fluid *(F)* and echogenic (solid) component, mimicking the spleen with perisplenic fluid. *B,* Computed tomography shows the fluid/fluid level in the stomach as well as the very posterior location of spleen *(Spl)* and kidney *(K). C,* Repeat ultrasound from very posteriorly correctly identifies the normal spleen and kidney, with no fluid.

7. Which transducer is used for trauma ultrasound?

For most trauma ultrasound, the best transducer is a routine abdomen probe, preferably with multifrequency function and a small face. These two features are useful because wounds body access limit and because of patient immobility. Low frequency may be needed to penetrate deeply enough to visualize the posterior regions where fluid accumulates.

8. How does one best visualize pelvic fluid and distinguish it from the bladder?

The biggest error in trauma ultrasound is missing pelvic fluid behind gas in the bowel. Filling the bladder retrograde via a Foley catheter displaces the bowel and permits visualization of the fluid. It also identifies the bladder, to be sure one does not mistake the bladder for fluid.

9. How does one deal with a poor image?

There is a misconception that "if you can't see, use more gel." This is not always the answer. Trauma ultrasounds are more difficult than is implied by the lay term of "fast" scan. These patients have a higher incidence of multiple injuries and are not usually fasted. Turn the lights down in the room and adjust the gain appropriately. Use a large field of view (FOV). If scanning from the front, the FOV should be 20 cm in order to see behind the liver and spleen and deep in the pelvis. Less may be needed if you can approach the quadrants from the flank. Insist that the patient's bladder be full and be sure to scan the right side of the patient.

10. Can the patient be moved to scan?

Most trauma patients cannot be moved. Many people are usually working on them at once. To gain access to the upper quadrants, especially the left, the patient's arms can usually be moved, and the patient scanned from the left. Scan from the sides of the patient as well as from the front.

11. How does one work around chest tubes?

Chest tubes are one of the biggest obstacles to scanning the upper quadrants. Although the tubes cannot be moved, the dressings can be pulled back to gain access. Ask for help from the other medical staff.

12. Is a trauma ultrasound effective later when fluid is not seen in the acute setting?

Yes. Often fluid accumulates as the patient is hydrated (resuscitated) and the blood pressure stabilized.

13. What is the value of serial scanning and when should it be performed?

Serial scans can be repeated as often as every 30 minutes, but they can also be repeated at the request of the referring clinician. Amounts of free fluid can change rapidly, especially with aggressive intravenous hydration and normalization of blood pressure. Serial ultrasound scans in patients with deteriorating clinical status can reduce the false-negative rate of ultrasound by as much as 50%.

BIBLIOGRAPHY

1. Chiu WC, Cushing BM, Rodriguez A, et al: Abdominal injuries without hemoperitoneum: A potential limitation of focused abdominal sonography for trauma (FAST). J Trauma 42:617–625, 1997.
2. Fernandez L, McKenney M, McKenney K, et al: Ultrasound in blunt abdominal trauma. J Trauma 45:841–848, 1998.
3. Henderson SO, Sung J, Mandavia D: Serial abdominal ultrasound in the setting of trauma. J Emerg Med 18:79–81, 2000.
4. Lentz KA, McKenney MG, Nunez DB, et al: Evaluating blunt abdominal trauma: Role for ultrasonography. J Ultrasound Med 15:447–451, 1996.
5. McGahan JP, Wang L, Richards JR: Focused abdominal US for trauma. Radiographics 21:191–199, 2001.

6. McGahan JP, Richards J, Gillen M: The focused abdominal sonography for trauma scan: Pearls and pitfalls. J Ultrasound Med 21:789–800, 2002.
7. McKenney MG, Martin L, Lentz K, et al: 1,000 Consecutive ultrasounds for blunt abdominal trauma. J Trauma 40:611–612, 1996.
8. McKenney KL: Ultrasound of blunt abdominal trauma. Radiol Clin North Am 37:879–893, 1999.
9. Miller TM, Pasquale MD, Bromberg WJ, et al: Not so fast. J Trauma 54:52–60, 2003.
10. Richards JR, McGahan JP, Jones CD, et al: Ultrasound of blunt splenic injury. Injury 32:95–103, 2001.

V. Organ Transplant Evaluation

25. LIVER TRANSPLANTATION

Deborah J. Rubens, M.D., Labib Syed, M.D., and David A. Dombroski, M.D.

1. What are the indications for liver transplantation in adults?

These include cirrhosis from chronic liver disease (e.g., hepatitis, alcohol abuse, primary biliary cirrhosis, primary sclerosing cholangitis, hemochromatosis, Wilson's disease, and Budd-Chiari syndrome), hepatocellular carcinoma (HCC), acute liver failure from drugs or viral causes, or congenital causes of liver failure including Caroli's disease or polycystic liver disease.

2. How do these differ from the indications in children?

Children are transplanted mostly for biliary atresia (50% of cases), metabolic diseases (20%) including alpha$_1$ antitrypsin deficiency and glycogen storage disease, and the remainder for tumors (HCC or hepatoblastoma) or acute liver failure.

3. Are there any contraindications for liver transplantation?

These include advanced cardiac or pulmonary disease, extrahepatic malignancy, portomesenteric vein thrombosis (portal, superior mesenteric, and splenic veins), active drug or alcohol abuse, and known cholangiocarcinoma. Cholangiocarcinoma is present occultly in as many as 10% of patients with primary sclerosing cholangitis, which makes sclerosing cholangitis a contraindication for transplant at some centers.

4. What is the success rate of liver transplantation?

Current 1-year survival is > 85%. Some chronic diseases persist despite transplantation, such as recurrent cirrhosis from hepatitis C (10–28% at 5 years) or hepatitis B graft reinfection (incidence of 80% without antiviral therapy).

5. What are the anastomotic sites in orthotopic liver transplantation?

These are the suprahepatic inferior vena cava (IVC), the infrahepatic IVC, the main portal vein, the hepatic artery, and the common bile duct.

6. Are all the anastomoses performed into the same recipient structure?

No. The common bile duct may also be anastomosed to a Roux-en-Y loop (a loop of jejunum) and the IVC of the donor liver may be ligated to perform a "piggyback" anastomosis. In this situation, the end of the donor suprahepatic IVC is attached to the side of the recipient IVC. The latter is left intact within the patient instead of being removed with the native liver.

7. Are there any contraindications for liver transplantation in a patient with HCC?

Contraindications include a primary tumor > 5 cm, more than three tumors, or metastatic disease, either local or distant.

8. What types of transplantation are performed?

The most common is cadaveric allograft, in which the entire donor liver is used to replace the recipient's liver. Living-related donor allograft involves resection of the right or left lobe (or the lateral segment of the left lobe, which is used in pediatric transplants) from a living donor and transplanting the resected portion into the recipient.

9. What happens to the gallbladder of the donor?
This is always removed to avoid potential gallbladder complications (stone disease, infection) in a nonfunctioning, denervated gallbladder.

10. What is the sensitivity for ultrasound detection of HCC in the cirrhotic liver?
This has been disappointingly low, with most series reporting 50–80% detection of primary lesions and as little as 15% of secondary lesions or tumor spread. This is in part due to variability of HCC ultrasound appearance, ranging from hypoechoic to hyperechoic masses, to diffusely infiltrating tumors; limited detection may also be due to the heterogeneous background of the cirrhotic liver, which makes it harder to discriminate subtle tissue differences. Computed tomography (CT) and magnetic resonance imaging (MRI) are much more sensitive, with detection rates of 80–100%, based primarily on arterial phase intense vascular enhancement.

11. What is the role of preoperative ultrasound in the recipient?
This is performed to exclude focal liver lesions and assess vessel patency, particularly the portal vein and splenic vein.

12. What is the function of preoperative ultrasound of the donor?
Mainly this is performed to assess the hepatic veins, and their number and size. In particular, one searches for the presence of a dominant right lobe branch off the middle hepatic vein that would be transected during a right lobe resection, for accessory right lobe branches that would require separate anastomoses, and for a conjoined left and middle hepatic vein trunk that would require transection for a left lobe harvest.

13. What are the main postoperative complications of liver transplantation that ultrasound may identify?
The major categories include vascular abnormalities, biliary tract complications, and localized fluid collections (abscess, hematoma, bile leak).

14. What is the major ultrasound-identifiable complication that threatens allograft survival?
The most significant complication is hepatic artery thrombosis (HAT), because it provides oxygenations for the entire donor biliary system. Loss of hepatic arterial perfusion results in biliary stenosis or necrosis with bile stasis, abscess formation, and sepsis. The reported mortality rate without retransplantation is 50–80% for acute HAT.

15. What is the incidence of hepatic artery thrombosis after liver transplantation in pediatric and adult populations?
This is 5% in adults and 9–18% in pediatric patients, and is most common in the first 6 weeks. Consequently, standard surveillance Doppler ultrasound is performed within the first 24 hours, and at some centers such surveillance is done frequently up to discharge. Thrombosis or stenosis may be diagnosed by ultrasound in as many as 10% of patients before any clinical symptoms are apparent.

16. What are the ultrasound findings of hepatic artery thrombosis?
This is defined as absent color and spectral Doppler flow. If collateral flow has developed, it may be detected as a tardus parvus waveform with a blunted upstroke and increased diastolic flow, mimicking hepatic arterial stenosis.

17. What are the clinical indications of hepatic artery (HA) stenosis or HAT?
These are usually signaled by deterioration of liver function tests, increasing AST, or bile leak. Specific presentations include massive hepatic necrosis, delayed biliary leak, or intermittent sepsis.

18. What is the significance of hepatic artery stenosis?
This also occurs in up to 5% of transplant recipients and is most common early after transplantation, but it may also occur several years later. Untreated severe stenosis can result in the same vascular and biliary complications of HAT.

19. What is the resistive index (RI)?
The RI is a ratio that assesses the amount of diastolic flow in a vessel. It is defined as peak systolic velocity minus end-diastolic velocity, divided by peak systolic velocity. Thus, an artery with an end-diastolic velocity of zero (very poor outflow) has an RI of 1.0. If the end-diastolic velocity is 75% of the systolic, the RI is 0.25.

20. What is acceleration time?
This is defined as the time from beginning of systole to peak systolic velocity. Acceleration time ≤ 0.08 second is normal.

21. How are the RI and acceleration time used to assess HA function?
The normal liver RI ranges from 0.6–0.7, higher numbers (0.7–1.0) are normal after eating, when blood flows away from the liver toward the mesenteric circulation. A low RI in the HA < 0.05) indicates abnormally high diastolic flow, usually due to relative ischemia from proximal stenosis or thrombosis. An RI < 0.05 or acceleration time > 0.08 is 73–81% sensitive to detect HA stenosis (Fig. 1).

22. Is a low RI specific for stenosis or thrombosis?
No. A low RI may also be caused by conditions that give rise to high diastolic outflow such as HA to pancreatic vein (PV), HA to hepatic vein (HV), or even HA to biliary fistulas. Intraparenchymal HA to HV shunting maybe also occur, especially in the early postoperative period up to 48 hours, so patients with a low RI with high-velocity systolic and diastolic flow and normal acceleration times should be followed up rather than being immediately sent to arteriography for suspected stenosis or thrombosis (Fig. 2).

23. Is there any other false-positive diagnosis for HAT?
Yes. Small, difficult to visualize HAs in edematous patients may result in nonvisualization of the vessels on color Doppler. This may be aided by administering ultrasound contrast media or by turning off the color or power Doppler and searching with spectral Doppler alone. Often a lower frequency Doppler (2.5 MHz) may be useful to detect flow deep in the patient.

24. Are there any false-negative diagnoses?
Yes. Rapid collateral formation and intrahepatic arteriovenous shunting may disguise a thrombosed or stenosed main vessel.

25. What is the significance of chronic (delayed) HAT?
HAT that occurs after the first 6 weeks is less likely to cause graft dysfunction because of the potential for collateral blood supply, especially if the thrombosis progresses gradually from a hepatic artery stenosis. Bile duct strictures, necrosis, and abscesses may still occur, depending on the degree of biliary duct oxygenation. Unlike early biliary strictures, these ischemic structures occur remotely from the anastomosis, often at the porta of the liver where the right and left ducts join.

26. What complications, if any, involve the IVC after transplantation?
Stenosis or occlusion (thrombosis) may occur at the (suprahepatic) anastomosis, but this is rare, occurring in < 1% of patients. Balloon angioplasty may be used to treat focal stenosis.

27. What are the ultrasound criteria for stenosis?
These include visible narrowing of the IVC with loss of cardiac pulsatility of the IVC proximal to the stenosis.

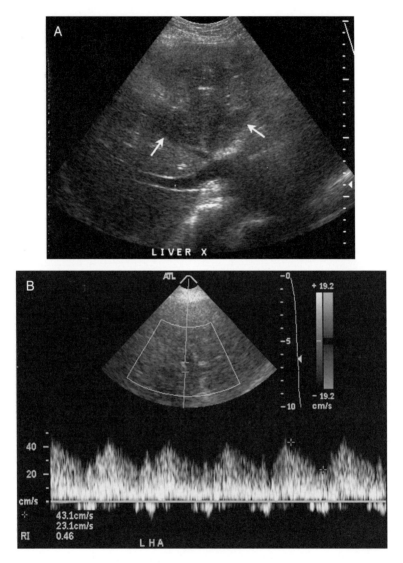

FIGURE 1. *A,* Liver infarct. Hepatic artery thrombosis with resultant left lobe infarct (*arrows*). *B,* Left hepatic artery. Left hepatic artery has a low-resistance waveform as indicated by resistive index < 0.05. This can be seen either with hepatic artery stenosis or due to collateral perfusion following hepatic artery thrombosis.

28. Is portal vein thrombosis or stenosis a significant post-transplant complication?

This is rare (less than 2%) and occurs most often in children, often with accompanying HA dysfunction. Abnormal turbulence at the portal vein anastomosis is common, but rarely results in a clinically significant stenosis with reduced portal flow (Fig. 3).

29. What are the ultrasound signs of portal or hepatic vein thrombosis?

These include internal echoes within the vein, expansion of the vein, and complete or partial loss of color Doppler signal within the main vein or its branches (Fig. 4).

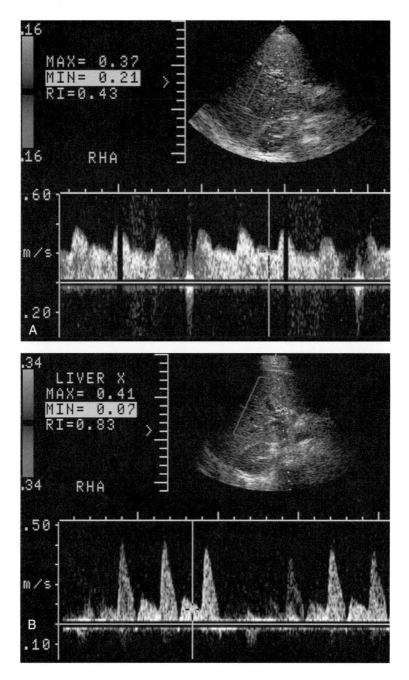

FIGURE 2. *A,* Immediate postoperative Doppler study shows a resistive index (RI) of 0.43, which is low. However, the systolic upstroke is brisk (acceleration time < 0.08 second) and velocity is high, suggesting that there is adequate inflow but too rapid outflow (shunting). *B,* One day later the RI has returned to normal at 0.83. No stenosis was present.

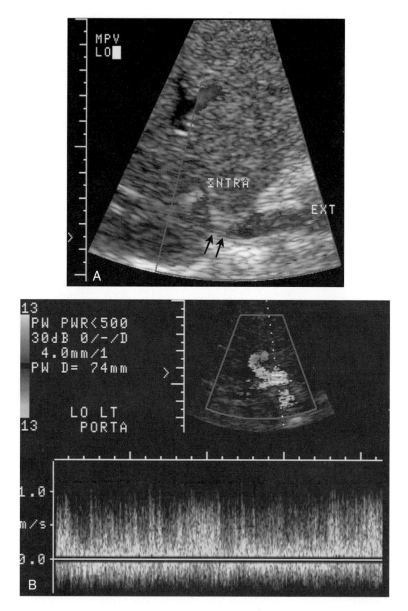

FIGURE 3. *A*, Portal vein stenosis. Note the narrowed portal vein lumen (*arrows*) in this pediatric transplant. *B*, Marked turbulence (mixed multicolored flow) is present just beyond the stenosis.

30. What are the major biliary complications after transplantation?
- Bile duct obstruction
- Bile leak
- Biliary duct necrosis

31. How common are biliary complications and when do they occur?
Complications of the biliary tract occur in up to 20% of patients, mostly in the first 2 months after transplantation. Biliary strictures, however, may present many years after transplant.

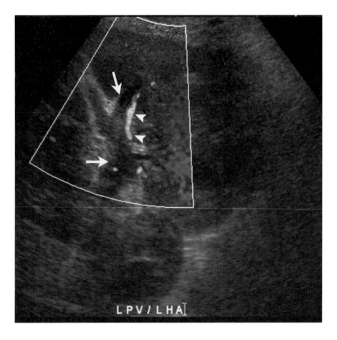

FIGURE 4. Portal vein thrombosis. The left portal vein (LPV) is avascular and hypoechoic (*arrows*). The adjacent hepatic artery (*arrowheads*) is patent. This patient had a left lobe infarct (*see* Fig. 1) with accompanying LPV thrombosis. (See also Color Plates, Figure 9.)

32. What types of strictures occur and what is their significance?

Anastomotic strictures occur as a result of technical complications of transplantation and occur early. These can often be treated with angioplasty. Nonanastomotic strictures are due to diffuse biliary injury, often from HAT, or prolonged cold ischemia time or incompatible donor blood types. These have a worse prognosis than anastomotic strictures.

33. What are the limitations of ultrasound in diagnosing biliary duct obstruction?

Intrahepatic duct dilation may not always be present when ducts are obstructed, especially with partial obstruction caused by stricture. If obstruction is expected clinically and ultrasound in nondiagnostic, then percutaneous transhepatic cholangiography (PTC) should be performed.

34. What is the utility of ultrasound in detecting bile leaks?

Ultrasound can detect fluid collections adjacent to allograft, but not their composition. Bile leak is diagnosed either by biliary scintigraphy or PTC. Leaks may be due to anastomotic complications. Leaks at the T-tube site or from biliary necrosis are due to HAT.

35. What is the significance of postoperative hematomas?

These are commonly detected as hypoechoic collections adjacent to the liver, posterior to the right lobe, or adjacent to the diaphragm. If the patient is asymptomatic, they can be ignored. They are usually clotted and drainage is unsuccessful as well as unnecessary (Fig. 5).

36. How common is abscess formation after liver transplantation? Where are abscesses located?

Abscesses occur postoperatively in up to 10% of patients. Most abscesses arise in preexisting collections such as hematomas or in bile collections, and they are located adjacent to the liver in the subphrenic or subhepatic spaces (Fig. 6).

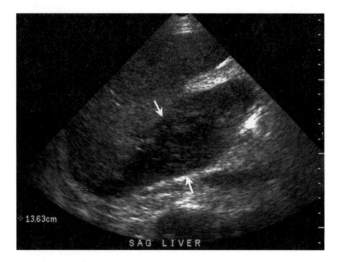

FIGURE 5. Hypoechoic collection (*arrows*) with internal echoes. Posterior to the right lobe of the liver is a typical appearance and location for a hematoma.

37. What modalities are used to diagnose abscess formation?

Ultrasound may be used to identify an abscess and to guide its drainage if warranted. Often the numbers and location of abscesses are underestimated by ultrasound, so CT is used in addition to ultrasound to monitor patients.

38. What is the most common complication affecting liver transplant survival?

Acute rejection occurs in as many as one third of all allografts. There are no diagnostic ultrasound criteria, although ultrasound is used to exclude other causes of graft dysfunction (vascular complications, biliary obstruction, or leak). Ultrasound is also used to guide liver biopsy.

39. How is rejection treated?

Rejection is treated by adjustment of immunosuppressive therapy.

40. What is PTLD?

Post-transplant lymphoproliferative disorder is a B-cell proliferation in lymph nodes or in solid organs. It is associated with Epstein-Barr (EB) virus infection and may progress to lymphoma.

41. What is the ultrasound appearance of PTLD?

Typically it is a hypoechoic (1–4 cm) mass that may be vascular. It can occur in the liver allograft or in a remote organ (e.g., bowel, kidneys, adrenals, spleen, retroperitoneal nodes). Alternatively, PTLD may occur diffusely in the liver or arise in the porta hepatis with subsequent biliary obstruction (Fig. 7).

42. What is the incidence of PTLD?

Incidence ranges from 2–10% in adults and from 3–19% in children. Children are thought to be at greater risk because they have less acquired immunity to the EB virus. Increasing PTLD has also been associated with the newer, more aggressive immunosuppressive drugs such as tacrolimus.

43. How is PTLD treated?

Initial treatment consists of reduction of immunosuppression. If masses resolve with this therapy, the prognosis is good. If they do not, more aggressive, systemic chemotherapy is required.

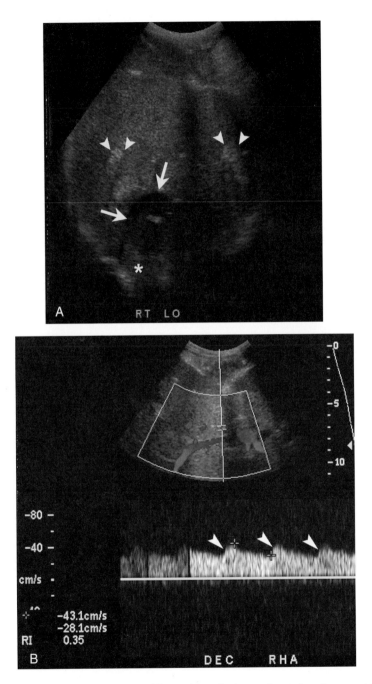

FIGURE 6. *A*, Hypoechoic mass (*arrows*) with some internal echoes and posterior enhancement (*asterisk*) typical of hepatic abscess. Rounded hyperechoic foci (*arrowheads*) represent biliary necrosis with echoes indicating debris in the duct spaces. *B*, Accompanying spectral tracing confirms the etiology of the abscess and biliary duct disease is poor oxygenation from hepatic artery stenosis or thrombosis. Note resistive index of 0.4 and classic delayed upstroke (*arrowheads*) characteristic of tardus/parvus waveform.

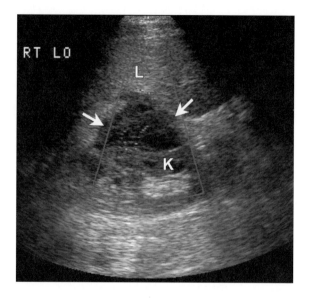

FIGURE 7. Right upper quadrant ultrasound demonstrates a hypoechoic 4-cm vascular mass (*arrows*) between the liver (*L*) and kidney (*K*). Histologically this was post-transplant lymphoproliferative disorder.

BIBLIOGRAPHY

1. DeGaetano AM, Cotroneo AR, Maresca G, et al: Color Doppler sonography in the diagnosis and monitoring of arterial complications after liver transplantation. J Clin Ultrasound 28(8):373–380, 2000.
2. Dodd GD, Memel DS, Zajko AB, et al: Hepatic artery stenosis and thrombosis in transplant recipients: Doppler diagnosis with resistive index and systolic acceleration time. Radiology 192:657–661, 1994.
3. Dharnidharka VR, Sullivan EK, Stablein EM, et al: Risk factors for posttransplant lymphoproliferative disorder (PTLD) in pediatric kidney transplantations: A report of the North American Pediatric Renal Transplant Cooperative Study (NAPRTCS). Transplantation 71:1065–1068, 2001.
4. Joynt LK, Platt JF, Rubin JM, et al: Hepatic artery resistance before and after standard meal in subjects with diseased and healthy livers. Radiology 196:489–492, 1995.
5. Garcia-Criado A, Gilabert R, Nicolau C, et al: Early detection of hepatic artery thrombosis after liver transplantation by Doppler ultrasonography: Prognostic implications. J Ultrasound Med 20:51–58, 2001.
6. Platt JF, Yutzy GG, Bude RO, et al: Use of Doppler sonography for revealing hepatic artery stenosis in liver transplant recipients. Am J Roentgenol 168:473–476, 1997.
7. Sakamoto Y, Harihara Y, Nakatsuka T, et al: Rescue of liver grafts from hepatic artery occlusion in living-related liver transplantation. Br J Surg 86(7):886–889, 1999.
8. Sidhu PS, Baxter GM: Ultrasound of Abdominal Transplantation. New York, Thieme, 2002.
9. Wolf R, Porte RJ, van der Vliet TM, Kok T: Development of intrahepatic arterial shunts in a transplanted liver: A potential pitfall for Doppler sonography. J Clin Ultrasound 29(7):406, 2001.

26. RENAL AND PANCREAS TRANSPLANTATION

Deborah J. Rubens, M.D.

1. What are some common indications for renal transplantation?
Renal transplantation is indicated for patients with chronic renal failure maintained by hemodialysis or peritoneal dialysis. The most common etiologies include diabetes and polycystic kidney disease, although other causes for chronic renal failure may result in transplantation as well.

2. What types of renal transplantation can be performed?
Three types of transplantation are possible. The most common in the United States is cadaveric renal transplant, which is a kidney donated by someone "brain-dead" who is unrelated to the recipient. The second most common donor type is a living-related donor. The third type of donor is a living-unrelated donor. The latter two types require the donor to give one of their two kidneys to the transplant recipient.

3. Is there a difference between the types of transplant in terms of patient outcome?
Overall, living-related donor kidneys perform better then cadaveric kidneys. Cadaveric kidneys have an 80% 1-year graft survival and 93% 1-year patient survival as opposed to living-related donors who have a 91% 1-year graft survival and 97% 1-year patient survival.

4. What are the differences between cadaveric and living donor transplants?
For cadaveric kidneys there is a greater delay between harvest and the actual transplantation period. Optimally, transplantation should be performed within 24 hours and no more than 48 hours from graft retrieval. There is a greater risk of acute tubular necrosis in cadaveric transplants due to longer warm ischemia time. Living-related donors have fewer complications because the kidney is fresher, being harvested within minutes to hours of transplantation into the recipient. Better human leukocyte antigen (HLA) locus testing can also be performed before transplantation, and pretransplantation anatomic imaging can be performed to assess for vascular supply and collecting system abnormalities.

5. What pretransplantation imaging is performed with living-related donors and living donors?
Traditionally, intravenous pyelography (IVP) and angiograms were performed; recently, however, cross-sectional imaging has been used. Ultrasound is often performed to detect stones or other renal pathology; however, magnetic resonance imaging (MRI) with angiography (MRA) or computed tomography (CT) with angiography can be a one-stop imaging examination to identify the number and locations of renal vessels; early branching of the renal artery, which creates difficult anastomosis; a retroaortic renal vein, which is important for laparoscopic retrieval; or a duplicated collecting system, which is important to recognize for ureteral anastomosis.

6. Are there any contraindications to living donor transplants?
Stone disease is a relative contraindication, but not an absolute one. Having an accessory artery to the lower pole of the potential transplant is an absolute contraindication because there is potential compromise of the ureteral blood supply, which arises from that lower pole artery. An accessory branch places the ureter at much greater risk of ischemia and necrosis. A renal tumor within the potential donor kidney is also a contraindication to transplantation.

7. What are the indications for post-transplantation renal imaging?
Routine surveillance, especially in the initial postoperative period, identifies asymptomatic fluid collections or obstruction. Most transplant imaging is performed for biopsy guidance to

diagnose rejection or drug toxicity. Scheduled biopsies also may be performed before adjusting medication, including reducing steroids. Transplant imaging is also used to screen for renal artery stenosis in patients with poorly controlled hypertension. Ultrasound is also useful to diagnose ureteral obstruction or fluid collections around the transplant.

8. Where is the transplantation performed?

Transplantation is usually performed in a retroperitoneal location, either in the right or left lower quadrant. The donor renal artery is anastamosed to the common or external iliac artery. The renal vein is anastamosed to the common or external iliac vein (Fig. 1).

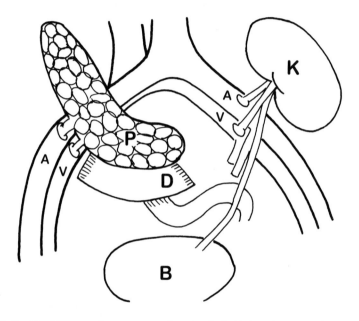

FIGURE 1. Combined kidney and pancreas transplantation. Left-sided renal anastomosis to the iliac artery (*A*) and iliac vein (*V*). The ureter is usually inplanted at the dome of the bladder (*B*). The pancreas (*P*) is transplanted with a segment of duodenum (*D*), then anastomosed to the bowel. The pancreatic vasculature is anastomosed to the right iliac artery and vein.

9. When will a peritoneal approach be used?

Intraperitoneal renal transplantation is done when a combined renal-pancreas transplantation is performed through a single incision. This permits placement of the pancreatic transplant in the right lower quadrant and the renal transplant in the left lower quadrant. The pancreas anatomy is better suited to the right lower quadrant then to the left. The renal transplant is more flexible and can be placed on either side (Fig. 1).

10. What is the normal protocol for imaging the renal transplant?

The transplant is imaged with grayscale ultrasound in a similar fashion to that used for the native kidney. A curved array or phased-array 3–5 MHz transducer may be used. The kidney size is measured in all three dimensions. The collecting system is imaged and assessed for hydronephrosis. Any fluid collections around the kidney are noted and measured (*see* Fig. 2A).

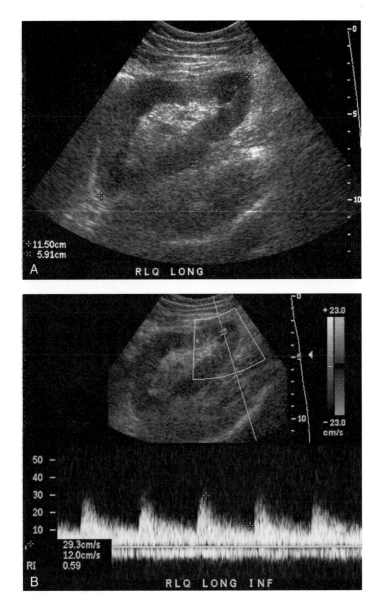

FIGURE 2. Normal renal transplant. *A,* Longitudinal ultrasound of a normal transplant (*cursors*) measuring length and anteroposterior dimensions. The kidney lies directly on the psoas muscle. *B,* Normal spectral tracing at the lower pole shows a normal resistive index of .59. Normal flow and spectral tracings should be obtained throughout the transplantation.

11. What causes enlargement of the renal transplant?

The transplant normally enlarges as much as 20%, especially if the donor is of pediatric age. Rejection causes enlargement in the renal transplant and occurs rapidly with volume increase of greater then 25% in less then 3 weeks. A rejecting renal transplant, however, is frequently normal in size. Other causes of renal enlargement include infection or renal vein thrombosis.

12. What might cause decrease in size of the renal transplant?
Ischemia or chronic rejection causes a decrease in the size of the renal transplant.

13. What vascular parameters should be obtained?
Color Doppler should be performed to assess for vascular supply throughout the kidney to exclude focal infarction. Resistive indices should be obtained at the upper, mid, and lower poles. Flow in the renal vein, renal artery, iliac artery, and iliac vein should be documented, as should velocity in the renal artery (*see* Fig. 2B).

14. What is the cause for an abnormally elevated resistive index?
This may be caused by rejection, acute tubular necrosis (ATN), drug toxicity, renal vein thrombosis, ureteral obstruction, or external pressure on the kidney, either from a fluid collection or from too much transducer pressure during the examination.

15. What is the cause of an abnormally low resistive index?
Ischemia from renal artery stenosis usually is the cause; however, a segmental low resistive index may be due to a fistula.

16. What abnormalities might be detected by ultrasound in the post-transplant period?
Ultrasound can identify anatomic abnormalities of the arteries or veins, the ureter, or peri-graft fluid collections such as urinoma, hematoma, lymphocele, or abscess. It can also identify mass lesions within the transplant kidney including tumors or abscesses.

17. What is the most common vascular abnormality in a renal transplant?
Renal artery stenosis is the most common vascular complication, occurring in up to 10% of cases and usually located at the anastomosis. Patients present with hypertension that is difficult to control, progressive renal failure, or both.

18. What is the diagnostic criteria for renal artery stenosis? Is it the same as for the native kidney?
The criteria for renal transplant artery stenosis is a peak systolic velocity of 2.5 m/sec or greater. It differs from the native renal artery stenosis criteria of 1.8 m/sec or a renal aortic ratio of ≥ 3.5 (Fig. 3).

19. When does renal artery stenosis occur?
Renal artery stenosis typically occurs within 2–3 years of transplant, although it may occur immediately after transplantation. Usually a high velocity at the anastomosis is secondary to edema in the early postoperative period and follow-up should be done.

20. Is ultrasound diagnostic of transplant renal artery stenosis?
Ultrasound is considered a screening modality, and stenosis should be confirmed angiographically or with MRA (*see* Figure 3B).

21. How does renal vein thrombosis present?
Typically, within the first week after transplantation, the allograft is tender and swollen, and there is no urine output.

22. What are the ultrasound criteria for renal vein thrombosis?
These criteria include absent venous flow on color flow Doppler, reversed diastolic flow in the intrarenal arteries, and a dilated renal vein, which contains thrombus. Occasionally, a severely compressed renal vein shows similar color and spectral Doppler findings to actual thrombosis. Patients with suspected renal vein thrombosis should be treated rapidly, because renal vein thrombosis is potentially reversible if detected early enough, and the transplant may be salvaged (Fig. 4).

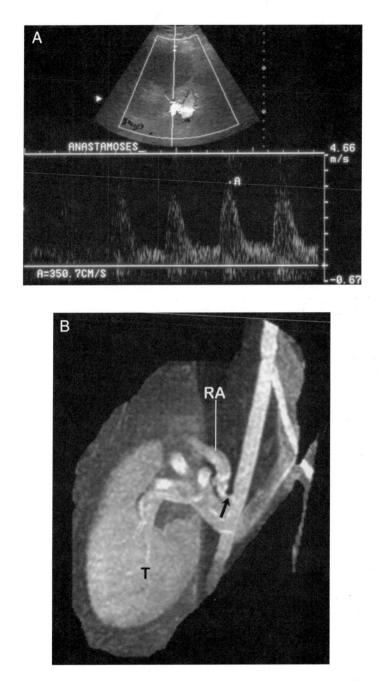

FIGURE 3. Renal artery stenosis. *A,* Spectral tracing at the anastomosis reveals a peak systolic velocity of 350 cm/sec. *B,* Reconstructed magnetic resonance angiography image shows the transplant (*T*) with narrowed renal artery (*RA*) at the anastomosis (*arrow*).

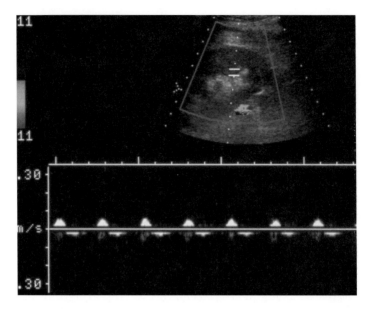

FIGURE 4. Renal vein thrombosis. Spectral Doppler tracing of an intrarenal artery demonstrates complete flow reversal during diastole.

23. How and when does renal artery thrombosis present?

Rarely, in the early post-transplant period (within the first week), patients are asymptomatic and present with a nonfunctioning graft.

24. Can renal artery thrombosis be treated?

No. The process is irreversible, resulting in graft infarction and transplant nephrectomy.

25. What causes renal artery thrombosis?

Predisposing factors include small arteries, either due to multiple renal arteries or a pediatric donor kidney. Atherosclerosis in either the donor or recipient also predisposes to renal artery thrombosis.

26. What are the characteristics of renal artery thrombosis on ultrasound?

Ultrasound shows renal artery occlusion. Spectral Doppler imaging of a renal transplant shows a transmitted "wall thump" pulsation of an occluded renal artery. Color Doppler through the renal transplant shows no vascular flow, indicating arterial thrombosis (Fig. 5).

27. What are other vascular abnormalities seen in transplant kidneys and what is their cause?

Transplants may exhibit arteriovenous fistulas or pseudoaneurysms secondary to renal biopsy. Arteriovenous fistulas have been reported in as many as 10% of patients undergoing renal biopsy.

28. How do arteriovenous fistulas present?

Patients may present with hematuria; however, most arteriovenous fistulas are small, asymptomatic, and resolve spontaneously.

29. How are arteriovenous fistulas diagnosed?

Diagnosis is based on color Doppler detection. The velocity scale should be set low to produce focal aliasing, which identifies the site where the highest velocity waveforms can be sampled. Typ-

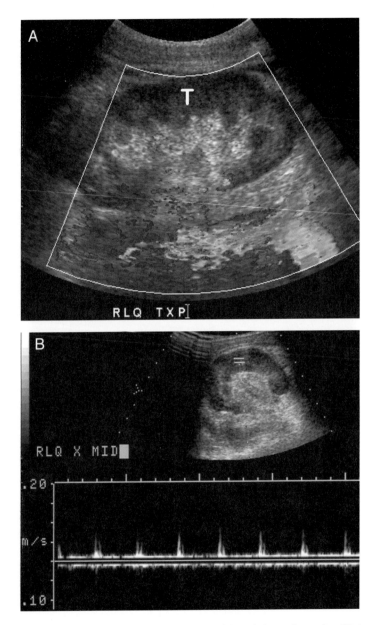

FIGURE 5. Renal artery occlusion. *A,* Longitudinal ultrasound through the renal transplant (*T*) shows no vascular flow, indicating arterial thrombosis. *B,* Transverse spectral Doppler image of the transplant shows a transmitted "wall thump" pulsation of an occluded renal artery.

ical fistulous flow should be detected as low-resistance, high-velocity flow. Ideally, if the arteriovenous fistula is central enough, arterialized flow can be identified within the renal vein (Fig. 6).

30. What other vascular pathology occurs in the transplants?

Infarcts may involve either the entire transplant or a portion of it. Infarcts most commonly occur as a consequence of rejection (Fig. 7).

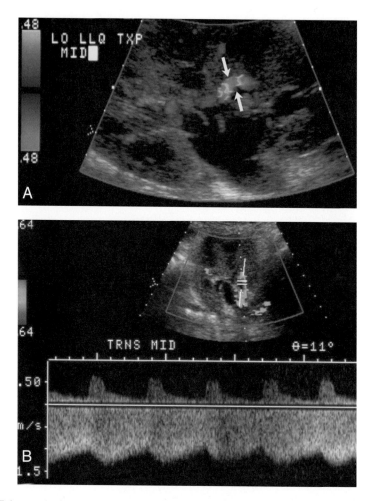

FIGURE 6. Area of aliased venous flow. *A*, Longitudinal color Doppler image reveals an area of aliasing (*arrows*) within a vessel with flow directed toward the renal hilum (a vein). *B*, Spectral tracing confirms high-velocity venous flow (below the baseline), which has an arterialized waveform, typical of an arteriovenous fistula.

31. What are causes of ureteral obstruction in renal transplants?

Early, ureteral obstruction may be due to edema, particularly at the anastomosis, or to blood clots. Later, the ureter is prone to distal stenosis. This is due to loss of a direct blood supply to the distal two thirds of the ureter during allograft harvest. Therefore, long ureters may have inadequate blood supply in the distal portion. The ureter also may be compressed externally from a fluid collection, either a hematoma or a lymphocele.

32. Does a dilated collecting system indicate obstruction?

A dilated collecting system of mild to moderate degree is not necessarily due to obstruction. The collecting system is denervated during allograft harvest and therefore has decreased tone. In particular, the ureter may not peristalse normally and a full bladder, which creates increased resistance to ureteral drainage, may result in a very full and distended ureter and pelvis. Transplants should be assessed after voiding to determine whether the hydronephrosis resolves.

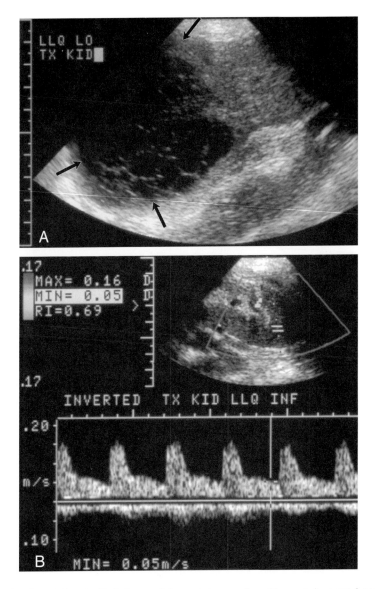

FIGURE 7. Infarct. *A,* Longitudinal ultrasound demonstrates an enlarged hypoechoic septated mass in this asymptomatic patient *(arrows).* This was a hemorrhagic infarct. *B,* Note normal vascular flow in the lower pole of this partially infarcted transplant.

33. What are the main post-transplant fluid collections that can be detected?

Hematoma is the most common fluid collection that occurs postoperatively or, rarely, secondary to infarction. Lymphocele is probably the second most common fluid collection. Urinoma and abscess also may be identified with ultrasound.

34. What is a urinoma and how does it occur?

Urinoma occurs in 3–10% of patients. It is usually due to disruption of the ureterovesical anastomosis from a vascular injury. Symptoms include pain or swelling over the graft and decreased urine output within the first month postoperatively. The diagnosis is suggested on ultrasound by a new or enlarged fluid collection, especially when associated with hydronephrosis. Ultrasound is not definitive, however, and a leak on either a nuclear medicine scan, a cystogram with leak, or an antegrade pyelogram with leak are specific (Fig. 8).

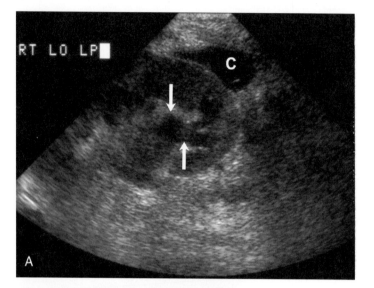

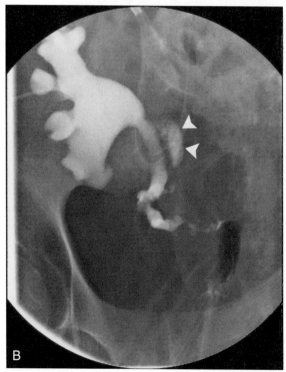

FIGURE 8. Urinoma. *A,* Longitudinal ultrasound shows mild to moderate hydronephrosis (*arrows*) and a post-transplant fluid collection (*C*). *B,* Antegrade nephrogram shows a contrast leak (*arrowheads*) adjacent to the transplant ureter.

35. How is the diagnosis of hematoma made by ultrasound?

Early postoperatively, hematoma is common, secondary to oozing in the surgical bed. The blood may originally be hyperechoic to isoechoic with the kidney and a hematoma is diagnosed as a result of displacement of the transplant kidney or external compression against the kidney (Fig. 9). As the hematoma progresses, it can become hypoechoic to anechoic, often containing internal septation (Fig. 10). At this point, it is easier to diagnose, and often hematomas are thought to be enlarging, whereas they are really becoming more visible. Most hematomas resolve spontaneously over several months and thus are not drained unless they are infected or are compressing or compromising the transplant.

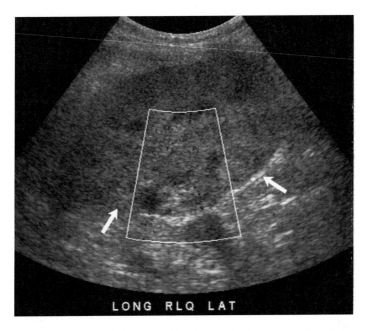

FIGURE 9. Hematoma Longitudinal ultrasound with color Doppler shows some echogenic hematoma with no flow on color Doppler. The hematoma deforms the normal contour of the kidney (*arrows*).

36. What is a lymphocele?

A lymphocele is a collection of lymph fluid caused by a surgical disruption of the lymphatic channels along the external iliac vein. These channels may reconstitute postoperatively, or they may obstruct, resulting in lymphatic fluid collection. These collections typically appear 6–8 weeks postoperatively. The characteristic appearance is a rounded or lobulated cystic mass, often with internal septations where it dissects the retroperitoneal space (Fig. 11). Frequently, normal vessels pass through without compromise. Complications include transplant ureteral compression or superinfection of the lymphocele.

37. What is the appearance of abscess in the renal transplant patient?

Abscesses are variable in appearance. They may range from septated fluid collections or fluid collections with debris (Fig. 12), to more solid material collections, to gas-containing collections (Fig. 13). Because renal transplant patients are immunocompromised, they are at increased risk for infection. In addition, secondary infection may occur in any preexisting stagnant collection such as a hematoma, lymphocele, or urinoma. Infection may also be introduced by drainage of noninfected collections, so small postoperative fluid collections are often left alone unless they are increasing in size or compromising the allograft. The ultrasound appearance of abscesses is

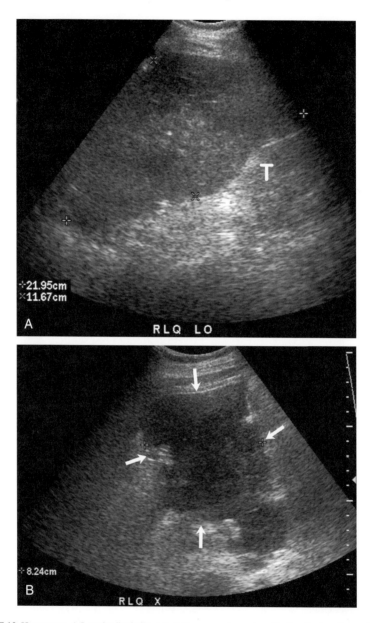

FIGURE 10. Hematoma. *A,* Longitudinal ultrasound shows an echogenic collection (*cursors*) superior and anterior to the renal transplant (*T*) and displacing the transplant posteriorly. *B,* Transverse image of the same left lower quadrant collection 10 days later (*arrows*). The collection has become hypoechoic with lysis of the blood.

nonspecific. CT may be helpful to show the enhancing rim of an abscess to differentiate it from a lymphocele.

38. What are the functional post-transplant complications?
Complications include rejection, ATN, and drug toxicity. Ultrasound is nonspecific to discriminate between these, and biopsy must be performed for final diagnosis.

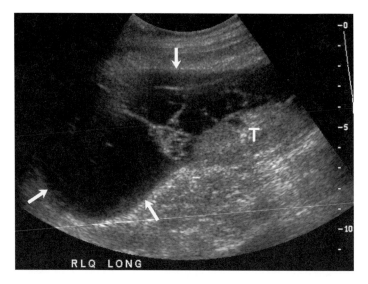

FIGURE 11. Lymphocele. Longitudinal ultrasound of a renal transplant (*T*) with a large septated collection (*arrows*) anteriorly and superiorly. This was eventually drained because of progressive enlargement and localized pain.

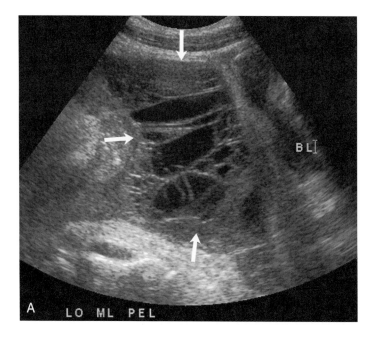

FIGURE 12. Renal transplant abscess. *A*, Multiseptated collection (*arrows*) just superior to the bladder (*BL*) in the midline. By ultrasound this is indistinguishable from a lymphocele. (*continued*)

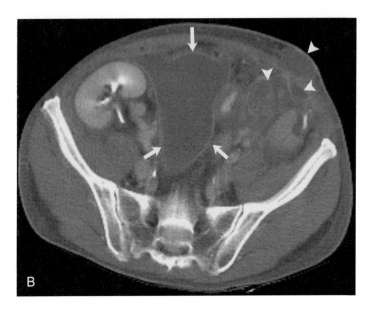

FIGURE 12. (*continued*) *B,* Computed tomography image of same patient. The abscess (*arrows*) has an enhancing rim, which differentiates it from a lymphocele. Note other abscesses as well, not seen on ultrasound (*arrowheads*).

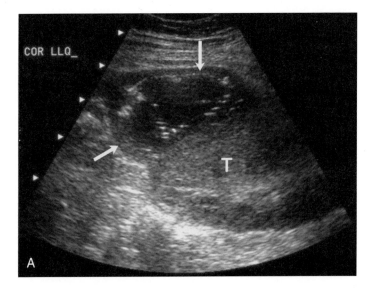

FIGURE 13. Abscess. *A,* Longitudinal ultrasound of a left lower quadrant renal transplant (*T*) shows a complex collection at the superior pole (*arrows*) containing internal echoes. (*continued*)

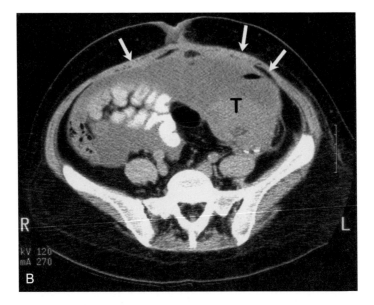

FIGURE 13. (*continued*) *B,* Computed tomography scan of same patient as in Figure 1A shows transplant (*T*) and gas-containing abscess (*arrows*). Note the abscess extends across the midline to the right lower quadrant, not appreciated by ultrasound.

39. What types of rejection can occur?

There are three types: hyperacute, acute, and chronic. Hyperacute rejection occurs within 24 hours, usually due to preformed circulating antidonor antibodies. This type of rejection is seen most often in patients undergoing retransplantation. With this type of rejection, the allograft never functions. Acute rejection is noted in up to 40% of patients, peaking at 1–3 weeks and is treated aggressively. Chronic rejection is a gradual deterioration, beginning at least 3 months postoperatively. It is denoted by interstitial fibrosis on biopsy.

40. What is acute tubular necrosis and how is it identified?

ATN occurs in 30% or more of patients after transplantation. It is more common with cadaver donors then with living-related donors. Between 10% and 30% of patients may require dialysis for short-term support after development of ATN. Spontaneous recovery usually occurs in 1–2 weeks.

41. Which drugs cause drug toxicity?

Cyclosporine and tacrolimus cause drug toxicity, which can be avoided to some degree by waiting to start these drugs until the second or third week after transplantation. Acute drug toxicity shows reversible renal vascular constriction in the parenchyma on biopsy. Interstitial fibrosis is seen long term.

42. When is renal transplant biopsy indicated?

Renal transplant biopsy is indicated for graft failure, including suspected rejection, ATN, and drug toxicity. It is also used to monitor therapy before changing steroid administration.

43. How is renal transplant biopsy performed?

This is an ultrasound-guided percutaneous procedure. Local anesthesia is used both in the skin and subcutaneous tissue down to the level of the renal capsule. Typically, two 18-gauge core biopsy samples are obtained, especially if light, immunofluorescence, and electron micropsy studies are to be performed. If only light studies are needed, a single core suffices. Tissue is taken from the peripheral cortex to sample the glomeruli. Images are obtained after biopsy check for bleeding.

44. What are major post-biopsy complications?

Hematoma is the most common post-biopsy complication. This is usually small and self-limited. Patients rarely exhibit hematuria, pain, or hemorrhage. Patients are kept at bed rest for 4 hours after biopsy. Arteriovenous fistulas are present in up to 10% of patients; however, they are usually self-limited and asymptomatic. Pseudoaneurysms are more rare, occurring in less then 1% of patients after biopsy; however, if not self-limited, they may require surgical therapy or percutaneous ablation.

45. What is post-transplant lymphoproliferative disorder (PTLD)?

PTLD is a prelymphomatous condition that may reverse if the patient's immunosuppressive therapy is stopped. PTLD is related to Ebstein-Barr virus infection and occurs in 1–2.3% of patients. It does not necessarily occur in the transplant organ and most often occurs 6–24 months after transplantation. The incidence of PTLD has increased over the past 10 years since introduction of new immunosuppressive drugs.

46. How does PTLD appear on ultrasound?

The lesions are solid, often hypoechoic and vascular. If they are homogenous, they may have enhanced through transmission (Fig. 14). Other organs, such as the liver or retroperitoneum and lymph node–bearing areas, should be monitored in addition to the transplant kidney. Decrease in immunosuppressive therapy may permit resolution of these lesions, and patients can be monitored with ultrasound for response.

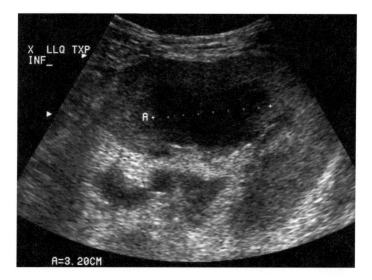

FIGURE 14. Post-transplant lymphoproliferative disorder. Transverse ultrasound through the lower pole of a renal transplant shows a hypoechoic mass measuring 3.2 cm. The patient was asymptomatic. After withdrawing immunosuppressive drugs for 2 months, the mass disappeared.

47. What are the indications for pancreas transplantation?

Pancreas transplantation is indicated when a patient has insulin-dependent diabetes and associated renal failure. Simultaneous renal and pancreas transplantation is performed.

48. Are there any contraindications to pancreas transplantation?

Contraindications to pancreas transplantation include the following complications of diabetes:
- Irreversible cardiac ischemia
- Severe peripheral vascular disease
- Previous stroke or transient ischemic attack
- Chronic sepsis

49. How is pancreatic transplantation performed?

The gland is harvested with a portion of the duodenum. The celiac and superior mesenteric artery remain attached to a piece of donor aorta. The arteries are anastomosed to the common or external iliac artery and the portal confluence to the accompanying iliac vein. The duodenal segment is anastomosed to the bowel or, less commonly, the bladder to allow drainage of the exocrine pancreatic enzymes (*see* Figs. 1 and 15).

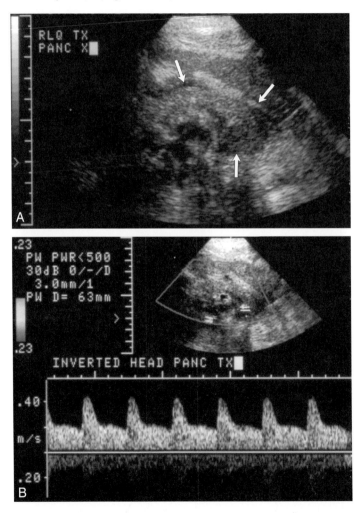

FIGURE 15. Pancreas transplant. *A,* Normal configuration of a pancreas transplant (*arrows*) in the lower quadrant. There are no fluid collections adjacent. *B,* Normal spectral tracing of the arterial inflow to the pancreatic transplant. (*continued*)

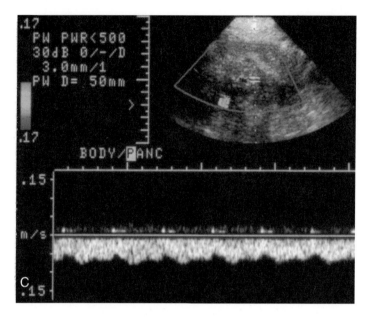

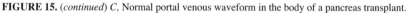

FIGURE 15. (*continued*) *C,* Normal portal venous waveform in the body of a pancreas transplant.

50. What are the outcomes of pancreas transplantation?

The patient survival rate at 1 year for pancreas transplantation is 95%, whereas allograft survival is 85% at 1 year for simultaneous kidney and pancreas transplantation.

51. How is ultrasound used in the post-transplant period?

Ultrasound can monitor the pancreatic vasculature and can assess for peripancreatic fluid collections, including pseudocysts or abscesses, which arise from pancreatitis.

52. What vascular complication can occur with pancreatic transplantation?

Vascular thrombosis occurs in 12% of patients, of which 5% are arterial and 7% venous (Fig. 16).

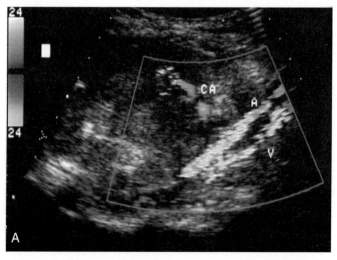

FIGURE 16. Pancreas transplant with venous thrombosis. Transverse (*a*) (*continued*)

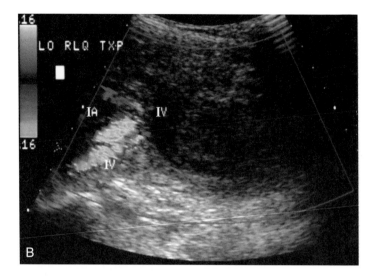

FIGURE 16. (*continued*) longitudinal (*b*) images show color flow Doppler signal in the celiac artery and in the adjacent iliac artery (*IA*) and vein (*IV*) but no flow in the anechoic vein (*V*) in the transplant. (See also Color Plates, Figure 10.)

53. How is arterial thrombosis manifested?

Arterial thrombosis is diagnosed by absent arterial flow throughout the allograft.

54. How is venous thrombosis diagnosed?

One may see reversed diastolic flow in the arterial spectral Doppler tracing and absent flow in the portal anastomosis. The distal third of the splenic vein is commonly thrombosed, because it is ligated and no longer drains the spleen.

55. How is rejection diagnosed?

The pancreas can be biopsied, much like the liver or the kidney. A site is selected without intervening bowel, and an 18-gauge core is obtained, avoiding major vessels.

BIBLIOGRAPHY

1. Baxter JM: Ultrasound imaging in renal transplantation. In Sidhu PS, Baxter GM (eds): Ultrasound of Abdominal Transplantation. New York, Thieme, 2002, pp 27–42.
2. Gottlieb RH, Voci SL, Cholewinski SP, et al: Sonography: A useful tool to detect the mechanical causes of renal transplant dysfunction. J Clin Ultrasound 27:325–333, 1999.
3. Gottlieb RH, Voci SL, Cholewinski SP, et al: Urine leaks in renal transplant patients: diagnostic usefulness of sonography and renography. Clin Imag 23:35–39, 1999.
4. Khanna A, Patel NH, Song Z, Jindal RM: Pancreas transplantation. In Sidhu PS, Baxter GM (eds): Ultrasound of Abdominal Transplantation. New York, Thieme, 2002, pp 125–130.
5. Jaques BC: Renal transplant surgery. In Sidhu PS, Baxter GM (eds): Ultrasound of Abdominal Transplantation. New York, Thieme, 2002, pp 23–26.
6. Maxwell H: Pediatric renal transplantation. In Sidhu PS, Baxter GM (eds): Ultrasound of Abdominal Transplantation. New York, Thieme, 2002, pp 43–54.
7. Moss JG, Edwards R: Interventional radiology and the transplant kidney. In Sidhu PS, Baxter GM (eds): Ultrasound of Abdominal Transplantation. New York, Thieme, 2002, pp 55–60.
8. Pozniak MA: Ultrasound evaluation of the transplant liver, kidney, and pancreas. In McGahan JP, Goldberg BB (eds): Diagnostic Ultrasound: A Logical Approach. Philadelphia, Lippincott-Raven, 1998.
9. Rodger RSC, Baxter GM: Chronic renal failure and pretransplantation assessment. In Sidhu PS, Baxter GM (eds): Ultrasound of Abdominal Transplantation. New York, Thieme, 2002, pp 13–22.

VI. Small Parts Sonography

27. SCROTAL SONOGRAPHY

Vikram Dogra, M.D., and Shweta Bhatt, DMRD, DMRE

1. What are the indications of scrotal sonography?

Epididymo-orchitis (acute or chronic), testicular torsion, testicular trauma, testicular tumors and torsion of testicular appendages are some of the major indications for scrotal sonography.

2. Describe the technique of scrotal sonography.

Scrotal sonography is performed with the patient lying in a supine position. High-frequency 8–14 MHz linear transducer is preferred for scrotal sonography. The testes are studied in long and transverse axes. The size and echogenicity of each testicle and the epididymis are compared with those on the opposite side. Color Doppler and pulsed Doppler are optimized to display low-flow velocities to demonstrate blood flow in the testis and surrounding scrotal structures. Power Doppler may also be used to visualize intratesticular flow in patients with an acute scrotum. Transverse images with portions of each testicle on the same image should be acquired in grayscale and color Doppler.

3. Describe the mediastinum testis.

The posterior surface of the tunica albuginea projects into the interior of the testis to form the incomplete septum, the mediastinum. The mediastinum testis is identified as an echogenic band of variable thickness and length extending in a caudocranial direction. If this is imaged at an oblique angle, it can be mistaken for a mass.

4. What is a mediastinal artery?

A transmediastinal artery branch of the testicular artery occurs in approximately one half of normal testes. It courses through the mediastinum, usually accompanied by a large vein. If this vessel is imaged at an angle, it resembles a hypoechoic lesion; this pitfall should be avoided.

EPIDIDYMO-ORCHITIS

5. Describe grayscale findings in epididymo-orchitis.

The epididymis is enlarged and has a heterogeneous appearance. The head of the epididymis measures > 17 mm. There may be hemorrhage within it. Other findings include reactive hydrocele and reactive skin thickening (Fig. 1).

6. Describe color Doppler findings in epididymo-orchitis.

Color Doppler reveals increased vascularity and increased concentration of the vessels within it. Hyperemia is the distinguishing characteristic of this disease, but normal blood flow can be seen in the epididymis with high-frequency transducer sonography; therefore, comparison with the other side is important. Visualization of blood flow within the epididymis is not equivalent to epididymitis (Fig. 2).

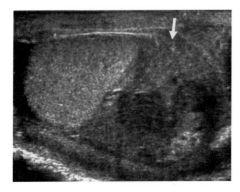

FIGURE 1. Clinically confirmed epididymo-orchitis. High-frequency sonographic image demonstrates a markedly enlarged epididymis with heterogeneous echo texture (*arrow*).

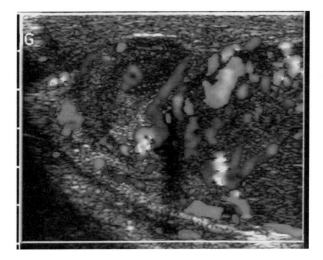

FIGURE 2. Clinically confirmed epididymo-orchitis. Color Doppler image demonstrates increased vascularity of epididymis and testis. (See also Color Plates, Figure 11.)

7. What part of the epididymis is commonly affected in epididymo-orchitis?

The tail of the epididymis is commonly affected first, extending to involve the body and head.

8. What percentages of patients with epididymitis have orchitis?

Orchitis develops in 40% of patients with epididymitis as a result of direct extension into the testis.

9. Describe sonographic findings in orchitis.

The testis is enlarged and has a heterogeneous appearance. This appearance is nonspecific and can be seen in many other conditions such as tumors, metastasis, and infarct. All patients with heterogeneous appearance of the testis should be followed up to demonstrate sonographic resolution after antibiotic treatment to exclude the possibility of tumor.

10. Describe other indirect signs of epididymo-orchitis.

A resistive index of < 0.5 and easy detectability of venous flow within the testis are suggestive of epididymo-orchitis. These findings are nonspecific and can be seen in tumors and metastasis, including lymphoma.

11. What tumor presentation can mimic orchitis?
Seminoma is most notorious; however, other germ cell tumors can also mimic this presentation.

12. What percentage of tumors present as epididymo-orchitis?
About 10% of tumors present with epididymo-orchitis.

13. Describe mumps orchitis.
Mumps orchitis is seen in 30% of patients with mumps and is bilateral in 10–30% of cases. The testis is enlarged and hypoechoic. Main complications are infertility and atrophy of the testis.

14. Name diseases resulting in granulomatous epididymo-orchitis.
- Tuberculosis
- Sarcoidosis
- Brucellosis
- Leprosy
- Syphilis

15. What is Prehn's sign?
While working with sailors at the Brooklyn Naval Hospital in 1934, D.T. Prehn observed that, in patients with epididymo-orchitis, elevation of the scrotum above the level of symphysis pubis resulted in relief of pain. This sign helps differentiate of testicular torsion from epididymo-orchitis during physical examination.

16. What is idiopathic granulomatous orchitis?
This is usually seen in middle-aged men. History of trauma is usually present. Sonographically there is intratesticular mass with peripheral hyperemia but no flow within it. Only histology can differentiate this from a testicular tumor.

17. What is the main differential diagnosis of epididymo-orchitis?
Testicular torsion is the main differential consideration.

18. What are the complications of epididymo-orchitis

Persistent pain	Infertility
Abscess	Atrophy
Pyocele	Gangrene
Infarction	

TESTICULAR TORSION

19. What is testicular torsion and how many types are there?
Testicular torsion is defined as the twisting of spermatic cord or of the testis itself on its attachments. Degree of ischemia is relative to the amount of twisting, beginning with venous compromise and progressing to arterial occlusion. A 360° twist may still have arterial inflow.

20. Testicular torsion is seen in what age group?
It is commonly seen in the 12–18-year age group, but it also occurs in neonates and patients older than 20 years of age.

21. Describe the conditions predisposing to testicular torsion.
Bell-clapper deformity and hypoplastic gubernaculum predispose to testicular torsion.

22. What is bell-clapper deformity?
When tunica vaginalis completely encircles the epididymis, distal spermatic cord, and the testis rather than attaching to the posterolateral aspect of the scrotal wall, it is called bell-clapper deformity. It is bilateral in most cases.

23. Describe the testicular salvage rate after torsion.

Salvage depends on the degree of torsion and the duration of ischemia. Salvage rate is nearly 100% within the first 6 hours after the onset of symptoms; 70% in 6–12 hours; and 20% in 12–24 hours.

24. Describe the grayscale findings of testicular torsion.

TYPE OF TORSION	FINDINGS
Acute torsion with viable testis	Normal appearance
Acute torsion with infarction	Hypoechoic pattern, which may be total or partial in the case of a partial infarct
Acute torsion with hemorrhagic infarction	Hyperechoic and heterogeneous pattern
Chronic torsion	Hypoechoic with small testis

25. What are the color and power Doppler findings in testicular torsion?
- Absent intratesticular arterial and venous flow
- Increased resistive index on affected side (diminished or reversed diastolic flow)
- Decreased flow velocity (difficult to measure due to small vessels and angle correction, but which may be subjectively inferred by relative difficulty in finding small, low-amplitude flow on symptomatic side)
- Peripheral reactive hyperemia (Fig. 3)

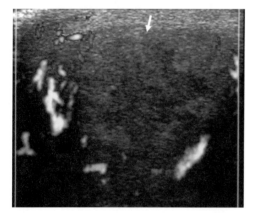

FIGURE 3. Surgically confirmed testicular torsion. Power Doppler image demonstrates absent intratesticular flow and variable echo texture of testis (*arrow*). There is peripheral hyperemia in the surrounding tunica. (See also Color Plates, Figure 12.)

26. What percentage of patients with testicular torsion have bilateral testicular torsion?

Bilateral torsion occurs in 2% of cases.

27. Does absence of flow in the testis always means testicular torsion?

Absence of flow in the testis usually means torsion; however, absence of flow in the testis can be seen secondary to faulty technique. External pressure from extratesticular hematoma or rapidly developing hydrocele can also result in absence of intratesticular flow. Conditions such as polyarteritis nodosa and lupus vasculitis can have a similar appearance.

28. Describe torsion-detorsion syndrome.

Intermittent torsion detorses itself. Patients usually present with pain. Sonography reveals increased hyperemia within the symptomatic testis. Such patients should undergo orchiopexy to prevent torsion.

29. What are testicular appendages?
These are müllerian duct and mesonephric duct remnants. There are four testicular appendages. The two that are clinically important are the appendix testis and appendix epididymis. Presence of minimal fluid facilitates their visualization.

30. What is the blue dot sign?
Physical examination reveals a small, firm nodule that is palpable on the superior aspect of the testis and exhibits a bluish discoloration through the overlying skin.

BENIGN TESTICULAR LESIONS

31. What is tubular ectasia of rete testis?
Tubular ectasia is a benign condition. It results from the ectasia of the rete testis. This process is usually bilateral but asymmetric, seen in men older than 45 years. Sonographically, it appears as tubular structure adjacent to the mediastinum testis in the posterolateral aspect (Fig. 4).

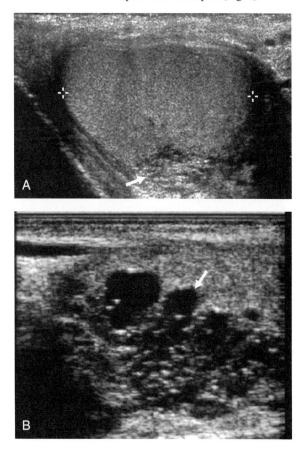

FIGURE 4. Tubular ectasia of rete testis. *A*, Mild grade of tubular ectasia. The longitudinal sonogram of the testis shows tubular structures in the posterolateral aspect of the testis (*arrow*). *B*, Severe grade of tubular ectasia. This sonogram demonstrates tubular structures (*arrow*) that are much bigger than in *A*.

32. Describe tunica albuginea cyst.
It is a benign cyst arising from the tunica albuginea. It affects patients 20–40 years of age. These patients always present with a palpable nodule. These cysts range from 2 to 5 mm in size and occur in the anterosuperior aspect (Fig. 5).

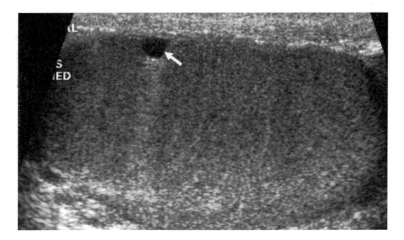

FIGURE 5. Surgically confirmed tunica albuginea cyst. The longitudinal sonogram demonstrates a cyst (*arrow*) arising from tunica albuginea in the upper anterior aspect of the testis with posterior acoustic enhancement.

33. What is an epidermoid cyst of the testis?

An epidermoid cyst is a benign intratesticular cyst that may be palpable. The sonographic appearance of epidermoid cyst varies with the maturation, compactness, and quantity of keratin present within the epidermoid cyst. The classic appearance is that of an "onion-ring" pattern with alternating layers of hyperechogenicity and hypoechogenicity. This onion-ring pattern is characteristic of an epidermoid cyst and corresponds to its natural evolution (Fig. 6).

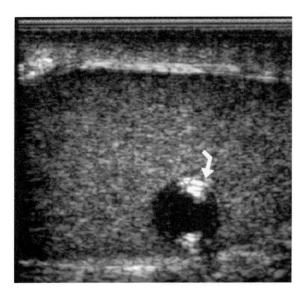

FIGURE 6. Surgically confirmed epidermoid cyst. The longitudinal sonogram demonstrates an intratesticular lesion with classic onion-ring pattern (*arrow*). (From Dogra VS, Gottlieb RH, Rubens DJ, Liao L: Benign intratesticular cystic lesions: US features. Radiographics 21:S273-S281, 2001, with permission.)

34. Describe simple testicular cysts.

Simple cysts of testis occur adjacent to the mediastinum and measure approximately 2 mm to 2 cm. They meet all the criteria of a simple cyst.

35. What do intratesticular varicoceles look like?

These have the same features as extratesticular varicoceles except where they occur. They fill up with color Doppler and demonstrate positive findings on Valsalva maneuver.

36. Describe the difference between spermatocele and epididymal cyst.

Both are benign cysts. The **spermatocele** occurs only in the head of the epididymis and contains spermatozoa. **Epididymal cysts** can occur in any part of the epididymis including body and tail.

TESTICULAR TUMORS

37. What are germ cell tumors?

Ninety percent to 95% of testicular tumors are derived from germ cells. They can be seminomatous or nonseminomatous.

38. Describe the features of seminomatous tumors.

Seminoma is the most common germ cell tumor affecting men in their 40s. The tumor marker alpha fetoprotein is always negative in these patients; however, elevated beta human chorionic gonadotropin may be present. Sonographically this tumor is hypoechoic and usually well circumscribed. Seminomas are usually confined by the tunica albuginea and rarely extend to the paratesticular structures. Lymphatic spread to retroperitoneal lymph nodes and hematogenous metastasis to lungs, brain, or both are present in about 25% of patients at the time of presentation.

39. What are some nonseminomatous tumors?

- Embryonal cell carcinoma
- Yolk sac tumor
- Choriocarcinoma
- Teratoma

40. What is a "burned out" tumor?

A burned out tumor occurs secondary to rapid tumor growth, resulting in the tumor outstripping its blood supply and in subsequent tumor regression. The sonographic appearance ranges from small echogenic foci to a relatively hypoechoic mass. In some cases, only retroperitoneal lymphadenopathy is seen and no testicular tumor is identified. These burned out tumors can calcify.

41. What are the sonographic findings in testicular lymphoma?

Testicular lymphoma is the most common tumor in men older than age 50 years. It can be bilateral in about 20% of cases. The testis is enlarged and reveals increased vascularity on color Doppler examination. Grayscale sonography shows a homogeneously hypoechoic testis or multifocal hypoechoic lesions of various sizes. Striated hypoechoic bands with parallel hyperechoic lines radiating peripherally from the mediastinum testis have also been described.

42. What is an adenomatoid tumor?

This benign tumor of the epididymis has variable echo texture on sonography (Fig. 7).

TESTICULAR TRAUMA

43. Describe the sonographic findings in testicular trauma.

- Interruption of tunica albuginea
- Heterogeneous testis with irregular borders
- Hematocele
- Direct visualization of fracture line (rare) in 17% of cases
- Interruption of tunica vasculosa (diagnostic)

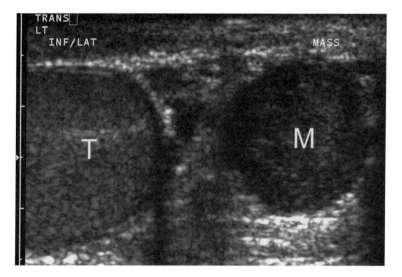

FIGURE 7. Surgically proven adenomatoid tumor. The transverse sonogram demonstrates an extratesticular hypoechoic mass (*M*) at lower pole of the testis (*T*). At surgery this mass was seen arising from the tail of the epididymis.

44. What percentage of a testis can be salvaged?

More than 80% of a ruptured testis can be saved if surgery is performed within 72 hours.

45. What percentage of tumors are brought to attention as a result of trauma?

Ten percent to 15% of testicular tumors first present after an episode of scrotal trauma. Therefore, all intratesticular abnormalities should be followed up if no surgical intervention is performed so that these tumors are not missed.

MISCELLANEOUS CONDITIONS

46. What is cryptorchidism?

Cryptorchidism is defined as complete or partial failure of the intra-abdominal testes to descend into the scrotal sac.

47. What are the common locations of undescended testes?

The most common location of an undescended testis is in the inguinal canal, followed by prescrotal and abdominal locations.

48. What is the sonographic appearance of an undescended testis?

The undescended testis is generally smaller and less echogenic than the normal testis.

49. What are the complications of cryptorchidism?

The major complications of cryptorchidism are malignant degeneration, infertility, and torsion.

50. What tumor is more common in cryptorchid testis?

Seminoma is more common with an 8–10% increase in its incidence.

51. Does orchiopexy change the incidence of malignant degeneration in a cryptorchid testis?

No. Orchiopexy does not change the risk of malignant degeneration of the once cryptorchid testis.

52. What is testicular microlithiasis (TM)?

TM is an uncommon condition, usually brought to attention when some other condition is being investigated. It is usually bilateral, asymmetric, and characterized by small, echogenic, non-shadowing foci scattered throughout the testis. Five or more foci per transducer field are required to make the diagnosis of TM (Fig. 8).

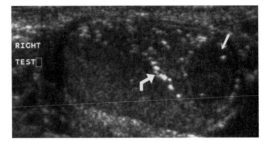

FIGURE 8. Testicular microlithiasis. The longitudinal sonogram shows multiple echogenic foci (*curved arrow*), with no posterior acoustic shadowing. The straight arrow points to a hypoechoic lesion, which was confirmed to be a seminoma after surgery.

53. Is TM a premalignant condition?

No. However, high association with malignancy has been reported.

54. Describe other conditions with which TM is associated.

Associations of TM with cryptorchidism, Klinefelter syndrome, infertility, male pseudohermaphroditism, and pulmonary alveolar microlithiasis have been reported.

55. Describe a primary varicocele.

Varicocele is an abnormal dilatation of the veins of the spermatic cord and is usually caused by incompetent valves in the internal spermatic vein. It is seen in 15% of men between 15 and 25 years of age.

56. Is there a relationship between infertility and varicocele?

The relationship between infertility and varicocele is controversial. Treatment of varicocele does result in improved sperm quality.

57. Describe the sonographic appearance of varicocele.

The sonographic appearance of varicocele consists of multiple, hypoechoic, serpiginous, and tubular structures of varying sizes > 2 mm in diameter.

58. What is a secondary varicocele?

Secondary varicoceles result from increased pressure on the spermatic vein produced by disease processes such as abdominal neoplasm. Neoplasm is the most likely cause of nondecompressible varicocele in men older than 40 years.

59. What is Fournier's gangrene?

It is a true urologic emergency. It is a polymicrobial infection, usually seen in diabetics manifesting as acute necrotizing fasciitis. This involves the perineum, and the scrotal and anterior abdominal wall. The testis and epididymis are usually spared because they have separate blood supply. These patients have a strong feculent odor that is characteristic of this disease. Crepitus is the hallmark of this disease. The crepitus (air) can be identified by ultrasound, computed tomography, or plain film.

BIBLIOGRAPHY

1. Bree RL, Hoang DT: Scrotal ultrasound. Radiol Clin North Am 34:1183–1205, 1996.
2. Dogra VS, Gottlieb RH, Oka M, Rubens DJ: Sonography of the scrotum. Radiology 227:18–36, 2003.
3. Dogra VS, Gottlieb RH, Rubens DJ, Liao L: Benign intratesticular cystic lesions: US features. Radiographics 21:S273-S281, 2001.
4. Dogra VS, Gottlieb RH, Rubens DJ, et al: Testicular epidermoid cysts: Sonographic features with histopathologic correlation. J Clin Ultrasound 29:192–196, 2001.
5. Horstman WG: Scrotal imaging. Urol Clin North Am 24:653–671, 1997.

28. THYROID, PARATHYROID, AND NECK LYMPH NODES

Patrick J. Fultz, M.D., and Jodie C. Crowley, B.S., RDMS

1. What are the indications for thyroid ultrasound?

These include but are not limited to:

- Diffuse enlargement on physical examination
- A palpable mass
- A nonpalpable mass seen on other imaging modality (computed tomography [CT] or magnetic resonance imaging [MRI])
- Nodule seen on nuclear medicine scan
- Abnormal thyroid function tests

2. Where is the thyroid in relation to other neck structures?

Two major vessels in the neck are used as landmarks for finding the thyroid. The thyroid is between the right and left common carotid arteries. The more lateral vessel next to the common carotid arteries are the internal jugular veins. The thyroid isthmus overlies the trachea.

NORMAL ANATOMY

- Location: See Figure 1.
- Appearance: echogenicity greater than strap muscles, very uniform, normal vessels may be seen (especially in lower poles).

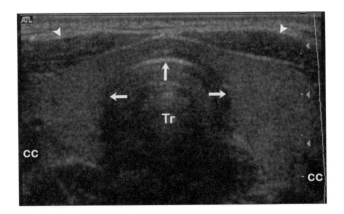

FIGURE 1. Normal thyroid. Transverse ultrasound image of normal thyroid (*arrows*) at level of isthmus. Note the relatively greater echogenicity of the thyroid with respect to adjacent muscles (*arrowheads*). CC, common carotid arteries; Tr, trachea.

3. What transducer is used for thyroid imaging?

- A linear array transducer is best, preferably with a vector format.
- The frequency should be at least 7 MHz or higher.
- For larger glands, one may need a larger field of view (wide), so a linear array with vector format or curved linear array probe is used.

4. How does one scan the thyroid?

Position the patient to best see the thyroid:

- Supine position
- No pillow
- Rolled towel behind neck with chin up to extend neck. *Do not hyperextend the neck.*

Turn the patient's head to left and right to see lower poles and substernal area. Angle down below the sternum or clavicle with a sector transducer.

Full sweeps of the thyroid should be done starting in the transverse plane. Begin midline transverse over the isthmus. Next, scan from superior to inferior on both the right and left lobes. Measurements should be taken at the middle portion of the thyroid. Longitudinal images of the right and left lobes, from lateral to medial, should be obtained next, again with measurements taken at the middle portion of each thyroid lobe.

5. What can be done to obtain an image of the whole length of the thyroid when it does not fit on the screen with a linear transducer?

With a linear array transducer, there is a split screen option, but this is accompanied by a large potential for error. To reduce this error, choose an area in the thyroid (e.g., a nodule or cyst) or an area outside the thyroid (e.g., muscle) that can be easily identified and matched.

One could also use a high-frequency curved transducer. A small footprint/high-frequency transducer is best because it fits on the neck.

6. Can harmonics help to visualize the thyroid?

Yes, but look at the thyroid without harmonics also. Some nodules are found with harmonics, but the image quality and sharpness of borders can decrease.

7. How can color Doppler help differentiate a cyst from solid thyroid lesion?

Color Doppler is a great tool to help differentiate between cystic and solid lesions in the thyroid. A purely cystic lesion does not have color flow. Color gain and other settings must be optimized correctly. A solid lesion can have a lot or a little color flow.

8. What is determined by a nuclear medicine scan of the thyroid?

Nuclear medicine scans of the thyroid are performed with various radiopharmaceuticals for a variety of purposes. These studies can be used to assist in evaluation of thyroid function and give information about whether nodules felt or seen in the thyroid are "hot" (hyperactive) or "cold" (hypoactive). Cold nodules have less uptake than the surrounding thyroid tissue, whereas hot nodules have greater uptake than the surrounding tissue.

Cold nodules have a 20% incidence of malignancy and generally need to be biopsied. Hot nodules are rarely involved by malignancy.

9. What are the various common types of generalized thyroid enlargement? Do they have distinguishing features on ultrasound?

Typically, the patient's clinical history and thyroid function chemistries help distinguish among conditions causing thyroid enlargement.

- Graves' disease (normal echogenicity with enlarged gland)
- Hashimoto's (hypoechoic, coarse heterogeneous echotexture; Fig. 2)
- Multinodular goiter (multiple nodules, often a combination of solid, cystic, and mixed solid and cystic nodules; Fig. 3)

10. What does a multinodular goiter look like on ultrasound?

Multinodular goiter can be difficult to scan and the split screen imaging function may be helpful (*see* Fig. 3). Multiple nodules on both sides can be simple to complex cystic and solid nodules. The most effective way to document these is to show the largest in each of the superior, mid, and inferior portions. It can be difficult to see normal thyroid tissue under these circumstances.

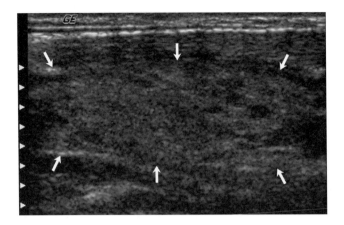

FIGURE 2. Hashimoto's thyroiditis. Longitudinal ultrasound image of right lobe in Hashimoto's thyroiditis. Note convex contours (*arrows*) of the hetergeneous gland with ill-defined nodular areas.

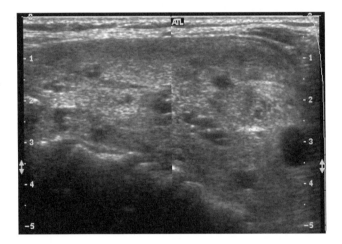

FIGURE 3. Multinodular goiter. Longitudinal dual image ultrasound of right lobe of a multinodular goiter. These nodules were a combination of solid, cystic, and mixed solid and cystic nodules.

11. What are the features of benign thyroid nodules?

There is no definite way to know whether a thyroid nodule is benign or not without a tissue sample. Colloid cysts are one of the most common types of benign thyroid nodules (Fig. 4). The more common characteristics of benign nodules are:

- Completely or nearly completely cystic, especially with echogenic foci with comet tail artifact
- Isoechoic to normal tissue
- A thin halo
- Well-described margin
- Rim calcifications

12. What are the features of malignant thyroid nodules?

Several sonographic features are seen more commonly in malignant thyroid nodules (Fig. 5):

- Microcalcifications with or without shadow

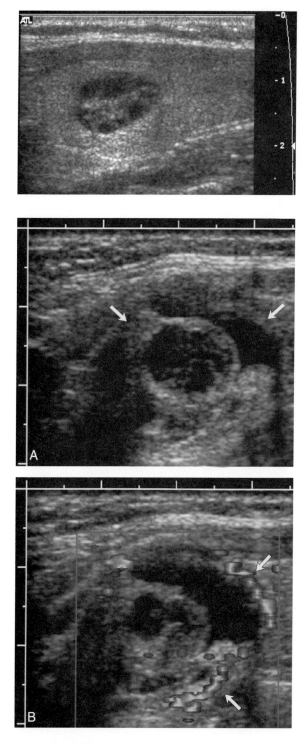

FIGURE 4. Colloid cyst. Longitudinal ultrasound image of left lobe reveals a mixed cystic and solid lesion, suggestive of a colloid cyst.

FIGURE 5. Papillary thyroid cancer. *A*, A longitudinal ultrasound image of cystic and solid thyroid cancer (*arrows*). *B*, Color Doppler imaging shows its hypervascular margin (*arrows*).

- Irregular or microlobulated margins
- Marked hypoechogenicity (with respect to background thyroid tissue)
- Taller than wide (this may indicate invasion into surrounding tissue)
- Hypervascularity

13. Does calcification in the thyroid lesion indicate it is benign or malignant?

This depends on the type of calcification. Large calcifications (> 2 mm) and rimlike calcifications are generally benign. Punctate calcifications are associated with malignancy, particularly papillary and medullary carcinoma. *Pitfall:* Cystic lesions with echogenic foci having a comet tail artifact can mimic calcifications. These foci usually indicate the lesion is a benign colloid cyst.

14. What is done for a patient with palpable thyroid nodules?

Generally, a history, physical examination, and thyroid function chemistries are initially done. Most palpable nodules can be needle biopsied with palpation guidance. Sometimes, nuclear medicine imaging or ultrasound is used, depending on results of the initial clinical evaluation.

15. What is done with an incidental (occult) nonpalpable thyroid nodule discovered by ultrasound, CT, or MRI performed for other reasons?

Most authorities agree that evaluation should include clinical history, physical examination, and thyroid function chemistries. Ultrasound-guided sampling of lesions ≥ 1.5 cm is usually recommended. For smaller nodules, sampling is sometimes recommended when there are risk factors for thyroid cancer (e.g., prior neck radiation) or the nodules have malignant features by ultrasound. Otherwise, small nodules can be followed by ultrasound or by serial palpation examination for interval growth.

16. What are some other lesions that may involve the thyroid?

- Metastases (e.g., lung cancer, renal cancers)
- Lymphoma

17. Where is the esophagus in relation to the thyroid and what can it be mistaken for?

The esophagus is situated midline and to the left in the neck (Fig. 6). In the transverse plane, it has a target appearance similar to other parts of the bowel and should move with swallowing. This should prevent it from being mistaken for an enlarged parathyroid gland.

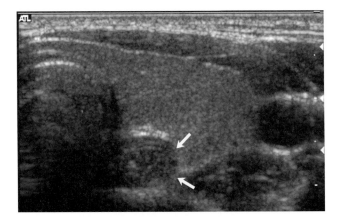

FIGURE 6. Esophagus mimicking a lesion. Transverse ultrasound image shows cervical esophagus (*arrows*) in its typical location on the left side. Note the esophageal wall layers.

18. What are the indications for parathyroid ultrasound?

Primarily it is to search for enlarged parathyroids (usually adenomas or hyperplasia) in patients with clinical evidence of hyperparathyroidism.

In addition, nuclear medicine parathyroid scans are sometimes used. CT or MRI may also be needed when there is a concern for parathyroid lesions (especially for lesions in ectopic glands).

19. Where are the parathyroids?

The parathyroids are usually located near the posterior thyroid margin, typically with two on each side. Usually it is the abnormal parathyroids that are seen with ultrasound. They can also be ectopic and lie anywhere in the anterior neck and even inside the chest.

20. How do parathyroids look on ultrasound?

Normal size is less than 6 mm. Echotexture is typically hypoechoic to isoechoic with respect to the thyroid. Their shape is elliptical, with greatest dimension craniocaudad. Abnormal parathyroids (adenomas and hyperplasia) tend to be hypoechoic and hypervascular on color Doppler imaging (Fig. 7).

21. How does one scan for parathyroids?

Scan transverse and longitudinal along the thyroid, beginning above the thyroid at the level of the mandible and inferiorly to angle down below the level of the clavicle. Search carefully in the tracheoesophgeal groove by turning the patient's head to the opposite side, angling in from a lateral approach, and having the patient swallow to identify the esophagus.

22. Where does one look for neck lymph nodes?

To look for lymph nodes, place the patient in the standard position for scanning the thyroid. Scan up and down the neck lateral to the common carotid arteries and internal jugular veins and laterally from the clavicle to the acromioclavicular joint. Most nodes are found in this area. Angle down in the supraclavicular fossa and medially to detect supraclavicular or infraclavicular lymph nodes.

23. What is the appearance of a normal lymph node?
- Size: less than 7 mm in short axis; less than 10 mm in long axis (except the jugulodigastric node, which can normally be up to 15 mm in long axis)
- Shape: generally "flat"; length-to-width ratio often ≥ 2:1
- Appearance: echogenic with convex "fatty" hilum and thin hypoechoic cortex

24. What do abnormal nodes look like?
- Size: generally ≥ 10 mm in length and ≥ 7 mm in short axis, with anteroposterior dimension approximately equal to length
- Appearance: often lacking echogenic hilum or with necrotic areas and possibly calcifications

25. What disease processes can present with lymph nodes in the neck?
- Infection
- Sarcoidosis
- Lymphoma
- Metastases from head and neck tumors (including thyroid cancer), or chest (Fig. 8), adrenal, or pelvic tumors

26. What are the size criteria for biopsying a neck node?

Various criteria have been proposed, but a good rule of thumb is to biopsy a known head and neck or chest primary malignancy that is ≥ 7 mm in short axis or ≥ 10 mm in long axis.

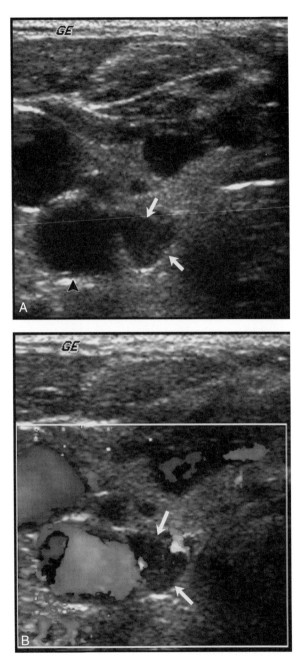

FIGURE 7. Parathyroid adenoma. *A,* Transverse ultrasound image of a hypoechoic parathyroid lesion (*arrows*) at the right thyroid lobe margin next to the right common carotid artery (*arrowhead*). *B,* Color Doppler image shows the typical hypervascular appearance of the parathyroid lesion (see also Color Plates, Figure 13).

27. **What other lesions can be found in the neck?**

Congenital lesions:

- Branchial cleft cyst
- Cystic hygroma
- Thyroglossal duct cyst

Miscellaneous lesions: Any structure in the neck can be a primary site for other types of tumors, such as the esophagus, trachea, muscles, connective tissues, bones, and nerves.

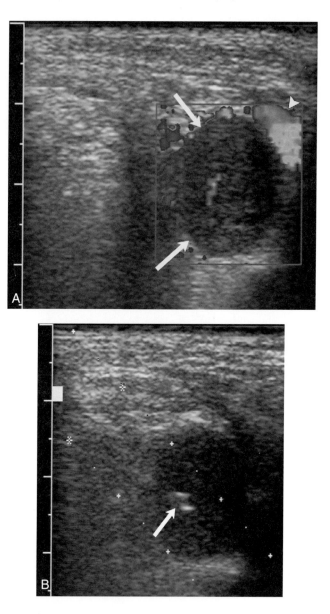

FIGURE 8. Lung cancer metastasis to supraclavicular lymph node. *A,* Transverse ultrasound image with color Doppler showing the enlarged lymph node (*arrows*) and adjacent right internal jugular vein (*arrowhead*). *B,* Ultrasound-guided needle biopsy (arrow on needle tip, which is only 2.5 cm from skin surface) yielded the diagnosis of metastatic lung cancer.

BIBLIOGRAPHY

1. Ahuja A, Chick W, King W, Metreweli C: Clinical significance of the comet-tail artifact in thyroid ultrasound. J Clin Ultrasound 24:129–133, 1996.
2. Bennedbaek FN, Hegedus L: Management of the solitary thyroid nodule: Results of a North American Survey. J Clin Endocrinol Metab 85:2493–2498, 2000.

3. Feld S: AACE Clinical practice guidelines for the diagnosis and management of thyroid nodules. Endocrine Prac 2:80–84, 1996.
4. Fultz PJ, Feins RH, Strang JC, et al: Detection and diagnosis of nonpalpable supraclavicular lymph nodes in lung cancer at CT and US. Radiology 222:245–251, 2002.
5. Kim EK, Park CS, Chung WY, et al: New sonographic criteria for recommending fine-needle aspiration biopsy of nonpalpable solid nodules of the thyroid. AJR Am J Roentgenol 178:687–691, 2002.
6. Tan GH, Gharib H: Thyroid incidentalomas: Management approaches to nonpalpable nodules discovered incidentally on thyroid imaging. Ann Intern Med 26:226–331, 1997.
7. Charboneau JW, James EM, Hay ID: The thyroid gland. In Rumack CM, Wilson SR, Charboneau JW (eds): Diagnostic Ultrasound, vol 1, 2nd ed. St. Louis, Mosby, 1998, pp 703–729.

29. BREAST SONOGRAPHY

Jeanne A. Cullinan, M.D.

1. When should breast sonography be performed?

The examination is performed in the assessment of an indeterminate abnormality identified on a mammogram. It is also used to evaluate palpable abnormalities to further characterize these lesions.

2. Who should have breast ultrasound?

Classic teaching is that ultrasound is used only for the evaluation of masses to determine whether they are solid or cystic. Recent work suggests an expansion of this role to include characterization of solid masses.

3. Is there a role for screening ultrasound?

Classic teaching is that screening ultrasound should not be performed. Recent articles suggest that given the decrease in mammographic sensitivity with increasing breast density, ultrasound might increase the detection of small cancers. This must be taken in the context of the potential for an increase in biopsies for benign disease. Recent investigations report that the cancer detection rate with whole breast ultrasound compares favorably to that of screening mammography.

4. Does ultrasound have a Breast Imaging Reporting and Data System (BIRADS) classification similar to mammography?

At present, there is no standard classification system, but it is anticipated that a system will be implemented.

5. Is there any standard for breast sonography?

The American College of Radiology has published standards for quality breast ultrasound evaluation. Attention to these standards is critical. Recent work suggests that a significant number of cases do not comply with these standards, which may result in an interpretation error or discrepancy.

6. What is the acoustic appearance of breast tissue?

Fat has a low acoustic impedance with the highest acoustic impedance seen in connective tissue. Glandular tissue as well as most tumors are of medium acoustic impedance.

7. How is the examination performed?

A high-frequency probe with color Doppler sonography, and possibly harmonics and compound imaging, is useful for evaluation of the breast. A dedicated focal zone is required for attention to the internal characteristics of these lesions.

8. How can one ensure that the ultrasound findings correlate with the mammogram?

Because findings are operator-dependent, it is critical to pay close attention to detail. The position of the mammogram must be mimicked. It is important to note the "o'clock" position as well as the distance from the nipple to the mass. One question is whether the lesion is concordant with the mammographic findings to determine whether the true lesion has been identified. The masses must be examined in all planes and a plan for follow-up determined based on the mammographic and sonographic findings.

9. Why do an ultrasound if the mass is palpable?

Ultrasound imaging allows better definition of the nature of the palpable mass and potentially detects second lesions.

10. What are some of the findings seen in benign masses?

Sonographic findings include a homogeneous circumscribed mass. It is usually hypoechoic and may have a thin, echogenic pseudocapsule. A few gentle lobulations may be seen.

11. What are the characteristic sonographic findings of the malignant mass?

The mass is irregular, angular, or micolobulated. It is often ill defined with spicules, with direct extension into surrounding tissue. It is often taller than wide. It may be hypoechoic with distal shadowing and punctate calcifications.

12. What are the sonographic findings of common breast lesions?

Cysts: A cyst appears as a circumscribed mass. It is anechoic with well-defined walls and through transmission. Given the improved resolution of the high-frequency probes, some cysts may be identified that have low-level echoes within them. A cluster of spongelike cysts is of concern and ultrasound core biopsy is recommended (Fig. 1).

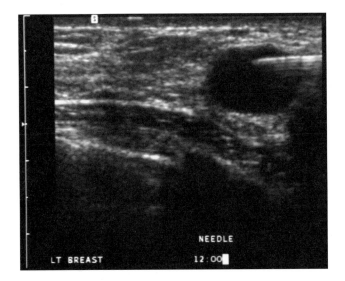

FIGURE 1. Cyst. An anechoic mass is seen. The tip of a needle is seen entering the mass before aspiration.

Infection: There is skin thickening with focal edema and hypoechoic areas coursing through the area of concern. A focal abscess may be identified. Ultrasound is useful for evaluating the infection as well as guiding therapy or intervention. Follow-up is mandatory to rule out the possibility of an inflammatory breast carcinoma.

Fibroadenoma: Classically, a fibroadenoma is longer than it is tall. The lesion has smooth borders and is of mixed echogenicity. More complex masses may require a biopsy to determine their benignity (Fig. 2).

Papilloma: The clinical finding is a bloody nipple discharge. Mammography is often nonspecific, although ductography is usually diagnostic. Alternatively, ultrasound can be performed to demonstrate the presence of a dilated duct with a solid intraductal mass (Fig. 3).

Galactocele: This finding is seen in the context of a lactating patient. The ultrasound findings are often that of a complex mass or a mass with a "ground glass" matrix.

Lymph nodes: A normal lymph node can be seen in the intramammary tissue as well as in the axillary tail. In general, they are hypoechoic with a characteristic echogenic fatty hilum (Fig. 4).

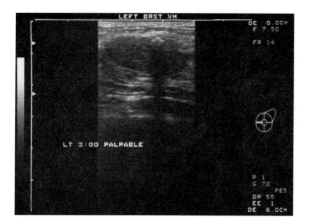

FIGURE 2. Fibroadenoma. An ovoid hypoechoic mass is identified. A coarse echogenic focus, which is the sonographic equivalent to a "popcorn" calcification, is seen along the superior edge of the mass.

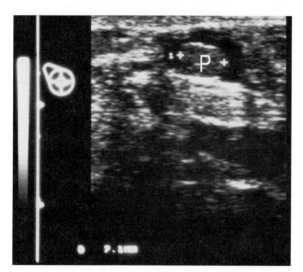

FIGURE 3. Papilloma. A hypoechoic mass is seen within a dilated duct.

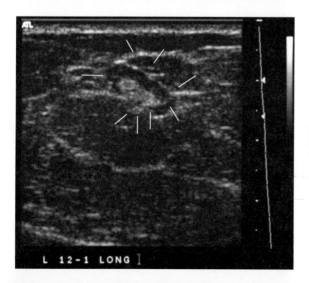

FIGURE 4. Lymph node. A hypoechoic kidney bean–shaped structure with an echogenic hilum is seen.

Fibrocystic changes: Ultrasound is usually not diagnostic in patients with fibrocystic changes. There may be an ill-defined mass or calcifications identified. The mammographic findings are superior in the evaluation of this process.

Breast cancer: The characteristic finding is that of a mass, which is taller than it is wide. The mass has irregular, angular tissue planes. It may demonstrate posterior shadowing and microlobulation. Some breast cancers are small, round, circumscribed, hypoechoic lesions and should not be confused with a cyst. If there is any doubt, biopsy is recommended (Fig. 5).

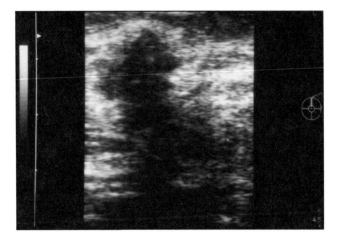

FIGURE 5. Cancer. An irregular hypoechoic mass with shadowing is identified.

13. Can the type of cancer be differentiated?

In general, ductal carcinoma in situ does not present with sonographic findings, although there are patients in whom a focal mass is demonstrated. Invasive ductal carcinoma is seen with the characteristic findings described.

Special cell-type tumors show similar sonographic findings to ductal carcinoma. The differentiation is best performed by pathology.

14. Can ultrasound be used to evaluate ductal carcinoma in situ?

Although some articles report the detection of calcifications on high-resolution sonography, the current recommendation is that ductal carcinoma in situ is best evaluated by mammography.

15. Can lesions be biopsied under ultrasound?

Ultrasound is an excellent tool for the assessment and evaluation of breast masses. Both spring-loaded and vacuum system devices are used with ultrasound. The technique involves placing the needle along the long axis of the transducer, parallel to the chest wall, with the needle placed just proximal to the lesion. Multiple core samples are obtained. The placement of the needle through the mass should be documented.

16. Can wire placement be done.

The technique is useful in patients in whom the mammographic findings may be subtle. The lesion is targeted. The needle with the wire is placed beyond the mass in question. Post-procedure mammograms are performed to assist the surgeon with spatial orientation in the operating room.

17. What is the major strength of ultrasound in breast sonography?
Ultrasound remains a valuable adjunctive tool to mammography. Its major strength is that it may convert a nondiagnostic mammographic examination into a diagnostic examination. One of the pitfalls is its limitation in the evaluation of calcifications.

BIBLIOGRAPHY

1. Baker JA, Soo MS: Breast US: Assessment of technical quality and image interpretation. Radiology 223:229–238, 2002.
2. Bassett LW: Imaging of breast masses. Radiol Clin North Am 38:669–691, 2000.
3. Kaplan SS: Clinical utility of bilateral-whole breast US in the evaluation of women with dense breast tissue. Radiology 221:641–649, 2001.
4. Kolb TM, Lichy J, Newhouse JH: Comparison of the performance of screening mammography, physical examination, and breast ultrasound and evaluation of factors that influence them: An analysis of 27,825 patient evaluations. Radiology 225:165–175, 2002.
5. Massengale JC, Brem RF: Use of ultrasound in breast disease. Ultrasound Q 18:149–159, 2002.
6. Moon WK, Myung JS, Lee YJ, et al: US of ductal carcinoma in situ. Radiographics 22:269–281, 2002.
7. Teboul M, Halliwell M: Atlas of ultrasound and ductal echography of the breast. The introduction of anatomic intelligence into breast imaging. Cambridge, MA, Blackwell Science, 1995.

30. ULTRASOUND-GUIDED BIOPSY

Deborah J. Rubens, M.D.

1. What are the factors in deciding to perform ultrasound-guided biopsies?
- The patient must be cooperative.
- There should be no undue risks to biopsy.
- The lesion should be accessible by ultrasound.

2. What are the advantages and disadvantages of ultrasound for biopsy compared to computed tomography (CT)?
In general, if you can see it by ultrasound, biopsy it by ultrasound. Ultrasound is done in real time, so the needle can be manipulated so that the target and needle are seen simultaneously. This makes each pass much faster; for abdominal biopsies, it is less than a breath-hold. Ultrasound allows one to choose the best plane or angle for entry, allowing double oblique approaches, which are difficult by CT. The disadvantages include limited ultrasound visualization through air (bowel gas, lungs) and bone. Ultrasound may not identify lesions discovered by CT or magnetic resonance imaging (MRI). Ultrasound may not visualize complications of biopsy.

3. What is required for patient cooperation?
The patient must be able to hold still, follow directions, and hold his or her breath. Anesthesia is generally used for severely mentally retarded patients or very young patients. For older children, deep conscious sedation with anesthesia standby is preferred. Most biopsies can be performed with local anesthesia, including anesthesia of the liver capsule or renal capsule. For patients who are apprehensive, a combination of analgesic and amnestic is used, commonly midazolam (Versed) and fentanyl.

4. Is consent important?
Yes. Patients should be assessed for consentability. If the patient cannot sign an informed consent, then consent must be obtained from a responsible guardian or a two-physician consent must be obtained.

5. What coagulation parameters are required and in which instances?
Coagulation parameters are required for all intrathoracic, intra-abdominal, and intrapelvic procedures. Prothrombin time (PT), partial thromboplastin time (PTT), platelet counts, and international normalized ratio (INR) should be drawn within the past month and more recently for patients with coagulopathies. A bleeding time measurement is recommended for patients coming off ticlopidine (Ticlid) or pentoxifylline (Trental).

6. What common medication history should be obtained and how long should medication be withheld?
- Lovenox (enoxaparin)—off for 24 hours
- Coumadin (warfarin)—usually discontinue for several days with PT rechecked
- Aspirin products—off for 1 week
- Persantine (dipyridamole)—off at least 7 days
- Nonsteroidal anti-inflammatory drugs (NSAIDs) (ibuprofen, Motrin, Advil, Aleve, naprosyn)—off at least 2 days
- Plavix (clopidogrel)—off at least 7 days
- Heparin—off 6 hours, then recheck INR, PTT
- Ticlid (ticlopidine)—off at least 7 days and check bleeding time on day 7
- Trental (pentoxifylline)—off at least 7 days and check bleeding time on day 7

- Screen for any other blood thinners
- Patients can take Celebrex (celecoxib) or Vioxx (rofecoxib)

7. When are coagulation studies not required?

Coagulation parameters are not required for superficial biopsies of superficial lymph nodes, thyroid, chest, abdominal wall, or extremity lesions. However, patients should be screened for medications and coagulopathies; the guidelines for those medications should be followed for any elective biopsy.

8. How are coagulation abnormalities corrected?

For an INR > 1.5 but < 2, the patient receives 2 units of fresh frozen plasma during the procedure. For an INR > 2, the patient receives 2 units of fresh-frozen plasma and then the INR is rechecked. Patients are transfused with two 5-packs of platelets when the platelet count is less than 50,000, immediately before the procedure and during it.

9. How can a lesion be biopsied when it is not easily seen by ultrasound?

Some lesions seen on CT or MRI are not readily visible by ultrasound; however, if anatomic landmarks such as portal vein, gallbladder, or hepatic veins can be used to localize the area for biopsy, then biopsy can still be performed. With the advent of ultrasound contrast material, lesions that had once only been visible on CT and MRI can now be seen with ultrasound during arterial phase imaging. Color Doppler can be used to identify abnormal areas for biopsy, particularly in the liver. Abnormal hepatic arterial flow indicates an area of tumor that may be diffusely infiltrating and invisible on grayscale alone.

10. What real-time lesion features are important to assess?

The lesions should be assessed for involuntary motion. Check for respiratory motion and also pulsatility if the lesion is near the heart. If the lesion is in an organ that moves or is in mobile tissue, such as breast tissue, it may be difficult to biopsy.

11. How small a lesion can be biopsied?

The size of the lesion is inversely proportional to depth. Very superficial small lesions can be biopsied, as small as 5-mm nodules in the thyroid or 7-mm lymph nodes in the neck; however, when these are attempted in a deeper organ with motion, such as the liver, small size biopsies can be nearly impossible. Whereas a superficial 1-cm lesion in the liver may be successfully biopsied, biopsying that same size lesion at a 10-cm depth is usually unsuccessful due to motion and bending of the needle.

12. What issues should be addressed regarding patient and transducer position?

- Can the patient be positioned adequately for the biopsy?
- Will there be bones, bowel, or other organs in the pathway?
- Will there be vessels in the pathway (color Doppler)?
- Can an alternate pathway be selected by changing transducer position, that is, by going from inferior to superior rather than right to left, or using an oblique path?
- In patients who cannot lie flat, can the biopsy be performed with the patient sitting up or lying on his or her side?

13. What are the major biopsy risks?

Bleeding and infection are the major biopsy risks. For bleeding, use color Doppler to identify any vessels that may cross the biopsy path en route to the target. Adjust needle position and orientation to avoid these vessels. For infection, inadvertent puncture of dilated biliary ducts or entering a dilated renal pelvis may result in sepsis. If infection is suspected, the patient should be placed on prophylactic antibiotics. Patients should be questioned for any susceptibility to infection, including heart murmurs and heart prostheses. Such patients should be placed on prophylactic antibiotics as determined by their individual situation. Transrectal biopsy of the prostate requires a preparatory enema as well as pretreatment with antibiotics. We commonly use ciprofloxacin, 500 mg, for 3 days, every 12 hours, starting the night before the procedure.

14. How common is needle track seeding?

This is rare, with an estimated frequency of less than 0.01%. Most reported cases of needle track seeding have been from pancreatic carcinoma and carcinoma of the prostate, with isolated cases reported of liver, kidney, pleura, breast, and eye.

15. What transducer should be used?

Choose the smallest footprint that provides access to the lesion and a transducer frequency that is low enough to penetrate. In the abdomen and pelvis, we generally choose a small footprint phased-array transducer rather than a larger and more limited footprint, linear array, or curved linear probe because of its flexibility and multiple windows and because of the ease of changing from transverse to long axis. Linear arrays are more useful in the neck, breast, and extremities.

16. When is a guide useful?

Guides are generally advantageous for deep abdominal biopsies and biopsies in which repeat samples must be obtained. We always use guides with core liver and renal biopsies. We generally use guides for chest and deep abdominal liver, pancreatic, and lymph node biopsies. Guides are routinely chosen with transvaginal and transrectal biopsies. Freehand biopsy is sometimes easier for small superficial lesions including breast. Thyroid nodules tend to be mobile and, therefore, we tend to use a guide. Deep lymph node cores are also better sampled with a guide.

17. Which type of needle should be used?

Needle choice depends on the pathologist's needs. Fine needle aspiration (FNA), which is evaluated by cytologic analysis, is usually preferred for evaluation of primary lung cancers, primary carcinomas, including pancreas, and any suspected metastases from carcinoma. Core biopsy, which provides tissue for histology, is performed for all liver or renal transplant evaluation, liver biopsy for cirrhosis or hemochromatosis, and any suspected lymphoma or sarcoma.

18. What needle is used for FNA?

A 22-gauge Chiba needle is used for most deep abdominal biopsies. We generally use coated needles for better visibility. For more superficial biopsies (< 10-cm needle required), we use spinal needles because they are less expensive. For thyroid aspiration, a 23- or 25-gauge needle can help reduce bloody samples. For liver or deep abdominal biopsies, 20-gauge needles are stiffer and track better for deep lesions, whereas a 22-gauge needle may bend.

19. How can needle tip visualization be improved?

- Turn the bevel up to improve scattering.
- Use etched or coated needles.
- Pump the inner stylet up and down within the needle. This moves gas inside the needle and improves needle contrast.
- Use color Doppler to detect tissue motion; however, the motion is often of the entire organ, not just the needle.

20. What needle size is used for core biopsies?

Eighteen-gauge core needles are sufficient for all except breast biopsy, for which our mammographers choose 14- or 11-gauge needles.

21. From what part of a lesion should a biopsy sample be obtained?

In general, blood is supplied to tumors from the periphery and biopsy is most viable there. We biopsy from the periphery of the lesion to avoid central necrosis (Fig. 1). For partially cystic

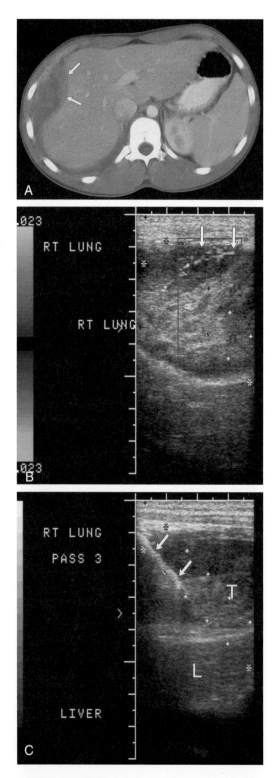

FIGURE 1. *A*, Lung biopsy. Computed tomography (CT) of a patient with a pleurally based mass indenting the liver (*arrows*) with peripheral enhancement. *B*, Ultrasound from a lateral approach shows a heterogeneous mass with peripheral vascularity (*arrows*) similar to CT. *C*, The 18-gauge core biopsy needle (*arrow*) is positioned in the peripheral (vascular) portion of the tumor (*T*), well away from the liver (*L*). Histopathology yielded metastatic Ewing's sarcoma.

and solid lesions, we biopsy the solid wall or nodule. If the cystic portion is encountered first, it is aspirated and the margin is biopsied on the second pass.

22. What are the indications for intraoperative brain ultrasound?

Ultrasound can be used to monitor deep biopsies with color Doppler to assess for bleeding that cannot be visualized from the surface or to permit biopsy through a smaller flap or burr hole.

Ultrasound also permits biopsy at angled approaches to avoid critical structures such as the motor strip or language centers. Brain mapping is performed with the patient awake, and ultrasound is used to angle around the critical areas into the area of the tumor.

23. How is a parotid biopsy performed?

Biopsy of the superficial portion of the parotid gland can be performed easily. This is generally an FNA biopsy for carcinoma. Color Doppler is used to identify the facial artery to avoid inadvertent biopsy of that artery or the adjacent facial nerve.

24. What are the diagnostic features of abnormal lymph nodes and what locations can be biopsied?

Abnormal lymph nodes are generally hypoechoic, round, and have lost their central echogenic hilum. Very small lymph nodes may be biopsied in the neck (Fig. 2). Nodes as small as 7 mm are biopsied in the supraclavicular region to obviate lung biopsy. As many as 25% of patients referred for supraclavicular node biopsy have their lung cancer diagnosed without a lung biopsy and have their cancer staged at the same time. Core biopsies are obtained for lymphoma. Additional sites include superficial neck, axillary, retroperitoneal, mesenteric, pelvic, and inguinal lymph nodes.

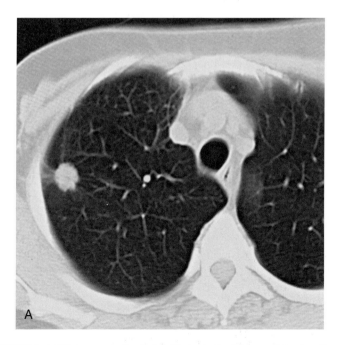

FIGURE 2. *A*, CT shows a small spiculated lesion in the right upper lobe. (*continued*)

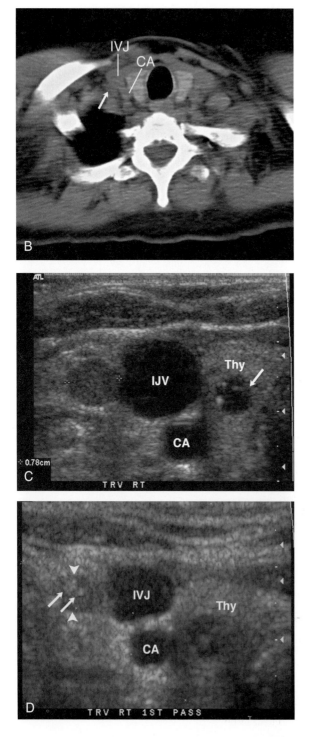

FIGURE 2. (*continued*) *B*, A small supraclavicular lymph node (*arrows*) behind the internal jugular vein (*IJV*) and the carotid artery (*CA*) suggests advanced disease. *C*, Transverse ultrasound image shows the 8-mm lymph node (*cursors*). A heterogeneous cystic mass (*arrow*) is incidentally noted in the thyroid (*Thy*). *D*, Transverse ultrasound imaging during biopsy with a 22-gauge needle (*arrows*). The needle samples the node (*arrowheads*) and the diagnosis was metastatic squamous cell carcinoma of the lung.

25. How is a thyroid biopsy performed?

A thyroid biopsy is performed with 22- to 25-gauge needles; spinal needles are adequate. Difficulties include avoiding the adjacent carotid and jugular vein. A guide is useful in that the thyroid is mobile, and with swallowing and breathing a freehand technique can be difficult unless the lesion is superficial. Other technical tips include the use of a long axis approach to help avoid vessels and an approach from lateral to medial to pin lesions against the trachea to decrease mobility, especially during aspiration.

26. What are the indications for mediastinal biopsy?

The usual request is to evaluate for lymphoma; therefore, a core biopsy is nearly always requested. As long as there is enough soft tissue lateral to the sternum (1 cm), a mediastinal biopsy can be performed. A fine needle biopsy is used for suspected metastatic carcinoma. Transducer choices include a sector with guide or endocavitary probes with endfire biopsy capability. Freehand biopsy can be performed with a small pediatric, 5- or 7-MHz footprint sector probe. Always identify the internal mammary arteries with color Doppler. Patient positioning can be supine, semierect, or upright (preferred for supraclavicular, superior mediastinum, and posterior mediastinal masses at the lung apex).

27. How can biopsy of pleural or parenchymal masses in the chest be obtained?

Be sure there is an adequate window between the ribs. Lung masses or pleural masses can be biopsied as long as there is enough contact with the pleural surface to ensure adequate visualization. FNA is generally sufficient, unless sarcoma is suspected, in which case core biopsy should be performed (*see* Fig. 1). Patients are frequently seated erect or leaning over a Mayo stand, unless the mass is anterior. Upright positioning permits access to the posterior and lateral chest and improves oxygenation in these patients who are frequently short of breath.

28. What are the general indications for liver biopsy?

- Cirrhosis evaluation (18 gauge, 2 cores)
- Transplant evaluation for rejection (18 gauge, 2 cores)
- Focal lesion evaluation (core biopsy for suspected hepatocellular carcinoma, FNA for all other lesions)

29. What are the general techniques for performing liver biopsy?

Frequently, better visualization of the liver can be obtained with a decubitus position. To perform a core biopsy (left lobe or subcostal right lobe), choose an approach that avoids major vessels, particularly portal veins. If hepatic veins are crossed, this is less of an issue.

Anesthetize the subcutaneous tissue and deep muscle as well as the liver capsule. Patients should be instructed for breath-holding during the procedure. Anesthesia of the liver capsule provides a practice run and helps ensure good localization. A subcostal approach avoids the pleural space; however, the intercostal approach is occasionally necessary for small cirrhotic livers or lesions near the dome.

30. What are the indications for renal biopsy?

- Renal transplant for rejection (18 guage, 2 cores)
- Native kidneys for disease etiology (18 guage, 2–3 cores)
- Localized and focal lesions: metastases, infection (FNA, 22 guage)

31. How is a renal biopsy performed?

Transplant and native biopsies for diffuse disease are performed in the lower pole. Choose a site without adjacent bowel. Localization can be performed in long axis or short axis (transverse). Choose a position that maximizes cortex that is in the outer 7 mm of the kidney rather than the medulla (Fig. 3). (The first 5–7 mm of the needle is dead space; be sure to allow for this when

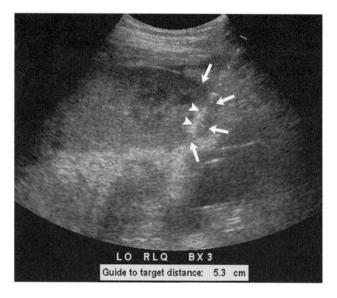

FIGURE 3. Renal transplant biopsy. The needle (*arrowheads*) passes peripherally through the lower pole (*arrows*) to obtain cortical tissue.

deciding when to fire the needle in relationship to the renal capsule.) Breath-holding is preferred for native kidney biopsy. Anesthesia is given subcutaneously and down to the renal capsule.

32. What are the indications and risks of pancreas biopsy?

Pancreatic biopsy is performed primarily for tumor diagnosis. The major risk is postbiopsy pancreatitis. A lesser risk is perforation of overlying bowel loops, leading to sepsis.

33. How is the pancreatic biopsy performed?

Use an FNA technique with local anesthesia. When biopsying for the head of the pancreas, multiple vessels need to be identified, including the superior mesenteric artery, superior mesenteric vein, and portal vein. With compression, bowel can usually be displaced or compressed so that it does not obscure access, and does not need to be transversed. A biopsy approach from inferior to superior generally avoids most vessels.

34. What is the differential diagnosis of cystic pancreatic masses and can it be determined by biopsy?

Pseudocyst, necrotic pancreatic carcinoma, and mucinous cystadenomas can be distinguished by high amylase content, columnar cells, and mucin, respectively.

35. Can adrenal biopsy be performed by ultrasound?

If the lesion can be well visualized, ultrasound-guided adrenal biopsy can be performed. Approach the adrenal posteriorly, with angling caudal to cephalad. Use a 22-gauge Chiba needle for FNA or a 20-gauge needle if a stiffer needle is needed. Adrenal biopsy is usually performed under CT due to limited visualization by ultrasound.

36. Which adrenal lesions should not be biopsied and why?

Benign lesions containing fat (myelolipomas) should be diagnosed by CT or MRI and require no biopsy. Similarly, adrenal cysts (usually post-traumatic pseudocysts) also require no biopsy. Pheochromocytoma biopsy may precipitate a hypertensive crisis. If pheochromocytoma is suspected, it should be established by laboratory testing, not by biopsy.

37. How are abdominal lymph node biopsies performed?

Retroperitoneal nodes and mesenteric nodes can be successfully sampled (Fig. 4). Bowel can be displaced by compression. Core biopsies can be obtained with a short throw if the node is small or a long throw if the nodal mass is large enough. The trick to these biopsies in particular is to use significant compression to decrease the space from the skin to the retroperitoneum and to displace the bowel.

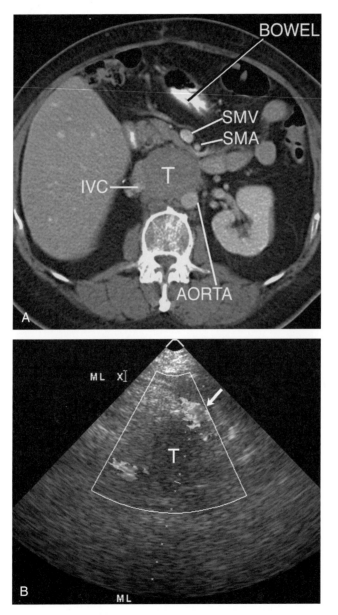

FIGURE 4. Retroperitoneal lymph node biopsy. *A*, CT shows a retroperitoneal tumor mass (*T*) surrounded by vessels. *B*, A transverse ultrasound approach using color Doppler identifies significant vessels in the biopsy path (*dotted line*). Note that the transducer pressure has decreased the distance from the skin to the tumor and has displaced the interposed bowel. (*continued*)

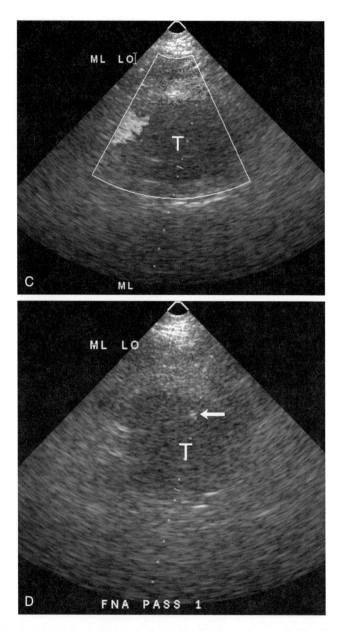

FIGURE 4. (*continued*) *C,* A longitudinal approach permits safe access to the mass. *D,* The 22-gauge needle tip (*arrow*) can be identified within the mass. Cytology yielded metastatic ovarian carcinoma.

38. Can the omentum be biopsied?

Omentum biopsy can be performed with either FNA or core biopsy. Good localization before biopsy with CT or MRI is critical to ensure that the same lesion is reproduced (Fig. 5).

Evaluation of the lesion is repeated over time to be sure that it is soft tissue and not bowel. Color Doppler can be used to evaluate for any large vessels to be avoided. An FNA is chosen for suspected carcinomas, core biopsy for sarcoma or lymphoma.

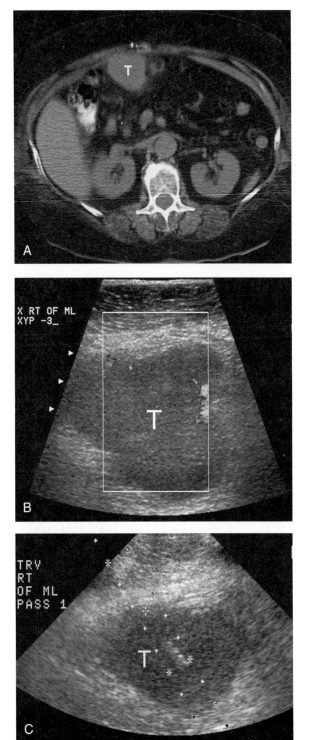

FIGURE 5. *A,* CT readily identifies a relatively superficial intraperitoneal tumor implant (*T*). *B,* Transverse ultrasound using the vector format of a high-frequency linear array identifies the tumor. Flow distinguishes this mass from bowel, as does its location, right of midline, 3 cm below the xiphoid. *C,* The biopsy needle (22-gauge spinal) passes between the guiding cursors to the center of the mass. Cytology yielded metastatic vulvar carcinoma.

39. When should ultrasound-guided bowel biopsy be performed and how?

Biopsies can be performed particularly for masses that are extraluminal and are difficult to obtain via gastroscopy or colonoscopy. Because these lesions are frequently carcinomas, fine needle is used first. Often these lesions are adjacent to bowel rather than behind bowel. Again compression is useful to displace gas that may be in the way. Needle passage through the bowel wall is generally safe for gastric or small bowel lesions, and no bowel prep or antibiotic prophylaxis is used.

40. Should the spleen be biopsied? If so, when?

The spleen is highly vascular and at greater risk for hemorrhage. Most often, patients with splenic lesions have other lesions in safer biopsy locations. Indications for splenic biopsy include isolated splenic lesions where the differential diagnosis is lymphoma versus metastasis. Biopsy may also be necessary to diagnose infection such as candida or tuberculosis.

41. What types of pelvic biopsies can be performed with ultrasound?

Masses or fluid collections can be approached transabdominally, transvaginally, transrectally, or transperineally. Transabdominal or transperineal biopsies are performed with 3–5 MHz curvilinear or phased-array transducers, with biopsy guides and 22-gauge Chiba needles for suspected carcinoma and 18-gauge core needles for suspected lymphoma or sarcoma (Fig. 6). Local anesthesia is used. Typical pelvic targets include soft tissue masses or nodes. Transperineal biopsy is usually of the prostate.

42. What are the indications for transvaginal ultrasound-guided biopsies?

This is commonly performed at the vaginal cuff to evaluate for recurrent disease, particularly ovarian carcinoma. The vagina is prepped with povidone-iodine (Betadine) and local anesthetic is given. Use color Doppler to identify increased arterial vascularity, which usually accompanies tumor recurrence. The transducer is an endocavitary endfire with a biopsy guide (the same as for prostate biopsies). The needle is usually a 20 cm, 22-gauge Chiba.

43. What are the indications for transrectal biopsy?

Transrectal biopsy is commonly performed for rectal or perirectal masses or prostate biopsy. The patient prepares the rectum with a sodium phosphate (Fleet) enema the day of the procedure and for prostate biopsy also an antibiotic prophylaxis (ciprofloxacin every 12 hours beginning the night before the procedure and 1 hour before the procedure on the day of the examination). Four doses of ciprofloxacin are continued after the procedure. No anesthesia is needed. An endfire transducer with a biopsy guide is used with an 18-gauge needle for prostate or suspected lymphoma; 22 gauge is used for other lesions. Six cores (minimum) are obtained of the prostate, three cores for other tissues. For FNA passes, two to three samples are usually sufficient.

44. Can ultrasound-guided biopsy be performed on the extremities?

Ultrasound can guide biopsy of primary or metastatic bone tumor, soft tissue tumors, or infection (pyomyositis, abscess). Lesions are usually hypoechoic, lacking the normal muscle signature. CT or MRI confirm the lesion location. Color Doppler may define margins (abscesses). For primary bone tumors, be sure to confirm the approach with the orthopedic surgeon so he or she can excise the tract if necessary.

45. How is the patient managed after biopsy?

Superficial biopsies (thyroid, breast, extremities, and palpable lymph node regions) require no postprocedure monitoring. Chest biopsies are followed by a post-procedure chest radiograph to exclude pneumothorax. If negative, the patient is discharged in an hour, as long as he or she remains asymptomatic. After FNA abdomen or pelvic biopsies, patients are monitored for 2 hours to ensure vital signs are stable and to be sure all effects of sedation have resolved before discharge. Core biopsies of liver, spleen, or kidney are monitored for 4 hours, with the patient kept at bed rest and frequent assessment made of vital signs (every 30 minutes).

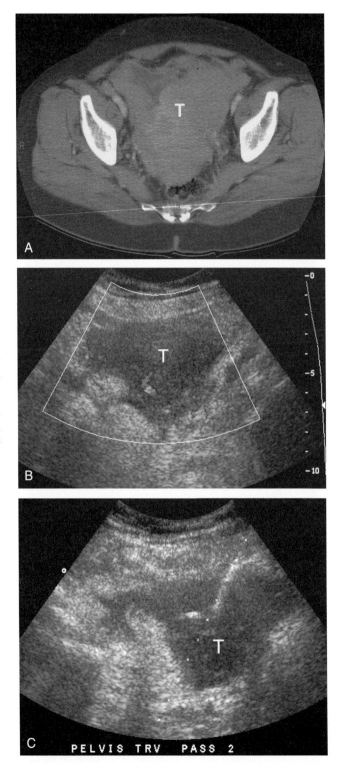

FIGURE 6. *A,* CT shows a large, enhancing soft tissue mass (*T*), which fills the pelvis. Recurrent lymphoma was suspected. *B,* Transverse ultrasound from the anterior abdominal wall identifies the tumor (*T*) with some vascularity. *C,* Core needle biopsy (18-gauge) into the solid mass yielded evidence of recurrent lymphoma.

BIBLIOGRAPHY

1. Burke BJ: Sonographic guidance for nonvascular interventions in the chest, abdomen, and pelvis. Ultrasound Q 16:185–202, 2000.
2. Caspers JM, Reading CC, et al: Ultrasound-guided biopsy and drainage of the abdomen and pelvis. In Rumack CM, Wilson SR, Charboneau JW (eds): Diagnostic Ultrasound, vol 1, 2nd ed. St. Louis, Mosby, 1998, pp 599–628.
3. Erturk E, Rubens DJ, Panner BJ, Cerilli JG: Automated core biopsy of renal allografts using ultrasonic guidance. Transplantation 51:1311–1312, 1991.
4. Gottlieb RH, Tan R, Widjaja J, et al: Extravisceral masses in the peritoneal cavity: Sonographically guided biopsies in 52 patients. Am J Roentgenol 171:697–701, 1998.
5. Memel DS, Dodd GD III, Esola CC: Efficacy of sonography as a guidance technique for biopsy of abdominal, pelvic, and retroperitoneal lymph nodes. Am J Roentgenol 167:957–962, 1996.
6. Rubens DJ, Gottlieb RH, Fultz PJ: Role of color Doppler imaging in interventional sonography. J Clin Ultrasound 27:259–271, 1999.
7. Rubens DJ, Strang JG, Fultz PJ, Gottlieb RH: Sonographic guidance of mediastinal biopsy: An effective alternative to CT guidance. Am J Roentgenol 169:1605–1610, 1997.
8. Snitzer EL, Rubens DJ, Fultz PJ, Lerner RM: Extrapelvic applications of endocavitary ultrasonographic transducers. J Ultrasound Med 16:261–263, 1996.

VII. Pediatric Sonography

31. PEDIATRIC NEUROSONOGRAPHY

Pranav Krishnakant Vyas, M.D.

1. What transducer is used for neurosonography?

A small-footprint, high-frequency sector transducer (typically ≥ 5 MHz) is used for the examination.

2. What acoustic window is used to perform a neurosonogram?

The usual acoustic window is the anterior fontanelle. However, in newborns and small infants, the posterior fontanelle can also be used.

3. What planes are recorded in the study?

Scanning is performed in coronal and sagittal planes. An axial image resembling a computed tomography (CT) scan image can be obtained from the mastoid fontanelle adjacent to the pinna of the ear.

4. How many images are obtained in a routine neonatal study?

Standard views include six coronal and five sagittal images. The six coronal images include from anterior to posterior:

    1. Frontal horns anterior to foramen of Monro (Fig. 1A)

    2. At the foramen of Monro (Fig. 1B)

    3. At the level of the thalami (Fig. 1C)

    4. At the level of the quadrigeminal plate cistern (Fig. 1D)

    5. Atria of the lateral ventricles (Fig. 1E)

    6. Posterior to the lateral ventricular system, encompassing the parietal and occipital cortex (Fig. 1F)

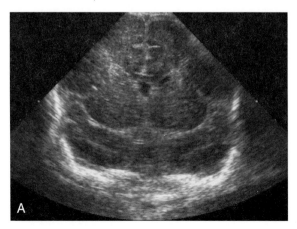

FIGURE 1. A 2-day-old ex-33-week premature infant examined with routine head ultrasound shows normal appearance of parenchyma for moderately premature patient. See text for level of images. (*continued*)

289

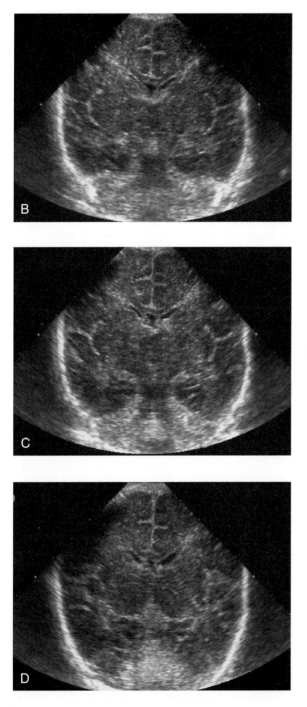

FIGURE 1. (*continued*)

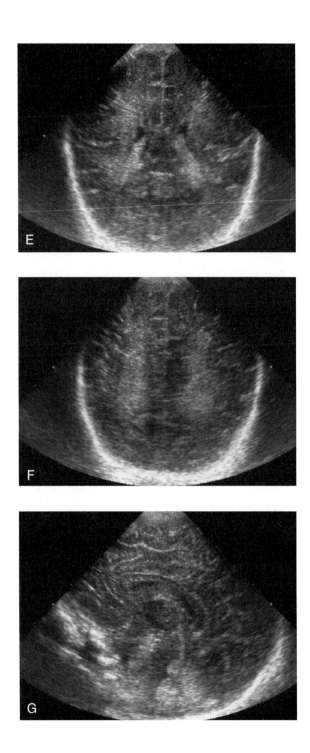

FIGURE 1. (*continued*)

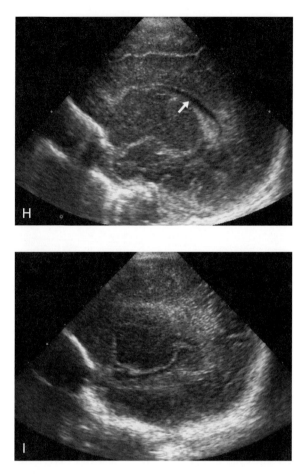

FIGURE 1. (*continued*)

The five sagittal images include a midline image (*see* Fig. 1G) and two parasagittal images on each side, including the caudothalamic notch (*see arrow* in Fig. 1H) and body of the lateral ventricle. A sylvian fissure is seen in Figure 1I.

5. What is the germinal matrix (GM) and why is it susceptible to hemorrhage?
The germinal matrix is a structure found before about 36 weeks of gestational age which houses immature neurons before they migrate out to the cortex. It is located in the subependyma, just deep to the junction of the thalamus and caudate head (caudothalamic notch). GM is susceptible to hemorrhage because of its rich vascular supply, which can easily be disrupted by changes in systemic blood pressure.

6. When is ultrasound obtained in a premature infant?
In an asymptomatic patient, a screening examination can be performed at 1 or 2 weeks of age. For symptomatic patients, neurosonograms are obtained as needed on a stat or urgent basis for apnea and bradycardia (As and Bs), neurologic compromise, or hematocrit drop.

7. When do most hemorrhages occur in premature infants?

Most cases occur within the first 4 days after birth, with the highest percentage occurring on the first day after birth. Small confined hemorrhages can be seen after the first week, but are usually not clinically significant.

8. What is the Papile system for grading intracranial hemorrhage and why is it important?

Papile grading of intracranial hemorrhage is a CT grading system, which has been adopted for use in ultrasound:

- Grade I: Hemorrhage is confined to the germinal matrix (also known as subependymal hemorrhage) (Fig. 2A)
- Grade II: Grade I hemorrhage with extension to lateral ventricle
- Grade III: Acute hyperechoic hemorrhage extensive enough to cause hydrocephalus caused by expansion by the bleed
- Grade IV: Grade III with an associated parenchymal hemorrhage (*see* Fig. 2B, C)

The significance of this grading system is its prognostic value when estimating the degree of neurologic compromise that the infant will sustain. Patients with grade I or II hemorrhage have substantially better long-term outcomes than those with grade III or IV.

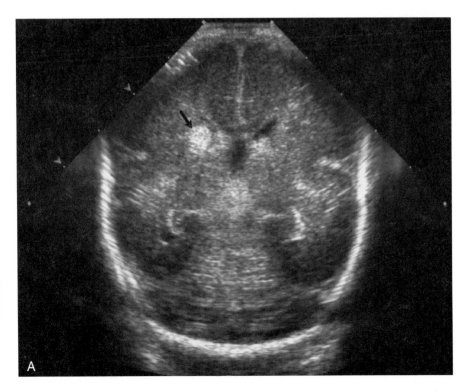

FIGURE 2. *A*, Premature infant sonogram demonstrates rounded hyperechoic focus (*arrow*) just inferior to the right frontal horn. (*continued*)

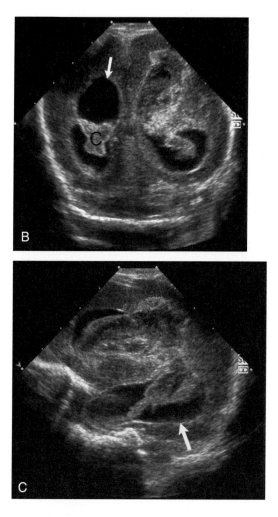

FIGURE 2. (*continued*) *B* and *C,* There is parenchymal hemorrhage seen adjacent to the superior aspect of the body of the lateral ventricle on the coronal (*B*) and sagittal (*C*) images. The right lateral ventricle (*B*) shows expansion and echogenic clot, which may reflect sequelae of previous grade II hemorrhage with subsequent ventriculitis, or, as in this case, it may be due to a grade III hemorrhage.

9. Describe the evolution of intraventricular hemorrhage.

With passage of time, intraventricular hemorrhage (grade II) can lead to ventriculitis (secondary to the blood products) and obstructive hydrocephalus. This should not be confused with grade III hemorrhage. The dilatation of the ventricles in grade III hemorrhage is not from obstruction but from an acute bleed of such sufficient size that it leads to acute distention of the ventricle with blood. A good rule of thumb is to evaluate the prior scan. If the present scan shows ventriculomegaly with old blood products and the previous showed acute blood without dilatation, grading remains stable at II.

10. Describe the neurosonographic appearance of premature brain.

Patients at 23–24 weeks of gestational age have a "simple" brain morphology, with almost no visible sulci. The exception is the prominent sylvian fissures adjacent to the temporal lobes. On a coronal section through these fissures, the brain has a "figure 8" type morphology (Fig. 3A). This should not be mistaken for lissencephaly ("smooth brain"), which is a developmental anomaly of migration of the neurons. In fact, patients with lissencephaly look like very premature infants on imaging, but the difference is in the gestational age. The mid-line cerebrospinal fluid (CSF) spaces between the lateral ventricles (cavum septum pellucidum anteriorly and cavum vergae posteriorly) are more prominent with younger gestational age (Fig. 3B).

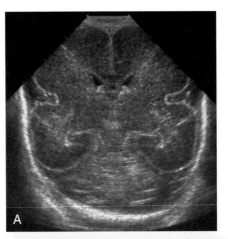

FIGURE 3. Matched coronal (*A*) and sagittal (*B*) sections from a 25-week premature infant. Arrow points to echogenic cerebellum.

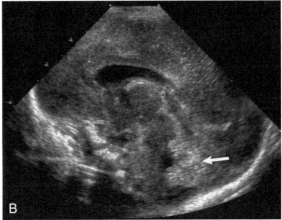

11. When does the anterior fontanelle normally close?

Anterior fontanelle closure starts at about 9 months of age and is usually completely closed by 15 months.

12. What is the periventricular "blush" or halo?

The periventricular (or peritrigonal) blush or halo is a roughly triangular shaped region of increased echogenicity just posterior and superior to the atrium of the lateral ventricle seen on all normal neurosonograms (Fig. 4). It is a normal finding and should not be confused with periventricular leukomalacia. Even though it is hyperechoic relative to the surrounding parenchyma, it should be less echogenic than the choroid plexus in the atrium of the ventricle.

13. What is periventricular leukomalacia (PVL)?

PVL is loss of white matter substance adjacent to the lateral ventricle, usually by the halo region or just superior to the frontal horn (Fig. 5). This is due to ischemia with or without associated hemorrhage. PVL represents the end stage of ischemia.

14. Describe the sonographic findings of PVL.

Early findings include increased echogenicity of the periventricular blush to equal or exceed that of the adjacent choroid plexus. As the lesion evolves, the increased echogenicity is replaced by cystic spaces filled with CSF, resulting in a "Swiss cheese" appearance.

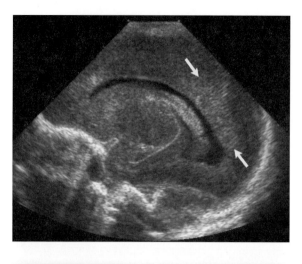

FIGURE 4. A 25-week premature infant. Parasagittal section at the level of the caudothalamic notch demonstrates triangular-shaped periventricular blush (*within arrows*) posterior to the trigone of the lateral ventricle. Note it is less echogenic than the choroid plexus in the adjacent ventricle.

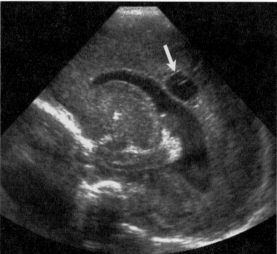

FIGURE 5. A 25-week premature infant. Left parasagittal image demonstrates large cystic area (*arrow*) within the periventricular halo.

15. What is ECMO?

Extra**c**orporeal **m**embrane **o**xygenation is a system of cardiopulmonary bypass. Blood is withdrawn from the right atrium via a large cannula threaded through the right internal jugular vein and oxygenated using a membrane oxygenator (which resembles a dialysis membrane) outside the body and then returned to the body via a cannula threaded through the right common carotid into the aortic arch. The entire system is heparinized to prevent clotting.

16. Can ECMO be performed in premature infants?

No. The heparinization needed with the ECMO system further increases the already significant chance of intracranial hemorrhage in premature infants.

17. What are the leading indications for ECMO?

The majority of ECMO patients either have congenital diaphragmatic hernia (CDH), meconium aspiration, persistent pulmonary hypertension of the newborn (PPHN), or neonatal pneumonia. ECMO is used in patients with reversible lung disease, to supply oxygenation for a limited period of time, until the lungs can recover spontaneously or after therapy. Since oxygenation can occur without ventilation, these patients can typically receive low-pressure mechanical ventilation, sparing delicate lung tissue the barotrauma associated with high insufflation pressures.

18. When are neurosonograms performed in patients on ECMO?

Preprocedure neurosonogram is performed to exclude preexisting intracranial (ICH) hemorrhage. Postprocedure ultrasounds are performed daily or every other day to detect ICH due to ECMO.

19. What are the sonographic characteristics of vasculopathy of prematurity and what is its clinical significance?

Vasculopathy of prematurity, or mineralizing vasculopathy, is seen as curvilinear regions of echogenicity on grayscale imaging within the basal ganglia and thalami. When Doppler is used, flow is noted in these areas, representing blood flow within the lenticulostriate vessels. The hyperechogenicity may reflect deposits within the walls of the lenticulostriate vessels and is a nonspecific finding seen with many different etiologies including TORCH infection, asphyxia, maternal cocaine use, encephalitis, ischemia, and trisomies 18 and 21.

20. Describe the sonographic findings of agenesis of the corpus callosum (ACC).

Widely spaced, vertically oriented lateral ventricles (sometimes referred to as a "bull's horns" appearance for the frontal horns) and distended posterior portions of the lateral ventricles (also known as colpocephaly) are characteristic features of ACC (Fig. 6). It is also possible for the corpus callosum to be hypogenetic, with partial absence.

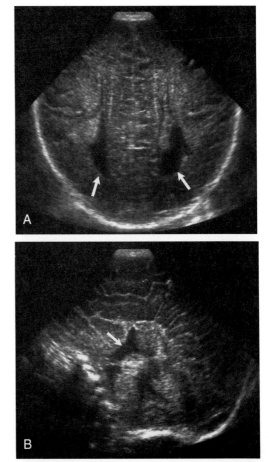

FIGURE 6. Full-term neonate demonstrates parallel ventricles (*arrows*) with prominence of the posterior portions of the lateral ventricles. The midline sagittal image demonstrates sulci extending to the margin of the third ventricle (*arrow*) and massa intermedia of the thalamus. This does not occur in the presence of corpus callosum.

21. What syndromes are associated with ACC?

ACC can be associated with a wide variety of other anomalies, including Dandy-Walker, Chiari II, and migrational anomalies.

22. What is a vein of Galen malformation (VGM, or VOG aneurysm)?

Abnormal arteries form fistulous connections with a primitive prosencephalic vein near the vein of Galen, resulting in arteriovenous malformation VGM.

23. Describe the sonographic findings of VGM.

VGM is seen as a large hypoechoic midline structure posterior to the third ventricle on sagittal view. Color Doppler evaluation shows a swirling, turbulent flow pattern.

24. How do the infants with VGM present?

The newborns are usually full term and present with cardiac failure and a loud bruit heard through the anterior fontanelle. They can also have hydrocephalus.

25. What are the sonographic findings of benign infantile hydrocephalus ?

Increased extra-axial fluid in an infant who is otherwise normal indicates benign infantile hydrocephalus (also called *benign macrocrania of infancy* or *benign hygromas of infancy*). These fluid collections usually resolve spontaneously by the time the patient is a toddler.

26. What is holoprosencephaly?

Holoprosencephaly is an anterior midline defect resulting in a series of induction malformations characterized by mild to severe midline facial and central nervous system (CNS) defects (Fig. 7). This is associated with trisomy 18 and 13.

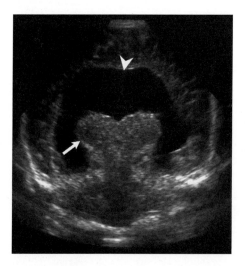

FIGURE 7. Full-term neonate with multiple anomalies. Coronal image reveals fusion of the thalami (*arrow*) with a monoventricle (*arrowhead*).

27. What are the types of holoprosencephaly?

- Alobar
- Semilobar
- Lobar

28. Describe the sonographic features of alobar holoprosencephaly

Alobar holoprosencephaly is the most severe form. It is characterized by:

- A single, undifferentiated monoventricle with a dorsal cyst

- Complete fusion of the thalami
- Absence of the interhemispheric fissure

Other features include anophthalmia, cyclopia , median and bilateral cleft lip and palate, and orbital hypotelorism.

29. Describe the features of semilobar and lobar holoprosencephaly ?

Features of semilobar holoprosencephaly are:
- Partially formed interhemispheric fissure posteriorly
- Partially fused thalami, flat nose, and orbital hypotelorism

The mildest is lobar, which has absence of only the anteroinferior portion of the interhemispheric fissure.

30. Describe the sonographic appearance of cerebral edema.

Findings on neurosonography include increased parenchymal echo texture with sulcus effacement and obliteration of CSF spaces. Cerebral edema is commonly seen in infants with acute asphyxia.

31. What are sonographic findings in hypoxic-ischemic encephalopathy (HIE)?

HIE demonstrates parenchymal volume loss with prominent CSF spaces.

32. What is hydrocephalus?

Hydrocephalus is an abnormal accumulation of CSF in the ventricles of the brain when the amount of CSF produced is more than is absorbed, causing pressure on the brain.

33. What are types of hydrocephalus?

1. **Communicating hydrocephalus.** The site of increased resistance to CSF drainage resides outside of the ventricular system in the subarachnoid space. Communicating means that the ventricles can pass along the CSF.

2. **Noncommunicating (obstructive) hydrocephalus.** The obstruction of the flow of CSF is within the ventricular system of the brain including the outlets of the fourth ventricle. The most common place for noncommunicating CSF obstruction is in the aqueduct of Sylvius (also known as aqueductal stenosis) (Fig. 8).

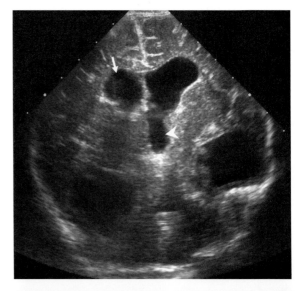

FIGURE 8. A 4-week-old infant with bulging fontanelle. Coronal image demonstrates enlargement of the lateral (*arrow*) and third ventricles (*arrowhead*), with an ovoid rather than slitlike appearance to the third ventricle.

34. What is a porencephalic cyst?

A cavity in the brain results from focal tissue destruction due to different causes, mainly ischemic but also posttraumatic.

In children, porencephaly is manifested by focal cavities with smooth walls and minimal surrounding glial relation. The distinction between porencephaly and encephalomalacia is possible because the mature brain reacts differently from the immature brain. In immature brain, there is almost no glial reaction and for this reason the destruction of brain results in a smooth, porencephalic cyst. In the mature brain, the resulting cavity contains septations and the wall is composed primarily by reactive astrocytes.

35. Describe Chiari II malformation.

It is characterized by:

Small posterior fossa	Enlarged massa intermedia
Downward displacement of cerebellum	Bat wing appearance of frontal horns
Small or absent fourth ventricle	Colpocephaly

36. What is hydranencephaly?

Hydranencephaly is characterized by the absence of both cerebral hemispheres. The cranium is filled with fluid and the falx is intact. Etiology is uncertain but believed to be secondary to complete occlusion of both internal carotid arteries.

37. Describe the sonographic findings in cytomegalovirus (CMV).

Periventricular calcifications have been considered a hallmark of congenital CMV infection. Diffuse pattern of cerebral calcifications is seen in toxoplasmosis, rubella, and congenital herpes simplex encephalitis.

The other findings of CMV include hydrocephalus, cortical atrophy, and cystic encephalomalacia.

BIBLIOGRAPHY

1. Barr LL: Neonatal cranial ultrasound. Radiol Clin North Am 37:1127–1162, 1999.
2. Enriquez G, Correa F, Lucaya J, et al: Potential pitfalls in cranial sonography. Pediatr Radiol 33:110–117, 2003.
3. Robertson RL, Ball WS, Barnes PD: Skull and brain. In Kirks DR, Griscom NT (eds): Practical Pediatric Imaging, 3rd ed. Philadelphia, Lippincott Williams & Wilkins, 1998, pp 65–200.
4. Siegel MJ: Brain. In Siegel MJ (ed): Pediatric Sonography, 3rd ed. Philadelphia, Lippincott Williams & Wilkins, 2002, pp 41–122.

32. THE PEDIATRIC HIP

Pauravi Shah Vasavada, M.D.

1. When is ultrasonography of the hip used?
Ultrasonography of the hip is used to evaluate developmental dysplasia of the hip (DDH) and to evaluate for joint effusions in children.

2. What is developmental dysplasia of the hip?
This is the preferred term used to describe the condition in which the femoral head has an abnormal relationship to the acetabulum. DDH includes frank dislocation, partial dislocation (subluxation), and instability wherein the femoral head comes in and out of the socket. It also includes a spectrum of radiographic abnormalities that reflect inadequate formation of the acetabulum.

3. What are the two major classifications of DDH?
DDH is classified into two major groups: teratologic and typical. Teratologic dislocations are less common and occur early in utero and often are associated with neuromuscular disorders such as arthrogryposis and myelodysplasia and with various dysmorphic syndromes. In the typical hip dislocation, the infant is otherwise normal and it may occur prenatally or postnatally.

4. What is the incidence of DDH?
The true incidence of DDH can only be presumed. It ranges from 1 in 100 (subluxation) to 1 in 1000 (dislocation) births. There is no single known cause.

5. What conditions predispose to DDH?
Conditions such as oligohydramnios or breech position predispose to DDH. Other risk factors include being the first born, having a positive family history, and being female. Girls are at higher risk for DDH because they are more susceptible to the maternal estrogens that may contribute to ligamentous laxity with resultant instability of the hip.

6. How is DDH diagnosed on clinical examination?
Evaluation of the hips for dysplasia is part of the routine clinical evaluation of the newborn. The Ortolani maneuver demonstrates a dislocated hip. With this maneuver, a dislocated hip is reduced by femoral abduction and flexion. As the hip reduces, a palpable jerk or clunk is heard as the hip slides back into the acetabulum. The Barlow maneuver demonstrates whether a hip is dislocatable. The femur is flexed and adducted while posterior pressure is applied. This displaces an unstable hip from the acetabulum. These are the most significant characteristics on examination. Other features that arouse suspicion include asymmetry of the thigh folds as well as a leg length discrepancy.

7. When is radiologic evaluation of the hips indicated?
The hips should be imaged if physical examination suggests that the hips are abnormal or if other risk factors are present.

8. Why is ultrasonography more advantageous compared with plain film for diagnosing DDH?
Plain film is difficult to accurately interpret until the patient is about 6–12 weeks of age because of difficulty in visualizing the cartilaginous femoral head. Also, the radiograph may be misleading because it is a single static image and only shows the position of this femoral head at the time the image is obtained. With ultrasonography, the cartilage can be visualized and the hip can be viewed while assessing the stability of the hip and the morphologic features of the acetabulum.

9. When is the ideal time to screen hips by ultrasound?
If the hips are normal at clinical examination, but there are risk factors present, sonography should be performed at 4–6 weeks. If there is abnormality on physical examination or a question, the hips should be studied at 3–4 weeks. In the instance of an unstable hip, the patient should be directly referred to an orthopedic surgeon.

10. Which techniques are used in pediatric hip ultrasonography?
Ultrasonography techniques include static evaluation of the morphologic features of the hip popularized by Graf versus dynamic evaluation of the hip as developed by Harcke.

11. How is Graf's technique different from Harcke's?
Graf's technique is aimed at morphologic assessment of the femoral head and the acetabulum. Using alpha and beta angles, the hip is classified according to the degree of development of the bony and cartilaginous components of the hip.

12. Which technique is more useful?
Dynamic ultrasonography yields more useful information because it allows one to determine the stability of the hip while using stress maneuvers. Many clinicians feel a combination of the two techniques may be best.

13. How are the alpha and beta angles obtained?
The alpha angle is created by two lines drawn on the coronal ultrasonographic image, one along the straight edge of the iliac bone, and one along the bony acetabulum roof. The beta angle is formed by the axis of the iliac bone and a line thru the axis of the labrum (Fig. 1).

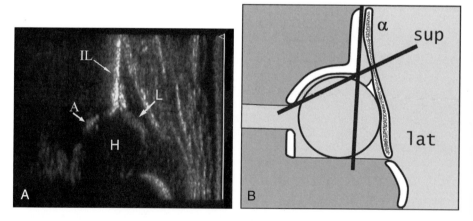

FIGURE 1. *A,* Sonographic anatomy of the hip. *B,* Graf technique. IL, Ilium; A, acetabulum; H, femoral head; L, tip of labrum. (Courtesy of H. Theodore Harcke, M.D.)

14. What are the alpha and beta angles as described by Graf?
The normal alpha angle is 60° or greater. The normal beta angle is less than 55°.

15. What type of transducer is used in hip sonography?
A high-frequency linear array transducer (5–7.5 MHz) is used.

16. Which views should be obtained in the dynamic standard minimum examination?

- Coronal neutral view in standard plane at rest or coronal flexion view in standard plane at rest. With both of these views, stress views and measurements are optional
- Transverse flexion view with stress.

The standard plane is a mid acetabular plane defined by a straight iliac line and the osilium (Fig. 2).

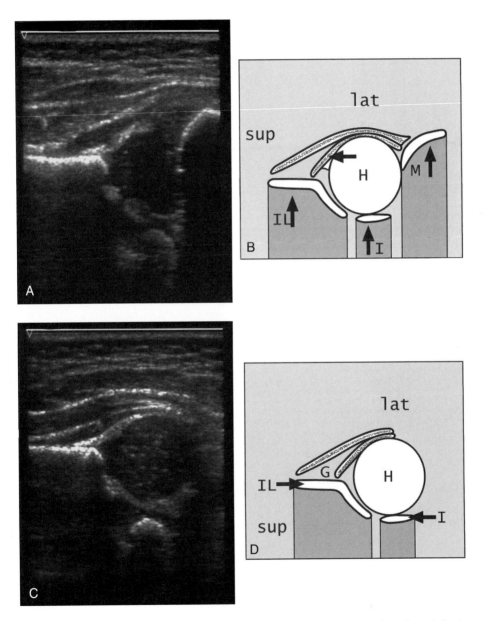

FIGURE 2. Normal sonographic relationships. *A,* Coronal neutral view. *B,* Corresponding schematic for *A.* *C,* Coronal flexion view. *D,* Corresponding schematic for *C.* (*continued*)

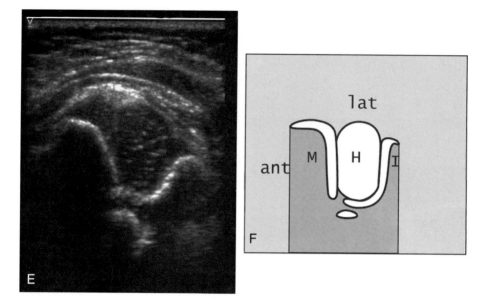

FIGURE 2. (*continued*) *E,* Transverse flexion view. *F,* Corresponding schematic for *E.* I, Ischium; IL, ilium; H, femoral head; M, femoral metaphysis; G, gluteal muscle. (Courtesy of H. Theodore Harcke, M.D.)

17. How are the hips and transducer positioned to obtain these views?
   With both the coronal neutral and coronal flexion views, the transducer is oriented in a coronal plane with respect to the acetabulum. With transverse flexion, the transducer is oriented in a transverse plane with respect to the acetabulum. With both flexion views, the hip is in 90° of flexion, whereas, in the neutral view, the hip is slightly flexed.

18. How is a stress maneuver performed?
   The hip is adducted and pushed posteriorly to provoke dislocation.

19. How does the appearance of a subluxed hip differ from a dislocated hip?
   Normally, the femoral head is seated within the acetabulum and acetabular configuration or coverage is satisfactory. With subluxation, the femoral head is partially displaced away from the acetabulum. In dislocation, the femoral head is lateral, superior or posterior to the acetabulum and the acetabulum is dysplastic (Fig. 3).

20. What is the initial treatment for a typical hip dysplasia?
   The hips are flexed and abducted and placed in an orthosis to maintain reduction. The Pavlick harness is the most commonly used orthosis in the United States.

21. At what interval should sonograms be obtained when a patient is in Pavlick?
   The frequency depends on the severity of DDH and is determined by the orthopedist. Generally, a dislocated hip in a Pavlick harness is studied weekly for 3–4 weeks to document improvement.

22. How successful is the Pavlick harness?
   Success is related to the age at diagnosis and severity of disease. Treatment has a higher success rate in a subluxed hip (96%) than in a dislocated hip (67%). In a child with a dislocated hip who is older than 3 weeks of age, the success rate is only 21%.

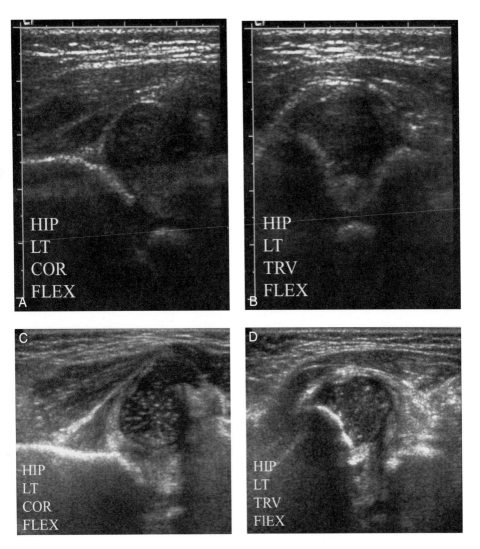

FIGURE 3. The subluxed hip versus the dislocated hip. *A*, Left coronal flexion of the subluxed hip. The femoral head is displaced laterally but has contact with the dysplastic appearing acetabulum. *B*, Left transverse flexion of the subluxed hip. The femoral head is displaced at rest but is still in contact with part of the acetabulum. *C*, Left coronal flexion of the dislocated hip. The femoral head is displaced posteriorly and superiorly and is not in contact with the markedly dysplastic acetabulum. *D*, Left transverse flexion of the dislocated hip. The femoral head is displaced and not in contact with the acetabulum.

23. What is the most common cause of hip effusion in children?
  Toxic synovitis.

24. In what plane should the hip be scanned to evaluate for joint fluid?
  Images should be obtained in the sagittal plane paralleling the femoral neck from an anterior approach with the patient supine and the hip in a neutral position (Fig. 4)

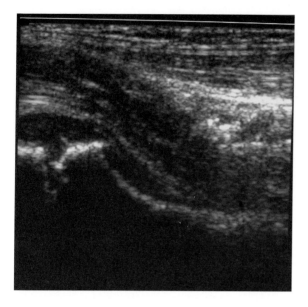

FIGURE 4. Normal hip capsule. The image that was obtained from an anterior approach shows a concave joint capsule paralleling the femoral neck.

25. What is the appearance of the abnormal hip when joint fluid is present?

When joint fluid is present, there is displacement of the capsule, which assumes a convex instead of a concave configuration (Fig. 5).

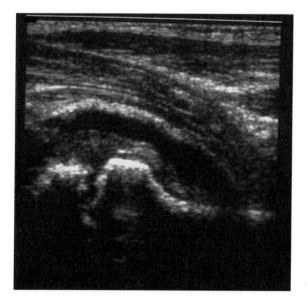

FIGURE 5. Joint effusion. Sagittal plane. The right hip capsule has a convex outer border as it is distended with fluid. This patient has toxic synovitis.

BIBLIOGRAPHY

1. ACR Standards of the Hip: ACR Standards. Revision 30, 1998, pp 27–29.
2. Clinical practice guideline: Early detection of developmental dysplasia of the hip. Pediatrics 105:896–905, 2000.

3. Harcke HT, Grissom LE: Infant hip sonography: Current concepts. Semin Ultrasound CT MRI 15:256–263, 1994.
4. Kruse RW, Bowen JR: Complications in the treatment of developmental dysplasia of the hip. In Bowen JR, Epps CH (eds): Complications in Pediatric Orthopedic Surgery. Philadelphia, Lippincott, 1995, pp 39–63.
5. Siegel MJ, McAlister WH: Musculoskeletal system and spine. In Siegel MJ (ed): Pediatric Sonography, 2nd ed. New York, Lippincott-Raven, 1996, pp 513–551.

33. APPENDICITIS IN THE PEDIATRIC PATIENT

Sheila C. Berlin, M.D.

1. On whom should imaging be performed in the setting of suspected acute appendicitis?
Imaging is reserved for the one third of patients with an atypical presentation. The usual presentation includes abdominal pain that may originate in the periumbilical region and migrate to the right lower quadrant, anorexia, fever, and leukocytosis. In these patients, prompt operative intervention is indicated. For all others, sonography can establish the diagnosis of appendicitis or help determine an alternate diagnosis.

2. How accurate is sonography in the diagnosis of acute appendicitis in children?
The sensitivity of sonography has ranged between 89% and 96% and the specificity has ranged between 89% and 98%.

3. How is graded compression sonography performed?
The technique of graded compression is accomplished using a linear transducer with the highest frequency able to penetrate the tissues of the deep right lower quadrant. Gradual and gentle but firm pressure is applied until the landmarks of the iliac vessels and psoas muscle are visualized. Graded compression clears the region of bowel gas and brings the transducer closer to the appendix, which should lie anterior to the iliac vessels and psoas muscle.

4. Where should I begin scanning?
Ask the child to point with one finger to where it hurts the most. If there is a sonographic McBurney's sign, it may guide the transducer directly to the inflamed appendix.

5. Should the bladder be full?
The bladder should be partially filled to provide a window for imaging the pelvic structures. However, a markedly distended bladder may shift the position of the cecal pole and appendix and compromise the graded compression of structures in the region of the appendix.

6. What does the normal appendix look like?
The normal appendix appears tubular, blind ending, and compressible. A characteristic inner hyperechoic line is surrounded by a hypoechoic outer zone, which represent the submucosa and muscularis propria, respectively (Fig 1.). Because it is often curved or tortuous, it may be impossible to visualize entirely in a single image.

7. Does the normal appendix show flow on color Doppler imaging?
No.

8. How commonly is the normal appendix seen?
In the pediatric population, the normal appendix is visualized in only one fourth to one half of cases.

9. To make the diagnosis of appendicitis, how large should the appendix be?
In acute, nonperforated appendicitis, the appendix should measure > 6 mm from outer wall to outer wall (Fig. 2). This measurement is used when optimum compression is applied and in context of a blind-ending structure in keeping with the appendix. A normal appendiceal diameter may be seen in the setting of ruptured appendicitis, so careful delineation of the entire appendix, incuding the tip, is necessary (Fig. 3).

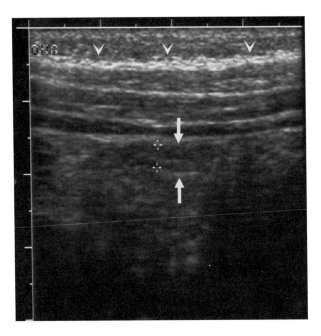

FIGURE 1. Longitudinal image of the normal appendix (*arrows*) with an inner hyperechoic submucosa surrounded by the hypoechoic muscularis propria. Note concavity of the abdominal wall resulting from graded compression (*arrowheads*).

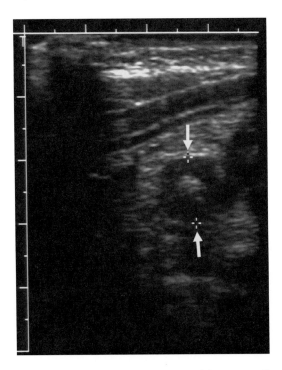

FIGURE 2. Transverse image of the enlarged appendix as measured from outer wall to outer wall (*arrows*). Note lack of compressibility.

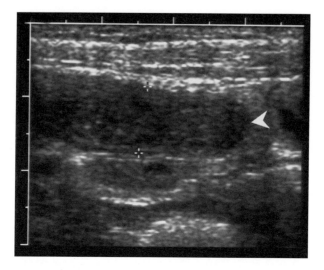

FIGURE 3. Longitudinal image through an enlarged appendix, showing the blind-ending tip (*arrowhead*).

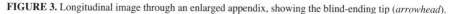

10. Does the size crtiteria for an enlarged appendix change with age?
   No.

11. Are there any additional sonographic signs of appendicitis?
   Increased flow in the appendiceal wall (in the nonperforated appendix) or periappendiceal fat may be seen using color Doppler sonography (Fig. 4). Periappendiceal inflammatory change, fluid, gas, or abscess may be found (Fig. 5). An echogenic, shadowing fecalith or increased number and size of mesenteric nodes can be seen (Fig. 6).

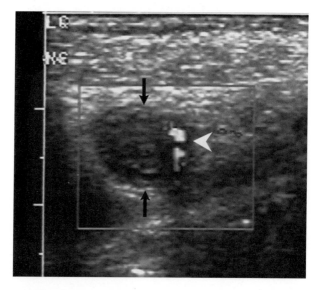

FIGURE 4. Transverse image through an inflamed and enlarged appendix (*arrows*) with increased flow in the appendiceal wall (*arrowhead*).

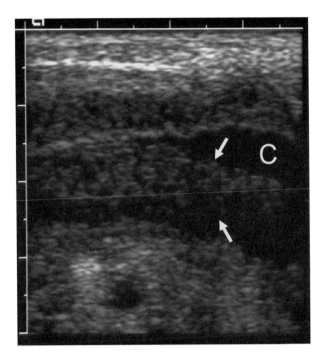

FIGURE 5. Longitudinal view of the right lower quadrant demonstrates an enlarged appendix (*arrows*) with a periappendiceal collection (*C*).

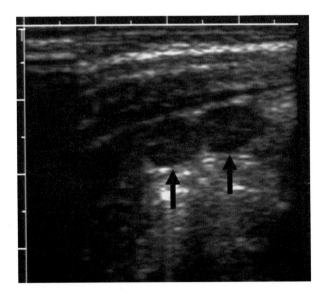

FIGURE 6. Transverse image through the right lower quadrant illustrates enlarged mesenteric lymph nodes (*arrows*).

12. Other than of the right lower quadrant, what other images should be obtained?

Images of the pelvis through an at least partially filled bladder are routinely obtained. If a normal appendix is found or if appendicitis seems unlikely, longitudinal images of each kidney should be obtained to exclude hydronephrosis.

13. Which childhood diseases can clinically mimic appendicitis?

Mesenteric adenitis, gastroenteritis, inflammatory bowel disease, ovarian torsion, and pelvic inflammatory disease are common mimickers of appendicitis. Less commonly, segmental omental infarction and renal stone or obstruction present with some clinical overlap.

14. How often does sonography define an alternate diagnosis?

Approximately, one fourth to one half of patients referred for sonography are found to have an alternate diagnosis.

15. What are some causes of nonvisualization?

- Inadequate compression of the right lower quadrant structures
- Atypical location of the appendix
- Appendiceal perforation

16. What are the disadvantages of sonography in the setting of suspected appendicitis?

Successful graded compression sonography is dependent upon the user's experience with this technique. Atypical location of the appendix and relative infrequency with which the normal appendix can be visualized in this population are limitations as well. Confusion between the terminal ileum and appendix can lead to a misdiagnosis of an enlarged appendix.

17. How does the appendix differ from a loop of collapsed ileum?

The appendiceal lumen has a more circular configuration when viewed along its short axis, whereas an ileal loop has a more flattened ovoid shape. The appendix lacks peristalsis.

18. When should CT be used for the diagnosis of appendicitis?

When operator dependency of the sonography team is a consideration, CT is an alternative means for imaging the child with suspected appendicitis. The reported sensitivity of CT for the diagnosis of acute appendicitis ranges from 87–100% and the specificity ranges from 89–98%. Reports have shown a decrease in the negative appendectomy rate in those undergoing CT for suspected acute appendicitis.

19. What are some additional advantages of CT?

Complications such as abscess and phlegmon are better defined with CT. CT images provide the anatomic detail of fluid collections requiring drainage.

BIBLIOGRAPHY

1. Callahan MJ, Rodriguez DP, Taylor GA: CT of appendicitis in children. Radiology 224:325–332, 2002.
2. Cohen HL, Sivit CJ: Fetal and Pediatric Ultrasound: A Casebook Approach. New York, McGraw-Hill, 2001.
3. Seigel MJ: Pediatric Sonography, 3rd ed. Philadelphia, Lippincott Williams & Wilkins, 2002.
4. Sivit CJ, Applegate KE: Imaging of acute appendicitis in children. Semin Ultrasound CT MRI 24(2):74–82, 2003.

34. INTUSSUSCEPTION

Melissa T. Myers, M.D.

1. What is intussusception?

This condition is characterized by bowel obstruction when a proximal segment of bowel invaginates into a more distal bowel segment and becomes "stuck" in that location.

2. What types of intussusception are there and which type is most common in children?

Intussusceptions are named for the portions of the bowel involved: colocolic, ileocolic, ileoileocolic, and ileoileal intussusceptions. More than 90% of intussusceptions are ileocolic in the pediatric population.

3. What are the causes of intussusception?

Most cases in children are idiopathic and are associated with enlarged lymph nodes in the right lower quadrant. Occasionally, a mass in the right lower quadrant acts as a lead point for the intussusception. The most common lead points in children include Meckel's diverticulum, non-Hodgkin's lymphoma, and bowel duplication cyst. Small bowel (ileoileal) intussusceptions may be seen in association with Henoch-Schönlein purpura, cystic fibrosis, and hemophilia.

4. What are the age range and clinical findings of patients with intussusception?

Idiopathic intussusception occurs in children between 6 months and 3 years of age. Those with a lead point can occur at any age. A child with intussusception generally appears ill. The symptoms include vomiting and crampy, intermittent abdominal pain. It is common for the patient to have blood and mucus in the stool, which is described as appearing like "currant jelly." There may be a palpable abdominal mass on physical examination.

5. How is the sonogram performed and what are the sonographic findings?

A high-frequency linear transducer is used to evaluate the abdomen. The entire abdomen should be imaged, specifically concentrating on the expected course of the large colon in a "picture frame" around the abdomen. The examiner should follow the colon with the transducer in the plane perpendicular to the bowel. The intussusception may be encountered anywhere within the abdomen and resemble a target (Fig. 1) or a pseudokidney (Fig. 2). The *target sign* refers to the transverse cross-section of the intussusception with concentric hyperechoic and hypoechoic rings of the bowel. In the longitudinal plane, the intussusception may resemble a kidney (the pseudokidney sign). The *pseudokidney sign* refers to the same alternating layers of bowel in the longitudinal plane. In the right lower quadrant, one might also see a mass with echogenic mesenteric fat and lymph nodes centrally with edematous hypoechoic bowel wall around it.

6. When is sonography used in the evaluation of a patient with suspected intussusception?

Patients for whom the diagnosis is uncertain benefit most from ultrasonography. Patients who have classic clinical findings and are in the appropriate age group for intussusception do not need a sonogram at all; they should proceed directly to treatment. Ultrasonography has a reported 100% sensitivity for intussusception and 100% negative predictive value. A negative ultrasound essentially eliminates the concern for that diagnosis, whereas a positive ultrasound indicates the need for immediate therapy.

7. What is the treatment for intussusception and what are the risks of the procedure?

The treatment of choice for intussusception is reduction by enema using either liquid contrast material or air. The fluid or air is administered per rectum under pressure to reduce or "push back"

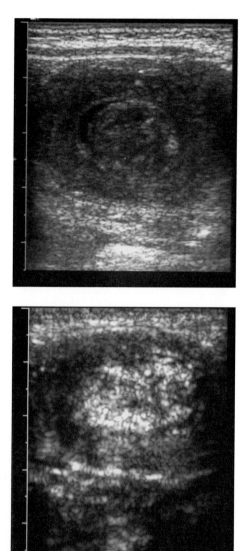

FIGURE 1. Transverse image in the right lower quadrant shows the concentric layers of bowel creating a target appearance of intussusception.

FIGURE 2. Oblique-longitudinal image shows the pseudokidney sign of intussusception.

the intussuscipiens. The risk is bowel perforation. If the effort is unsuccessful or if there is a perforation, surgery is required.

8. What sonographic features are associated with failed hydrostatic reduction?

Various authors have indicated that certain imaging features may be associated with unsuccessful attempts at enema reduction. These findings include lack of color Doppler flow to the bowel wall involved in the intussusception, free fluid, and loss of alternating bright and dark layers in the bowel wall. Other authors have disproved these associations. These findings are not considered contraindications to attempted hydrostatic reduction in stable patients. Free intraperitoneal air on the radiograph is the only absolute contraindication to fluoroscopic reduction. In general, a surgeon should be consulted before reduction in all patients because there is potential risk of perforation.

Practitioners may proceed with the enema in stable patients with intussusception and no free air on abdominal radiograph. If the attempt is unsuccessful, surgical intervention is necessary.

9. Can reduction be monitored by sonography?

A number of authors have concluded that intussusception reduction by fluid or air may be monitored by ultrasonography to reduce radiation exposure. The disadvantages of this method are that perforation is difficult, if not impossible, to detect at sonography, and it is sometimes difficult to differentiate between a swollen ileocecal valve and a small, residual intussusception. At our institution, monitoring is still done by fluoroscopy because of the higher confidence level of the examiner using fluoroscopy.

BIBLIOGRAPHY

1. Jamieson D, Stringer DA: Small bowel. In Stringer DA, Babyn PS (eds): Pediatric Gastrointestinal Imaging and Intervention, 2nd ed. Hamilton, Ontario, BC Decker, 2000, pp 421–434.
2. Sambasiva KR, Stringer DA: The stomach. In Stringer DA, Babyn PS (eds): Pediatric Gastrointestinal Imaging and Intervention, 2nd ed. Hamilton, Ontario, BC Decker, 2000, pp 275–281.
3. Sivit CJ, Siegel MJ: Gastrointestinal tract. In Siegel MJ (eds): Pediatric Sonography, 3rd ed. Philadelphia, Lippincott Williams and Wilkins, 2002, pp 339–344, 355–357.

35. HYPERTROPHIC PYLORIC STENOSIS

Melissa T. Myers, M.D.

1. What are the age range and the classic presentation of hypertrophic pyloric stenosis (HPS)?

Symptoms of HPS may be present from birth, but children generally come to medical attention between 2 weeks and 2 months of age. Children with pyloric stenosis have a prolonged history of nonbilious vomiting that gradually worsens to projectile vomiting. Boys are affected more frequently than girls. There also appears to be a familial predisposition.

2. What is the pathophysiology of this disease?

HPS is characterized by a failure of relaxation and hypertrophy of the circular muscle layer of the pylorus. The muscle thickens in the transverse dimension and elongates in the longitudinal dimension, leading to progressive gastric outlet obstruction.

3. How is the diagnosis of HPS made clinically?

When a child of the proper age presents with projectile, nonbilious vomiting, one should consider HPS. On physical examination, one may be able to palpate the enlarged, hypertrophied pyloric muscle. The examiner may feel a firm mass in the right upper quadrant, which is similar in size and shape to an olive. Hyperperistalsis of the stomach may also be visible on the abdomen. The child may be dehydrated and may have a metabolic alkalosis from prolonged vomiting.

4. What imaging modalities may be used to assess the patient with vomiting and what are the advantages and disadvantages of each?

Imaging is often necessary to differentiate between pyloric stenosis and pylorospasm, malrotation, and gastroesophageal reflux. The infant may be assessed by an upper gastrointestinal (UGI) barium study or by ultrasonography. This author recommends ultrasonography when pyloric stenosis is thought to be the most likely diagnosis and UGI when an alternate diagnosis is being considered more strongly.

The advantages of ultrasonography are that it is well tolerated, the baby does not need to drink contrast material, and there is no ionizing radiation. The examination is performed quickly and the pylorus can be directly visualized. The disadvantage is that the other potential causes of vomiting cannot be detected. With UGI, malrotation or gastroesphageal reflux can be detected. A disadvantage of UGI is that it may take a long time to perform in patients with gastric outlet obstruction. The duodenum may fill slowly or not at all, and the examiner may not be completely confident with the diagnosis because the pylorus is not directly imaged.

5. How is the ultrasound performed?

A high-resolution linear transducer is used to examine the right upper quadrant of the abdomen. The baby is placed in the right posterior oblique position so that gastric fluid can fill the antrum of the stomach. The child may be given clear glucose solution to drink to distend the stomach, which helps distinguish between collapsed stomach and pyloric channel.

6. What are the imaging features of a patient with pyloric stenosis?

The stomach, seen in the left upper quadrant, is often full of fluid and is hyperperistaltic. The enlarged pylorus is generally encountered in the right upper quadrant. In the transverse plane, it demonstrates a target appearance in which the thickened pyloric muscle is uniform and hypoechoic and surrounds the central echogenic mucosa (Fig. 1). In the longitudinal plane, the thickened muscle layers appear as parallel hypoechoic lines separated by echogenic mucosa.

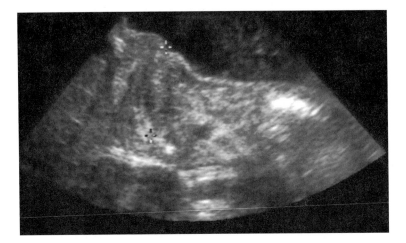

FIGURE 1. Longitudinal image of the pylorus (*within calipers*) in a patient with HPS. The parallel hypoechoic lines represent thickened muscle on either side of the lumen, whereas the central echogenic lines represent the mucosa of the pyloric channel.

In normal patients, the pylorus opens frequently to allow passage of gastric contents through the pyloric channel. This finding is helpful in excluding the diagnosis. The opening and closing of the pylorus can be seen readily at sonography in patients who do not have HPS (Fig. 2).

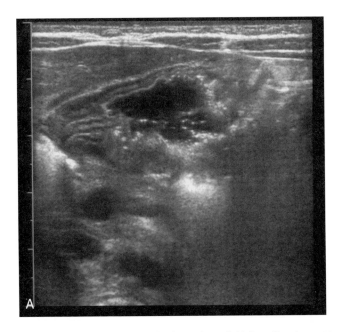

FIGURE 2. *A*, Longitudinal image of the normal pylorus shows fluid distending the gastric antrum and a closed pyloric channel. (*continued*)

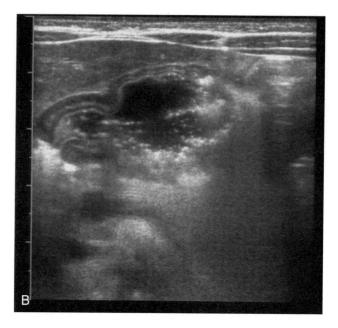

FIGURE 2. (*continued*) *B,* Several minutes later, the channel opens and the gastric fluid passes through the channel.

7. What are the dimensions of the normal pylorus and the hypertrophied pylorus?

The muscle thickness of the normal pylorus is generally less than 2.0 mm on one side of the lumen and the length is less than 14 mm. An experienced sonographer can diagnose pyloric stenosis without actually measuring muscle thickness or width; however, when the length and width exceed certain limits, the level of confidence increases. In general, the longer the channel is and the thicker the muscle is, the greater the confidence in the diagnosis. The measurement of muscle thickness is thought to be more important than length.

If the length (Fig. 3) is greater than 16 mm and the muscle thickness (Fig. 4) is greater than 3.0 mm on one side of the lumen, one can be fairly confident that the patient has pyloric stenosis. The measurements can vary, however, depending on patient age and size at presentation. Borderline measurements may be seen in younger children with HPS or with pylorospasm at any age.

8. What if the pyloric measurements are borderline?

To avoid unnecessary surgery, one should not diagnose HPS when the imaging findings are equivocal. A repeat scan may be performed the following day if the patient's symptoms do not resolve spontaneously. HPS persists, whereas pylorospasm may resolve.

9. What is the appropriate therapy for pyloric stenosis?

In most medical centers in the United States, the treatment for pyloric stenosis is surgery (called *pyloromyotomy*). A longitudinal incision is made in the pyloric muscle.

10. Does the pylorus return to normal immediately after surgery?

No. Although the operation relieves the gastric outlet obstruction, a reduction in pyloric muscle length or thickness is not seen immediately. It may take several months for the muscle measurements to return to normal.

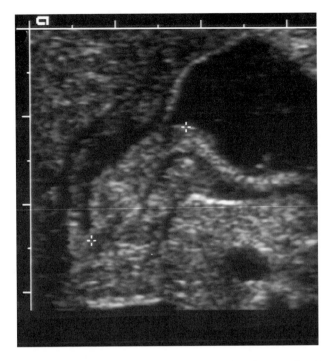

FIGURE 3. Longitudinal image of the pylorus shows caliper position for measuring channel length.

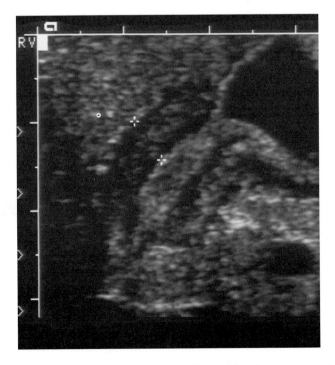

FIGURE 4. Longitudinal image of the pylorus shows caliper position of measuring muscle thickness.

BIBLIOGRAPHY

1. Jamieson D, Stringer DA: Small bowel. In Stringer DA, Babyn PS (eds): Pediatric Gastrointestinal Imaging and Intervention, 2nd ed. Hamilton, Ontario, BC Decker, 2000, pp 421–434.
2. Sambasiva KR, Stringer DA: The stomach. In Stringer DA, Babyn PS (eds): Pediatric Gastrointestinal Imaging and Intervention, 2nd ed. Hamilton, Ontario, BC Decker, 2000, pp 275–281.
3. Sivit CJ, Siegel MJ: Gastrointestinal tract. In Siegel MJ (eds): Pediatric Sonography, 3rd ed. Philadelphia, Lippincott Williams and Wilkins, 2002, pp 339–344, 355–357.

36. THE PEDIATRIC SPINE

Sheila C. Berlin, M.D.

1. In which patient groups can spinal sonography be performed?
Young infants up to about 6–8 months of age can be scanned easily. After this time, the acoustic window is smaller and imaging becomes more difficult. It is also possible to obtain good images in patients with laminectomy defects.

2. Why are the intraspinal contents of an infant so much easier to evaluate?
Incomplete ossification of the cartilaginous posterior elements allows for a large, unobstructed acoustic window.

3. Which transducer is best for spinal sonography?
In early infancy, a high-frequency linear transducer allows for the largest field of view. A sector transducer may be necessary in the older patient, because the ossified posterior elements permit a smaller acoustic window.

4. How is the patient positioned for scanning?
The infant is positioned prone with a small, rolled towel under the upper abdomen and lower chest. This position straightens the lumbar lordosis, allowing for maximum contact with the transducer. With a relative kyphosis, the posterior elements are splayed, opening the window to the canal contents.

5. Which views are routinely obtained?
Longitudinal and transverse planes through the lumbosacral spine are obtained in the routine evaluation of the infant spine. Most scans in this age group are performed for the evaluation of occult spinal dysraphism, requiring precise localization of the conus medullaris.

6. What is the sonographic appearance of the normal conus medullaris?
A longitudinal image through the midline of the conus medullaris resembles a tadpole's tail. The spinal cord appears as a relatively hypoechoic structure with echogenic walls (Fig. 1A). The

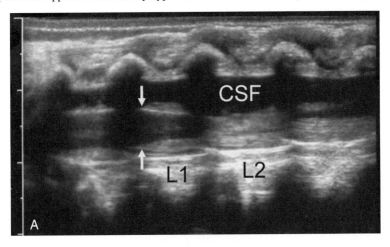

FIGURE 1. *A*, Longitudinal image through the distal cord. The cord (*arrows*) floats freely in the thecal sac, bordered posteriorly by cerebrospinal fluid (*CSF*) in the subarachnoid space. (*continued*)

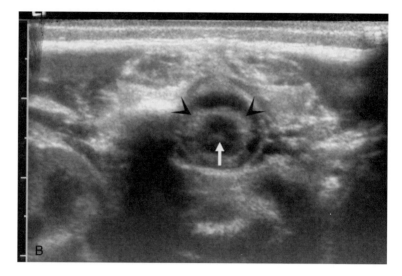

FIGURE 1. (*continued*) B, Transverse image through the distal cord demonstrates the central echogenic complex (*arrow*). Note the echogenic nerve roots suorrounding the cord (*arrowheads*).

echogenic line in the center of the cord represents the tissue between the ventral white commissure and the central portion of the anterior median fissure (*see* Fig. 1B).

7. Should the cord move?

Yes. Real-time images demonstrate vascular pulsations. In addition, the cord should gently thump in the thecal sac in an anteroposterior motion with respirations. Lack of motion suggests cord tethering. Cord motion is best seen with the infant prone and is accentuated by crying.

8. At what level should the conus terminate?

The tip of the normal conus medullaris lies above the superior aspect of the L3 vertebra. Cord tapering occurs normally at about the first lumbar vertebral body. The tip of the conus medullaris is continuous with the filum terminale, an echogenic stringlike structure extending into the sacral canal. The filum terminale is surrounded by echogenic nerve roots, comprising the cauda equina (Fig. 2). The cord is considered tethered when the cord lies below the superior aspect of L3, there is a thickened filum, and movement is absent with repirations or crying (Fig. 3).

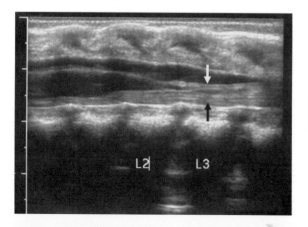

FIGURE 2. Longitudinal image through the echogenic nerve roots of the cauda equina (*arrows*).

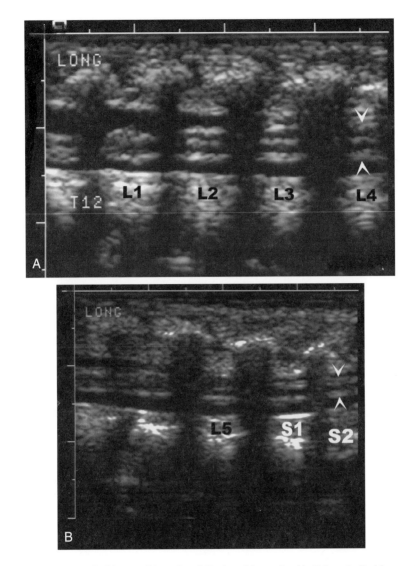

FIGURE 3. *A,* Longitudinal image of the tethered distal cord (*arrowheads*). *B,* Longitudinal image of the conus medullaris (*arrowheads*) terminating in the sacrum.

9. How is the vertebral level determined?

The easiest method for assigning vertebral body level is by counting cranially from the sacral segments. This method assumes a normal number of sacral segments. There are five sacral segments. In the newborn period, the coccyx is also visualized as the most inferior segment and should not be mistaken for a sacral segment. An alternative method of level confirmation is to identify the twelfth rib sonographically and count segments caudally.

10. What are the sonographic appearances of occult spinal dysraphism?

Findings other than a low-lying conus are present with occult dysraphic lesions. These include a dorsal location of the cord within the bony canal, a nontapered, bulbous appearance of the conus, a patulous distal thecal sac (Fig. 4), a thick filum, and solid or cystic mass (Fig. 5) in the distal canal.

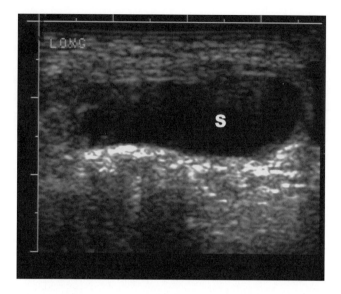

FIGURE 4. Longitudinal image through the enlarged, patulous distal most thecal sac (*S*).

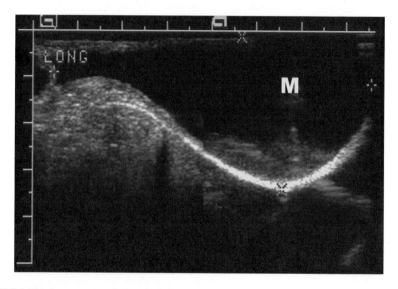

FIGURE 5. This large cyst seen in a sagittal view of the sacrum was associated with a tethered cord. It represents a meningocele (*M*).

11. What are the findings on physical examination that warrant a screening sonogram for occult spinal dysraphism?

Infants are referred for spinal sonography if they have a lumbosacral skin dimple (usually below the gluteal crease), skin appendage, hair patch, or mass. They may also present with lower extremity weakness.

12. Is sonography the imaging study of choice for primary evaluation of such patients?

In infants, sonography is the preferred screening study.

13. Is a small syrinx in the distal cord normal?

The ventricullus terminalis, or "fifth ventricle," is a normal anatomic variant seen from time to time in term infants. The sonographic appearance is a small hypoechoic region that appears to "split" the central echo complex of the conus medullaris (Fig. 6). It represents the ependymal lined residual lumen of the cauda equina.

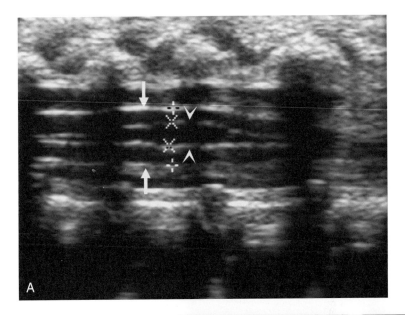

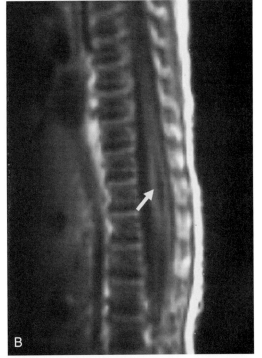

FIGURE 6. *A,* The distal cord (*arrows*) is "split" by the hypoechoic terminal ventricle (*arrowhead*) on this sagittal view at the lower lumbar level. *B,* Correlative sagittal T1-weighted image through the thoracolumbar spine also shows the terminal ventricle (*arrow*).

14. Which occult dysraphic lesions are much better seen with magnetic resonance imaging?
A small dorsal dermal sinus can be difficult to detect with sonography; however, there is often a coexistent low-lying cord. A fatty filum can be missed if careful attention is not paid to detect this thickened echogenic, fixed-appearing structure.

15. Other than spinal dysraphism, what other conditions can be evaluated with sonography?
Diastematomyelia, or splitting of the cord, can be detected. Cord tumors may be seen in the infant. Intraoperative sonography has been used to determine the precise location of an intramedullary tumor, arteriovenous malformation, or syringomyelia.

BIBLIOGRAPHY

1. Korsvik HE, Keller MS: Sonography of occult spinal dysraphism in neonates and infants with MR imaging correlation. Radiographics 12(2):297–306, 1992.
2. Kriss VM, Kriss TC, Babcock DS. The ventriculus terminalis of the spinal cord in the neonate: A normal variant on sonography. Am J Roentgenol 165(6):1491–1493, 1995.
3. Rohrschneider WK, Forsting M, Darge K, Troger J: Diagnostic value of spinal US; Comparative study with MR imaging in pediatric patients. Radiology 200(2): 383–388, 1996.
4. Seigel MJ: Pediatric Sonography, 3rd ed. Philadelphia, Lippincott Williams & Wilkins, 2002.

37. PEDIATRIC KIDNEYS AND BLADDER

Pranav Krishnakant Vyas, M.D.

1. What is the normal renal size in newborns?

Mean newborn renal length is about 4.5 cm, with 2 standard deviations being about 0.6 cm. A good rule of thumb is about 1 mm of length for each gestational week.

2. Rank the echogenicity of renal cortex in relation to liver in otherwise normal premature, full-term, infant, and pediatric kidneys.

Normal premature:	kidney > liver
Normal full-term:	kidney = liver
Normal infant:	kidney ≤ liver
Normal child:	kidney < liver

3. How can one distinguish between medullary pyramids and hydronephrosis in infants and neonates?

Infants and neonates have prominent, hypoechoic medullary pyramids. A hydronephrotic collecting system should be even more hypoechoic than the pyramids and demonstrate connections between the calices, whereas pyramids do not show hypoechoic connecting structures (Fig. 1). In suboptimal studies, however, the distinction may be difficult. In these patients, prone scanning with a high-frequency (≥ 8 MHz) linear or curved transducer may be helpful to rule out or confirm the presence of hydronephrosis.

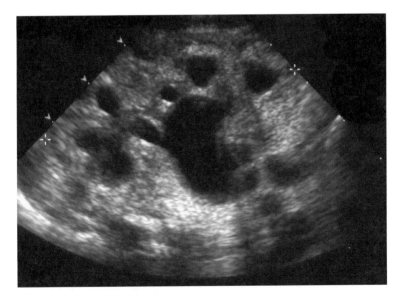

FIGURE 1. Longitudinal view of right kidney in a newborn with posterior urethral valves demonstrates moderate hydronephrosis. Note the connection of dilated upper pole major calyx with central renal pelvis.

4. In neonates, what are common reasons for increased medullary echotexture?

Many otherwise normal neonates can display transient idiopathic echogenicity (also known as *stasis nephropathy*) of the pyramids; this finding resolves by the second postnatal week (Fig. 2).

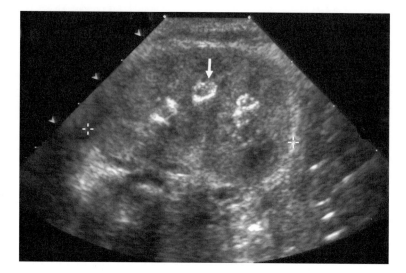

FIGURE 2. Longitudinal view of right kidney in premature infant demonstrates multiple hyperechoic pyramids (*arrow*), which resolved on follow-up examinations.

Premature infants or those with heart disease on diuretic therapy with furosemide (Lasix) commonly have increased medullary echogenicity.

5. What are the most common causes for antenatal hydronephrosis?
- Ureteropelvic junction obstruction (UPJ)
- Vesicoureteral reflux (VUR)
- Ureterovesical junction obstruction (UVJ)
- Posterior urethral valves (PUV)
- Other etiologies include primary megaureter, prune belly syndrome, and obstructed duplication anomalies of the collecting system.

6. Describe the sonographic features of UPJ.
Sonographic signs include pelvicaliectasis with a disproportionately large renal pelvis and without evidence of ureteral dilatation.

7. How is VUR graded?
This grading system is based on the voiding cystogram.

GRADE OF REFLUX	DESCRIPTION
I	Contrast refluxes into the ureter only.
II	Contrast reaches the renal pelvis, which is not dilated.
III	Contrast reaches the renal pelvis, with mild dilatation of the ureter and pelvicaliceal system (IIIA) or moderate dilatation with early forniceal blunting (IIIC).
IV	Moderate pelviureteroectasis with obliteration of the forniceal angles but preservation of the papillary impressions.
V	There is moderate to severe pelviureteroectasis with near-complete or complete obliteration of the papillary impressions. The latter may be associated with severe or extreme collecting system dilatation.

8. What modalities are used to diagnose VUR?
VUR may be demonstrated by fluoroscopic voiding cystourethrogram (VCUG) or voiding radionuclide cystography (sometimes designated RNC). European investigators have diagnosed

VUR using contrast-enhanced sonography, with better results obtained by harmonic imaging. VUR may be unilateral, bilateral, or intermittent. Pediatric cases of lower grades of primary VUR can often be successfully managed with medical treatment, with spontaneous resolution as child grows. Other children may require surgery.

9. Is the presence of VUR reliably excluded by a normal renal ultrasound?

No. Patients can have no visible hydronephrosis or hydroureter and still have significant reflux. Alternatively, patients with a full bladder or in the prone position can have some mild distention of the collecting system, especially centrally, and have no pathology. Ultrasound can diagnose VUR if contrast (such as Levovist) is used, but this is still in the clinical research stage.

10. When should a postnatal ultrasound be obtained to evaluate a patient with antenatal hydronephrosis?

In the immediate postnatal period, the neonate is relatively dehydrated, so a false-negative scan may be obtained. Waiting a week or so after birth decreases the chance of a false-negative result.

11. What is the natural history of VUR?

Most cases of VUR in infants resolve by early childhood, with patients with low grades (I–III) by VCUG having a better chance of resolution than those with grade IV–V. Ultrasound is often used to follow up patients on conservative medical therapy (usually antimicrobial prophylaxis) on a yearly basis. As long as renal growth documented by ultrasound is proceeding normally, without evidence for scarring, many clinicians will continue conservative treatment.

12. What is a STING procedure?

STING is a cystoscopic technique that involves the subureteric injection of Teflon or other biochemically inert material by the ureteral orifice to eliminate VUR. On imaging, an echogenic hillock of material is seen intramurally within the posterior bladder wall (Fig. 3). Failures of this procedure are manifested by absence of the hillock, representing migration of the injected material. It can also rarely migrate up the ureter into the kidney, where it appears as echogenic material within the collecting system with posterior shadowing.

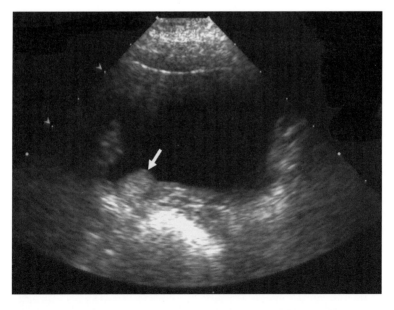

FIGURE 3. Transverse view of bladder in preschooler after right STING procedure (*arrow*).

13. What are the sonographic features of pyelonephritis?

Ultrasound signs include renal swelling, focal hyperechoic regions, loss of corticomedullary differentiation, and collecting system wall thickening. Sensitivity of ultrasound is about 50%. Use of power Doppler may increase this sensitivity by showing a region of relative ischemia. Contrast-enhanced computed tomography (CT) or magnetic resonance imaging (MRI), or scintigraphy with DMSA all have 90% or better sensitivity for this diagnosis.

14. How is reflux nephropathy diagnosed?

Cortical thinning, especially at the poles, and lack of normal renal growth over time are the primary sonographic features. Reflux nephropathy leads to scarring and decreased size of the involved kidney with potential serious long-term sequelae, including hypertension and renal failure.

15. What are the mimics of renal scar?

A scar is characterized by a "divot" in the renal cortex, with its apex over a medullary pyramid. The following can mimic a scar:

- **Fetal lobulation:** Fetal lobulation is usually much more uniform, with a scalloped border around both kidneys, rather than more focal, and is seen predominantly in infants and small children.
- **Junctional parenchyma:** Presence of a linear hyperechoic junctional parenchymal defect between the upper and mid poles of the kidney can be mistaken for a scar. Unlike a scar, there should not be any associated volume loss.

16. How is a duplicate collecting system discovered?

Usually it is an incidental finding. Many children have a duplicated collecting system, ranging from an incomplete duplication of the intrarenal collecting system, all the way to two different renal pelves, ureters, and ureteral orifices in the same kidney. Even though it is often of no clinical consequence, documentation of a duplicated collecting system by ultrasound is important, because duplicated systems can have a number of serious complications.

17. What is the Weigert-Meyer rule?

In patients with complete duplication of the collecting system:

- The upper pole moiety usually obstructs. The ureter inserts medially and inferiorly.
- The lower moiety refluxes and ureter inserts superiorly and laterally (normal insertion).

18. What is a ureterocele?

A ureterocele can exist in a nonduplicated system but is more common in duplex systems. In contrast to the small "cobra-headed" ureteroceles seen commonly in older females without a duplicated system ("simple ureterocele"), the ectopic ureterocele is often large, causing obstruction to the upper pole moiety if a duplex system is involved and sometimes causes bladder outlet obstruction. If a sonogram shows a duplication with hydronephrosis of the upper pole, an ectopic ureterocele should be sought in the bladder (Fig. 4). In patients with bilateral duplications with bilateral ectopic ureteroceles, these can approximate in the midline of the bladder, often causing bladder outlet obstruction ("kissing" ureteroceles). Ureteroceles can also prolapse and are a cause for a mass presenting at the introitus in young females.

19. What is autosomal recessive polycystic kidney disease (ARPCKD)?

ARPCKD was previously known as infantile polycystic disease, and most patients are affected during childhood, although not always in infancy. There is dilatation of the renal collecting tubules, as well as periportal fibrosis within the liver. There is usually an inverse relationship in terms of severity of the kidney and liver pathology.

20. Describe the sonographic findings of ARPCKD?

Imaging characteristics include bilaterally large, hyperechoic kidneys with lack of corticomedullary differentiation (Fig. 5). Differential considerations for this appearance include auto-

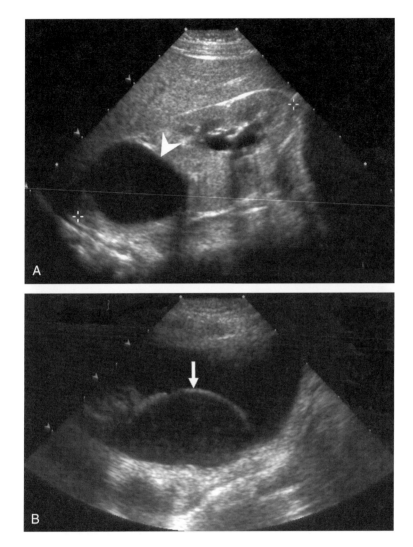

FIGURE 4. *A,* Longitudinal right kidney in infant shows marked hydronephrosis in upper pole moiety of duplicated system (*arrowhead*). Note the mild prominence of the central collecting system of the lower pole moiety, which was due to vesicoureteral reflux (Weigart-Meyer rule). *B,* Transverse view of the same patient's bladder reveals a large obstructing ectopic ureterocele arising from right of midline (*arrow*).

somal dominant PCKD (ADPCKD) and glomerocystic disease, which is sporadic in nature. Discrete macrocysts are sometimes present in ARPCKD.

21. What are the clinical and sonographic findings of ADPCKD?

ADPCKD was previously known as adult polycystic disease, but this is a misnomer, as is infantile polycystic kidney disease, because ADPCKD can have manifestations in childhood and infancy. Macroscopically visible cysts are present within the cortex and medullary portions of the kidney, and cystic changes can be seen commonly within the liver and pancreas. Liver cysts are present in 70–75% of cases. There is also an association with saccular aneurysms within the cerebral vasculature. Imaging findings include diffusely enlarged hyperechoic kidneys in infants, which can resemble ARPCKD, and multiple large parenchymal macrocysts in older children.

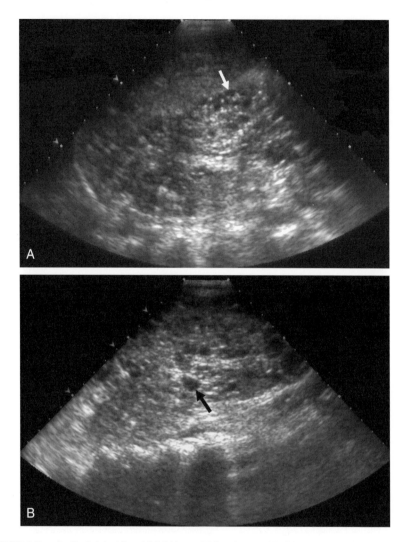

FIGURE 5. Longitudinal right (*A*) and left kidneys (*B*) in a 9-year-old with autosomal recessive polycystic kidney disease. Note multiple small cysts (arrows) with poor corticomedullary differentiation and overall hyperechoic parenchyma.

22. What is multicystic dysplastic kidney (MCDK)?

MCDK is one of the most common masses in infants. MCDK can affect only a segment of the kidney or one moiety of a duplex kidney, but usually it affects the entire organ. It is characterized by multiple cystic structures of varying size, which do not communicate. The more common type has the largest cyst in a noncentral position (Fig. 6). The renal artery is absent or atretic. The ureter normally does not communicate with the pelvis. This kidney is nonfunctional.

23. What distinguishes MCDK from hydronephrosis?

Imaging with scintigraphy, either furosemide renography with MAG3 or cortical scintigraphy with DMSA, can be helpful in many cases by showing no activity in the involved renal unit, which is diagnostic of MCDK. Activity with delayed drainage by furosemide renography or diminished but not absent uptake by cortical scintigraphy strongly suggests hydronephrosis from a UPJ obstruction.

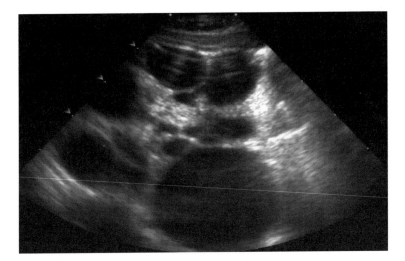

FIGURE 6. Longitudinal view of the right kidney in an infant reveals multiple noncommunicating cysts consistent with multicystic dysplastic kidney.

24. In what age group is a Wilms' tumor common?

Wilms' tumor (nephroblastoma) is a malignant neoplasm of primitive cells presenting in early childhood (peak age of 3 years).

25. Describe the sonographic features of Wilms' tumor.

A large mass usually presents within the kidney with heterogenous echotexture (Fig. 7). A rim of increased or decreased echotexture peripherally can be present, which reflects a pseudo-capsule. A sonographic finding that should be sought is extension to the ipsilateral renal vein or beyond into the inferior vena cava.

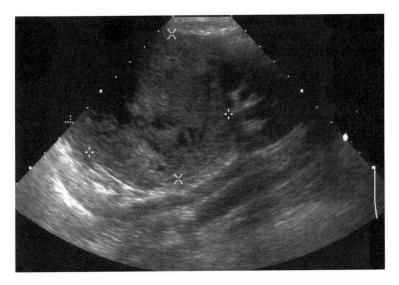

FIGURE 7. Longitudinal view of the left kidney in a 4-year-old girl reveals a large hyperechoic mass (within calipers) replacing the superior half of the kidney, which was a Wilms' tumor at resection.

26. What tumors resemble Wilms' tumor?

Clear cell sarcoma and rhabdoid tumor of the kidney resemble Wilms' sonographically, although rhabdoid tumor can also have an associated peripheral fluid collection.

27. Name five conditions that can predispose a child to Wilms' tumor.

1. Nephroblastomatosis: Nephroblastomatosis is a premalignant condition.
2. Sporadic aniridia
3. Beckwith-Wiedemann syndrome
4. Hemihypertrophy
5. Drash syndrome

28. What is Beckwith-Wiedemann syndrome?

This rare disorder with multiple anomalies can include omphalocele, macroglossia, and gigantism, along with an increased incidence of neoplasms, including Wilms'.

29. Describe Drash syndrome.

Drash syndrome is a rare syndrome in which patients are XY in phenotype but are pseudohermaphrodites with ambiguous genitalia and glomerulonephritis.

30. What systemic disorder is associated with angiomyolipoma of the kidney?

Tuberous sclerosis is associated with angiomyolipoma, which is characterized by cortical hyperechogenicity due to fat content and which is often multiple and asymptomatic, although it can cause hematuria or mass effect.

31. What are imaging findings associated with *Candida* infection?

Candida infection can cause nephromegaly with increased echotexture as well as echogenic mycetoma ("fungus ball") formation within a dilated collecting system, which can lead to obstruction.

32. Describe the progression of imaging findings with renal vein thrombosis.

Renal vein thrombosis acutely causes swelling of the affected kidney with increased echotexture, which then resolves over the course of a few weeks, with the kidney becoming hypoechoic or heterogenous in echotexture. The chronic appearance can be near normal or that of a small shrunken hyperechoic structure. Thrombus with either partial or total venous occlusion should be sought, as should elevated arterial resistive index.

33. How does a newborn with PUV present?

A newborn male with a posterior urethral valve presents with a history of prenatal hydronephrosis and oligohydramnios.

34. Describe the findings in PUV.

Obstructing folds of tissue occur within the posterior urethra. Sonographic findings include hydronephrosis, either bilateral or unilateral (so-called pop-off mechanism, with one renal unit severely damaged and the other relatively spared), hydroureter, bladder wall thickening, and increased renal echogenicity. Urinary ascites can sometimes be present. A dilated posterior urethra can sometimes be visualized using a transperineal approach, although definitive diagnosis is made with a voiding cystourethrogram.

35. A large heterogenous soft tissue mass is found within the kidney of an infant. What is its most likely etiology?

Mesoblastic nephroma is the most likely cause. This tumor may resemble Wilms' with homogenous increased echotexture or increased heterogenous echotexture, but it is more common in the infant age group, with peak incidence of Wilms' being about 3 years of age. Multilocular cystic nephroma (MCN) can also present as a large renal mass within the kidneys of infants, but as suggested by its name, presents with large cystic spaces, with small amounts of intervening stroma. A rare tumor that is not distinguishable from MCN on sonographic grounds is cystic partially differentiated nephroblastoma, which is a borderline malignant variant of MCN.

36. What is a neurogenic bladder?

Neurogenic bladder is characterized by small size and significant bladder wall thickening (normal being about 5 mm or less, depending on bladder distention). To decrease complications such as infection and reflux, many patients have bladder augmentation with portions of small bowel or colon, which produce mucus that can cause echogenic debris. The Mitrofanoff stoma is formed by intussuscepting the appendix and using it to bridge the augmented bladder and the abdominal wall. This technique allows for continent, clean intermittent catheterization of the bladder without need for a stoma bag.

37. How does an infant with patent urachus present?

An infant presents with an inflamed umbilical region. The caregiver mentions that the area appears constantly wet. The urachus is an embryologic communication between the dome of the bladder and the umbilicus. This usually closes within the second trimester. If it persists after birth, it can lead to periumbilical inflammation and infection.

38. Describe the sonographic findings in patent urachus.

Sonography in the sagittal plane can demonstrate a narrow fluid collection extending from the dome of the bladder to the superficial aspect of the umbilicus. Other developmental anomalies involving this structure include midline urachal cysts located between the bladder dome and umbilicus (which can be anechoic or contain debris if infected), urachal sinus (Fig. 8), and urachal diverticulum, which is a fluid-filled structure adjacent to the bladder dome.

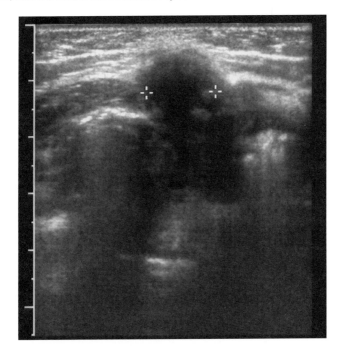

FIGURE 8. Transverse view of an infant infraumbilical region with a linear transducer reveals fluid-filled channel (*within calipers*), which approaches the dome of the bladder on the longitudinal view (not shown) but could not definitely be connected on sonography, suggesting a urachal sinus.

39. How is cystitis differentiated from rhabdomyosarcoma of the bladder?
Cystitis usually presents with relatively uniform bladder wall thickening without a focal mass, whereas rhabdomyosarcoma usually presents as a focal mass with grapelike echogenic or heterogenous clusters or fronds. Cystitis can be focal and tumefactive, however, and rhabdomyosarcoma may manifest as more diffuse bladder wall infiltration, so history and cystoscopic evaluation may be necessary in difficult cases.

40. Describe pyonephrosis.
Pyonephrosis is infected material in an obstructed renal collecting system. The most common cause is *Escherichia coli*. Pyonephrosis is an emergency that requires decompression, usually via a percutaneous nephrostomy, which can be ultrasound or fluoroscopically guided. Noninfected patients can present with the same sonographic findings, so history and laboratory findings are important to differentiate between the two conditions.

41. What is prune belly syndrome?
Eagle-Barrett syndrome (prune belly syndrome) manifests as hypoplasia or aplasia of the anterior abdominal wall, various urinary tract anomalies, and bilateral cryptorchidism. On inspection, the infant's abdominal wall has a wrinkly or prunelike appearance.

Urinary tract anomalies include marked hydroureter and moderate pelviectasis with mild or minimal caliectasis in severely affected infants. Megaurethra (urethral ectasia) and presence of a utricle (midline cystic-appearing müllerian remnant between the bladder and rectum) are seen. Urinary bladder has markedly enlarged capacity with thickened wall and may show an hourglass configuration on VCUG.

42. What is bladder exstrophy?
Bladder exstrophy is a congenital condition in which the bladder lies exposed on the lower abdominal surface through an anterior abdominal wall defect. The incidence is about 1 per 10,000 live births. The diagnosis is instantly obvious after delivery; boys have associated epispadias. The pubic symphysis is always widened with diastasis of the rectus muscles. Vertebral anomalies are sometimes associated. Surgical reconstruction of the bladder is often feasible and bladder augmentation or diversion procedures are sometimes necessary.

BIBLIOGRAPHY

1. Avni FE, Hall M, Damry N, Schurmans T: Vesicoureteric reflux. In Frotter R (ed): Pediatric Uroradiology. New York, Springer Verlag, 2002, pp 121–144.
2. Barnewolt CE, Paltiel HJ, Lebowitz RL, Kirks DR: Genitourinary tract. In Kirks DR, Griscom NT (eds): Practical Pediatric Imaging, 3rd ed. Philadelphia, Lippincott-Raven, 1998, pp 1010–1161.
3. Siegel MJ: Urinary tract. In Siegel MJ (ed): Pediatric Sonography, 3rd ed. Philadelphia, Lippincott Williams & Wilkins, 2002, pp 385–474.
4. Swischuk LE, John SD: Differential Diagnosis in Pediatric Radiology, 2nd ed. Baltimore, Williams & Wilkins, 1995, pp 182–183.

VIII. Vascular Sonography

38. LOWER AND UPPER EXTREMITY DEEP VENOUS THROMBOSIS EVALUATION

Christopher Bang, D.O.

1. How common is venous thromboembolic disease (deep venous thrombosis; DVT)?

Venous thromboembolism (VTE) is a common problem that affects up to 70 per 100,000 patients per year in the United States, accounting for up to 250,000 hospitalizations and nearly 50,000 deaths per year.

2. What is the major complication associated with DVT?

The major cause of mortality is due to pulmonary embolism (PE). More than 50% of patients with a lower extremity DVT have a PE. The actual prevalence is likely to be higher because the disease is undiagnosed or misdiagnosed in many cases. Other complications include recurrent DVT (20%) and post-phlebitic syndrome.

3. What are the major risk factors for development of VTE?

Many studies have shown that age older than 60 years, major surgery or trauma, history of VTE, malignancy, pregnancy, and use of oral contraceptives are among the major acquired risk factors for VTE. Orthopedic and abdominal surgery or trauma pose higher risks, with general anesthesia, immobility, and premorbid and perioperative complications increasing the risks. Inherited hypercoaguable conditions such as protein S and protein C deficiency, antithrombin III deficiency, and factor V Leiden mutation are uncommon causes of VTE but are clinically significant in the context of an associated major risk factor. Medical conditions such as myocardial infarction, congestive heart failure, cerebrovascular event, spinal cord injury, and nephrotic syndrome have been associated with increased risk of VTE.

4. Which vessels are commonly involved?

The deep veins of the lower extremities above the knees include the common femoral veins, superficial femoral veins (SFVs), deep femoral veins, and popliteal veins (Fig. 1). Below the knees, the calf veins include the posterior tibial and peroneal veins. DVT rarely involves the anterior tibial veins. The saphenous veins are not considered deep veins, but may be a thromboembolic source for PE. More proximal disease may involve the iliac veins or inferior vena cava.

5. What is May-Thurner syndrome?

May-Thurner syndrome obstructs the left common iliac vein, frequently causing DVT in the left iliofemoral system. It is also known as iliac compression syndrome or pelvic venous spur. It is more common in females.

6. What is the clinical presentation for lower extremity DVT (LEDVT)?

Clinical findings are neither sensitive nor specific, and accuracy of clinical diagnosis approaches only 50%. The signs and symptoms include erythema, warmth, swelling, and pain in the

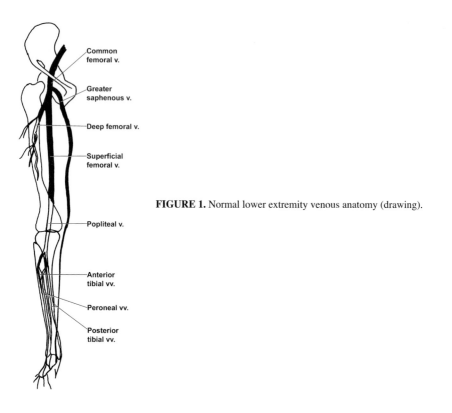

FIGURE 1. Normal lower extremity venous anatomy (drawing).

affected limb. Symptoms often increase with ambulation and may progress proximally (i.e., from the calf to the thigh). Ileofemoral DVT (10% of all DVTs) presents with pain in the buttocks or groin and associated thigh or entire leg swelling.

7. What conditions can mimic DVT clinically?

Baker's cyst, hematoma, superficial thrombophlebitis, cellulitis, abscess, myonecrosis, soft tissue tumor, arterial disease, venous scarring, and chronic venous insufficiency should all be considered as possible etiologies of the patient's symptoms.

8. How accurate is ultrasound in the diagnosis of lower extremity DVT?

Real-time ultrasonography is very sensitive and specific, exceeding 95% and 98%, respectively, for femoral-popliteal DVT in symptomatic patients. Results are more variable for calf DVT.

9. What other imaging modules are used to image DVT?

Other modalities include conventional venography, impedance plethysmography, computed tomography (CT) and CT angiography (CTA), magnetic resonance imaging (MRI) and MR angiography (MRA), nuclear medicine, and D-dimer assays. Conventional contrast venography is considered the gold standard for diagnosis of DVT.

10. What are the disadvantages of conventional venography?

The procedure is invasive and uncomfortable for patients. Potential contrast reactions include renal failure and allergic reactions. Local reactions such as extravasation and phlebitis may occur. Radiation exposure is also a factor.

11. What are the limitations of ultrasound with respect to the diagnosis of DVT?

It is operator dependent, and appropriate technique and equipment are critical for accurate diagnosis. Disease location (i.e., pelvic or calf veins), body habitus, and swollen limbs are limiting factors for image resolution, especially of small vessels. Sensitivity is less for asymptomatic patients because of small clot size and noncontiguous thrombi. Anatomic variants such as duplicated segments (SFV 20% and popliteal vein 35%) and collateral veins may lead to false-negative results. It may be difficult to distinguish between acute versus chronic DVT.

12. Why is ultrasound considered the initial modality of choice for diagnosis of DVT?

Real-time duplex (B-mode with pulsed Doppler) ultrasound is cost effective, noninvasive, highly accurate, and easy for the patient, and it provides both anatomic and physiologic information, as well as quantitative and qualitative information. It has a high negative predictive value and is useful to diagnose other causes of leg pain and swelling.

13. Should asymptomatic high-risk patients be screened with ultrasound?

DVT in high-risk patients such as postoperative and pregnant patients tend to occur in the calf and pelvic veins, respectively, and the sensitivity of ultrasound is decreased in these situations. Screening ultrasounds for asymptomatic patients (i.e., without leg symptoms) is not currently recommended.

14. Which lower extremity vessels are examined?

The LEDVT examination includes examination of the following veins: the common femoral vein (CFV) just below the inguinal ligament, the profunda femoris vein just as it branches from the CFV, the superficial femoral vein (SFV), the popliteal vein, and, if indicated, the calf veins (anterior tibial, posterior tibial, and peroneal veins) and the muscular veins (gastrocnemius and soleus)

15. Which transducers are ideal for lower extremity Doppler ultrasound?

A 5-MHz or higher frequency linear array transducer is ideal for most patients for grayscale imaging. Lower frequencies may be used with color Doppler ultrasound.

16. How is the patient positioned during the examination?

The patient is supine with the leg slightly flexed, abducted, and externally rotated, and the transducer is coursed along the medial aspect of the thigh and behind the knee. For the popliteal vein behind the knee and calf veins, the knee may be slightly flexed; or, the patient may be placed in the prone position or have the leg hanging over the side of the bed while in the sitting position.

17. How is the examination performed?

The examination starts with visualization of the common femoral vein just below the inguinal ligament with transverse compression along the vein in a stepwise fashion every 1–2 cm, through the superficial femoral vein to the distal popliteal vein. The profunda femoris at the junction of the SFV is identified and compressed, and the origin of the greater saphenous vein is also identified and compressed. Color and spectral Doppler are then used to interrogate the same vessels, documenting color fill in the veins and response of the veins to augmentation.

18. If the SFV in the distal thigh does not initially compress, what should be done before the diagnosis of a DVT is made?

It is helpful to compress the SFV in the distal thigh by placing one hand directly under the distal thigh and compressing the vessel with the transducer from the anteriolateral direction. This maneuver can be recorded using a cine loop feature or videotape.

19. Should the asymptomatic leg be examined?

Only the spectral Doppler waveform of the asymptomatic CFV is routinely evaluated. When there are positive findings in the symptomatic leg, then the other leg should be evaluated for venous access for possible filter placement by way of the common femoral vein. Both legs are evaluated if they are both symptomatic.

20. When should the calf veins be evaluated?

If symptoms are focal to the calf region, then the calf veins should be evaluated, with more emphasis on the posterior tibial and peroneal veins, because anterior tibial vein DVT is rare. The asymptomatic calf is not routinely evaluated. Calf veins are evaluated primarily with compression. Color Doppler can be used to locate the veins and confirm absence of flow in a noncompressible vein.

21. What can be done if the calf veins are difficult to see?

If possible, scan with the patient sitting up with the calves dangling over the edge of the stretcher. This position allows blood to pool in the calf veins, making visibility easier.

22. What is the role of serial ultrasound?

If the initial ultrasound is negative but clinical suspicion is high and symptoms persist, then a follow-up ultrasound evaluation is recommended in 5–7 days. Otherwise, serial ultrasound is unnecessary. If there is a low pretest probability and the initial ultrasound is normal, then the presence of a DVT can be reliably excluded.

23. What are the diagnostic features of a DVT on ultrasound?

Incomplete coaptation of the vein walls, direct visualization of the thrombus, vein distention, and abnormal flow dynamics with either absent flow or disturbed flow around a thrombus are seen on ultrasound.

24. Which diagnostic feature is the most sensitive for DVT?

Incomplete compressibility of the vein is the most sensitive and specific finding for DVT. Visualization of the thrombus is very specific but not a very sensitive finding for acute DVT (Figs. 2 and 3).

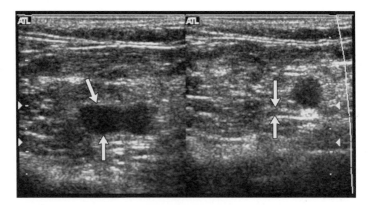

FIGURE 2. Transverse image of normal common femoral vein (*arrows*) without (*left*) and with (*right*) compression. The vein disappears with compression and only the artery remains.

25. How can acute DVT be distinguished from chronic DVT?

The acute thrombus tends to be more homogeneous and hypoechoic to isoechoic within a focally distended vein. The thrombus usually becomes more echogenic over time, and the wall of the vein becomes thick, irregular, and echogenic, with decreased lumen diameter or atretic segments. Collateral veins also develop over time (Fig. 4).

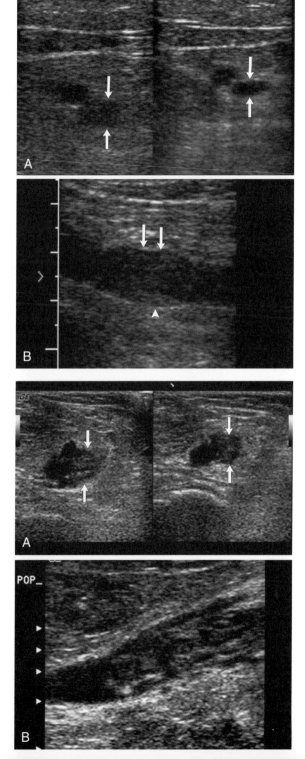

FIGURE 3. Transverse (*A*) and longitudinal (*B*) images of acute DVT (*arrows*) in superficial femoral vein. Note incomplete coaptation of venous walls in compression image and focal distention.

FIGURE 4. Transverse (*A*) and longitudinal (*B*) images of chronic DVT in popliteal vein. Note incomplete coaptation of irregular venous walls (*A*) (*arrows*) and echogenic thrombus (*A* and *B*).

26. Does color Doppler add anything for the diagnosis of DVT?

Color Doppler is a useful adjunct especially when compression cannot be performed because of profound swelling or deep vessel depth, such as in the proximal thigh and pelvis. Deeper veins can be identified by using a lower frequency Doppler (Figs. 5 and 6).

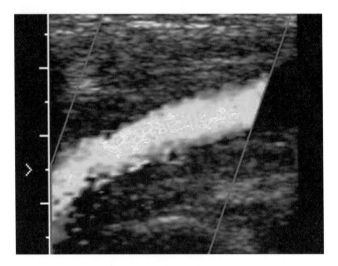

FIGURE 5. Color Doppler image of normal common femoral vein.

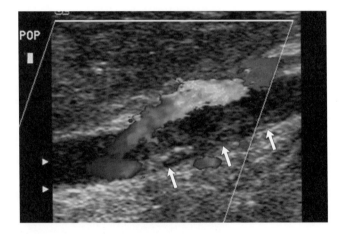

FIGURE 6. Color Doppler image of DVT in popliteal vein. Note incomplete color filling of vein lumen and echogenic thrombus (*arrows*). (See also Color Plates, Figure 14.)

27. How sensitive is color Doppler for detection of DVT?

In a patient in whom compression cannot be used, color Doppler is 95% sensitive for DVT from the groin to the knee; it is much less useful from the calf.

28. What is the significance of Doppler spectral waveform analysis?

One of the advantages of duplex sonography is the ability to demonstrate normal respiratory phasicity of venous flow. The physiology may be altered by patient positioning, slow blood return, hypovolemia, and heart failure, but monophasic waveforms suggest more proximal disease either within the veins or compressing the iliacs or IVC.

29. What is the purpose of the Valsalva maneuver?

A normal venous response to Valsalva maneuver is transient flow reversal, followed by cessation of flow from increased intra-abdominal pressure and then a surge of antegrade flow with release of the maneuver. The lumen diameter should also increase by at least 15%. This response is lost or diminished with proximal disease involving the iliacs or IVC (Figs. 7 and 8).

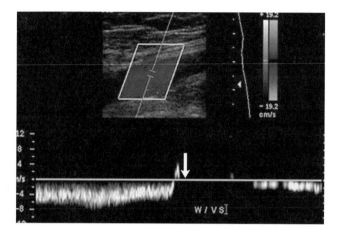

FIGURE 7. Normal venous response to Valsalva maneuver with complete cessation of spontaneous flow in the common femoral vein (*arrow*).

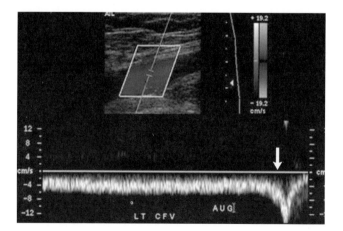

FIGURE 8. Normal venous response to augmentation maneuver with increased flow (*arrow*) following calf augmentation.

30. What is the purpose of the augmentation maneuver?

Squeezing the calf should normally increase venous flow at the segment being evaluated, indicating venous patency proximally and distally. Loss of this normal response may indicate an obstructing thrombus.

31. What are the pitfalls of these maneuvers?

Patient symptoms, body habitus, and leg edema may not permit such maneuvers to be performed. Non-occlusive thrombus and collaterals may also give a false-negative response.

32. What is the role of D-dimer assay in the diagnosis of DVT?

D-dimer is a fibrin degradation product that is formed as a thrombus is produced and degraded. It is sensitive but not very specific, in that there are many other conditions in which levels are elevated such as acute myocardial infarction or cerebrovascular accident (CVA), sepsis, disseminated intravascular coagulation, malignancy, postsurgical status or trauma, and liver disease. Thus, in the appropriate clinical context, it may be used to exclude DVT in conjunction with other modalities such as ultrasound.

33. What are the main goals of DVT treatment?

The goals are to prevent a pulmonary embolism, to restore venous patency and valvular function, and to prevent post-phlebitic syndrome.

34. What are the treatment options for DVT?

Anticoagulation with intravenous or subcutaneous injections of unfractionated heparin, or subcutaneous injections of a low-molecular-weight heparin, and initiation of oral warfarin is the initial management for acute femoral-popliteal DVT. Calf vein DVT may also be treated this way, or it may be treated conservatively with no medical therapy. Catheter-directed thrombolysis and surgical thrombectomy are other treatment options for extensive thrombosis. IVC filter placement is an option when there is a contraindication to anticoagulation or disease recurs despite anticoagulation. Prophylactic treatment, either medically or mechanically, is recommended for patients at risk for DVT.

35. How common is upper extremity deep venous thrombosis (UEDVT)?

UEDVT is reported to account for 4% of all DVTs. DVT in the upper extremities is much less common than in the lower extremities, primarily because of better flow dynamics, fewer venous valves, less hydrostatic pressure, and extensive collateral circulation. The uncommon primary (or spontaneous or effort-induced) UEDVT accounts for only about 2% of all DVTs. Secondary UEDVT resulting from catheters, intravenous lines, or pacer wires accounts for most of the clinically evident cases.

36. What is Paget-Schroetter syndrome?

Also known as idiopathic, primary, traumatic, spontaneous, or effort-induced thrombosis of the axillosubclavian vein, Paget-Schroetter syndrome is more common in younger males and usually involves the right arm.

37. Which vessels are involved in UEDVT?

The deep veins of the arm include the brachial, axillary, and subclavian veins. The basilic and cephalic veins are superficial veins, which actually account for most of the upper extremity venous return. More proximal disease may include the innominate veins, internal jugular veins, and SVC (Fig. 9).

38. What are the common etiologies?

The uncommon primary UEDVT may occur spontaneously, but it may also be associated with repetitive motion of the dominant limb, or it may be due to prolonged fixed position of a limb. Approximately 30–60% of the more common secondary type is attributable to indwelling central venous catheters and transvenous pacemaker wires, especially in the subclavian vein. Other causes include trauma or postoperative state, intravenous drug abuse and repetitive venipuncture, intravenous irritants (contrast, chemotherapy, drugs), and radiation-induced fibrosis. Thoracic outlet syndrome leads to vascular stasis and impingement. External irritation and compression by a mass or inflammation may be a cause. Hypercoaguable states such as malignancy, congestive heart failure, sepsis, and recurrent LEDVT are also risk factors.

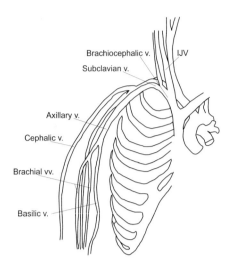

FIGURE 9. Normal upper extremity venous anatomy (drawing).

39. What is a fibrin sheath?

This is a collection of fibrin, fibronectin, and platelets around the indwelling catheter tip. It is more common than a DVT. It is echogenic and does not permit complete coaptation of the vessel walls. Correlation with clinical history and visualization of a structure that looks like a piece of catheter (parallel echogenic walls) help confirm the diagnosis.

40. What is the clinical presentation of UEDVT?

Most cases of UEDVT are asymptomatic. The signs and symptoms are nonspecific and may include limb pain, swelling, erythema, and warmth, with functional impairment of the affected limb or neck. Dilated superficial veins and a palpable axillary cord may be present. Suspicion should also be raised in patients with indwelling catheters, or any other risk factors, who present with the scenario of pulmonary embolism, especially if LEDVT has been excluded.

41. What are some conditions that can mimic UEDVT clinically?

An extrinsic limb mass, hematoma, inflammation, infection, and lymphedema may have a similar presentation.

42. What are the potential complications?

Although UEDVT is less common than LEDVT and even though the upper extremities are less prone to complete venous obstruction than the lower extremities, serious complications such as PE and death can result. Up to one-third of UEDVTs are associated with PE; some are fatal. Other complications include septic thrombophlebitis, loss of limb function, and venous insufficiency.

43. How is the diagnosis of UEDVT made?

Contrast venography, ultrasound, CT, MRI, and nuclear scintigraphy are among the modalities that can be used. The gold standard for diagnosis is conventional contrast venography, which is limited by lack of venous access (these patients often have central lines for chemotherapy access) and which does not evaluate the internal jugular vein (IJV).

44. How accurate is ultrasound with respect to the diagnosis of UEDVT?

Duplex ultrasound with color Doppler has greater than 90% sensitivity and specificity when diagnosing UEDVT in the peripheral upper extremity veins, especially the axillary vein, and the lateral portions of the subclavian vein. It is more limited centrally, especially in the brachiocephalic veins and the superior vena cava (SVC).

45. What is the standard technique for ultrasound evaluation for UEDVT?

Bilateral imaging is performed initially, starting with the asymptomatic side. With the patient supine, color and spectral Doppler, and transverse compression with a 5 to 7-MHz linear array transducer are performed beginning with the IJV from the angle of the mandible to the junction of the subclavian or innominate veins. Having patients turn their head slightly away from the transducer may help visualize the more proximal portions. A lower frequency (5 MHz), smaller faced transducer is used with color and spectral Doppler to evaluate the innominate and proximal portions of the subclavian veins. A small footprint phased-array (2–4 MHz) transducer may be used to visualize the SVC. The lateral portions of the subclavian vein, the axillary vein, the brachial veins, the basilic vein, and the cephalic vein are examined with a linear (5–7 MHz) transducer. These vessels are examined with compression, color Doppler, and spectral Doppler. A higher frequency transducer may be needed to visualize the smaller arm veins.

46. How are follow-up examinations performed?

Follow-up examinations are of the affected limb only, with the asymptomatic contralateral IJV waveform included.

47. How is the patient positioned for the examination?

The patient is positioned supine. The head can be slightly elevated if necessary. Initially the head is turned away from the side being examined and the arm is resting at the side. To examine the axillary, brachial, and basilic veins, the arm must be abducted with the palm facing up.

48. What are the major limitations of ultrasound in evaluating for UEDVT?

Operator dependency, patient body habitus, extent of edema, and extensive collateral circulation are the main limitations. Visualization of the more proximal vessels such as the medial portions of the subclavian vein, innominate vein, and SVC are commonly obscured by the clavicle, as well being limited by transducer footprint size and depth of field. Mistaking a collateral vessel for a patent vein is more common in the upper extremity than in the lower extremity. Identification of the adjacent accompanying artery is helpful in these situations. The smaller peripheral veins such as the basilic, cephalic, and brachial veins may also be difficult to identify. Color Doppler is essential in these areas. Intravenous devices and scarring can be confusing.

49. Because the clavicle limits compression of the subclavian vein, how can it be evaluated for a non-occlusive thrombus?

The subclavian vein can be scanned with the transducer placed transverse to the vessel using color Doppler to make sure the vessel fills with color. It is necessary to angle the transducer toward the midline when using this technique, and the color sensitivity is maximized to fill the vessel, without inducing noise.

50. What do collateral veins look like?

Compared with normal veins, collateral veins are of smaller caliber, more tortuous, and usually displaced away from the accompanying artery.

51. Are the forearm veins routinely evaluated?

No. The radial, ulnar, and interosseous veins are evaluated only if indicated by clinical presentation. DVT involving these veins is rare.

52. What are the sonographic findings of UEDVT?

Loss of complete compressibility is the most specific finding associated with DVT, followed by incomplete vessel filing with color Doppler. Rapid inspiration or sniffing normally causes the IJV and subclavian veins to collapse, and loss of this phenomenon, wall motion abnormality, or no change in flow velocity may be a sign of an obstructing thrombus. Pulsed Doppler can demonstrate flow disturbance, defined as reduced cardiac pulsatility and respiratory phasicity, or absent flow (Figs. 10 and 11).

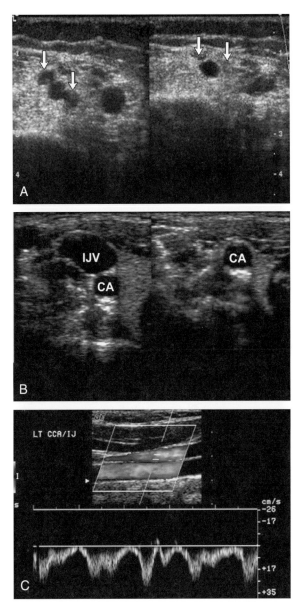

FIGURE 10. Transverse images of normal upper extremity vein (*A*) and normal internal jugular vein (IJV) (*B*). *C,* Color Doppler image of normal IJV in blue with carotid artery in red posteriorly. Note complete color fill of vein with normal spectral respiratory phasicity.

53. Can augmentation maneuvers be used?

The peripheral veins may respond to augmentation maneuvers, but smaller volumes and more elaborate collateral channels in the upper extremities may make it less apparent.

54. What are the treatment options for UEDVT?

Conservative treatment with elevation, rest, and heat, with removal or correction of the offending cause, is standard. Anticoagulation, thrombolysis, surgical thrombectomy, and SVC filter placement are not as well studied for UEDVT as for LEDVT, but they are reasonable options in the appropriate clinical context. Because of the risk of catheter-induced UEDVT, many centers recommend prophylaxis with warfarin or low-dose heparin for catheterized patients.

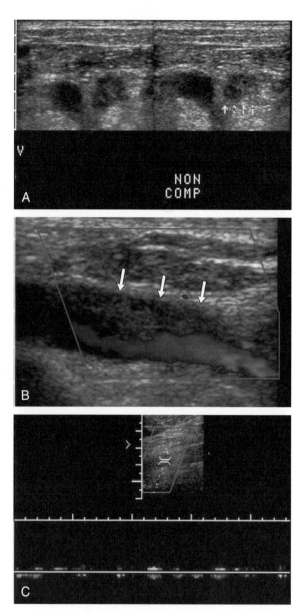

FIGURE 11. Transverse (*A*) and color Doppler (*B*) images of upper extremity DVT. Note noncompressibility and echogenic thrombus (*arrows*) (*A*), incomplete color fill-in, and abnormal waveform. With color Doppler (*B*) there is incomplete filling of the lumen because of marginal thrombus (*arrows*). Spectral tracing (*C*) in an area of complete occlusion shows no flow, only transmitted motion from the adjacent artery.

55. What is the evolution of DVT?

After treatment with anticoagulation, DVT will undergo complete resolution in approximately 60% of the patients. In 40% of the patients, some residual thrombus will remain. Six months after anticoagulation treatment, whatever changes are observed within the vein are permanent.

56. What are phlegmasia alba dolens and phlegmasia cerulea dolens?

These conditions result from acute massive venous thrombosis and obstruction of the venous drainage of an extremity. In phlegmasia cerulea dolens (PCD), the thrombosis extends to collateral veins, resulting in massive fluid sequestration and more significant edema. In phlegmasia alba dolens (PAD), collateral vessels are not involved.

PCD presents with the clinical triad of edema, agonizing pain, and cyanosis. Massive fluid sequestration may lead to bleb and bullae formation. The pain is constant, usually starting at the femoral triangle and progressing to the entire extremity. Cyanosis progressing from distal to proximal areas is the pathognomonic finding of PCD. This causes venous gangrene and ultimately results in a compartment-type syndrome and arterial compromise.

BIBLIOGRAPHY

1. Falk RL, Smith DF: Thrombosis of upper extremity thoracic inlet veins: Diagnosis with duplex Doppler sonography. Am J Roentgenol 149:677–682, 1987.
2. Fraser JD, Anderson DR: Deep venous thrombosis: Recent advances and optimal investigation with US. Radiology 211:9–24, 1999.
3. Gottlieb RH, Widjaja J, Mehra S, Robinette WB: Clinically important pulmonary emboli: Does calf vein US alter outcomes? Radiology 211:25–29, 1999.
4. Hirsh J, Hoak J: Management of deep vein thrombosis and pulmonary embolism. Circulation 93:2212–2245, 1996.
5. Lewis BD: The peripheral veins. In Rumack CM, Wilson SR, Charboneau JW (eds): Diagnostic Ultrasound, 2nd ed. St. Louis, Mosby, 1998, pp 943–958.
6. Lewis BD, James EM, Welch TJ, et al: Diagnosis of acute deep venous thrombosis of the lower extremities: Prospective evaluation of color Doppler flow imaging versus venography. Radiology 192:681–685, 1994.
7. Naidich JB, Torre JR, Pellerito JS, et al: Suspected deep venous thrombosis: Is US of both legs necessary? Radiology 200:429–431, 1996.
8. Polak JF: Venous thrombosis. In Peripheral Vascular Sonography: A Practical Guide. Philadelphia, Lippincott Williams & Wilkins, 1992, pp 155–214.
9. Wells P, Anderson DR, Bormanis J, et al: SimpliRED D-Dimer can reduce the diagnostic tests in suspected deep vein thrombosis. Lancet 351(9113): 1405–1406, 1998.

39. CAROTID ARTERIAL AND VERTEBRAL DOPPLER ULTRASOUND

Andrea Zynda-Weiss, M.D., and Nancy L. Carson, M.B.A., RDMS, R.V.T.

1. What are the clinical indications for carotid ultrasound?

Carotid ultrasound is used for the workup of ipsilateral stroke and transient ischemic attacks (TIA), amaurosis fugax, and carotid bruit. In addition, carotid ultrasound is used to follow up patients after carotid endarterectomy and follow the progression of known carotid atherosclerosis. Preoperative screening before cardiac or major vascular surgery is also an indication.

2. What is NASCET?

The North American Symptomatic Carotid Endartectomy Trial (NASCET) randomized patients to medical versus surgical management of symptomatic carotid stenosis. The measured outcome was reduction in death and hemispheric stroke. This study definitively showed that for symptomatic stenosis of greater than 70% diameter reduction, the long-term benefit of carotid endarterectomy was significantly greater than that of medical treatment. This study ensured the future of carotid ultrasound as a screening tool and helped standardize criteria to measure stenosis.

3. If emboli cause stroke, why measure stenosis?

Ninety percent of strokes are ischemic and the majority of ischemic strokes are due to emboli. Most ischemic strokes caused by carotid occlusion are due to emboli from plaques rather than decreased flow. It has been shown that, as the degree of stenosis increases, the risk of stroke increases.

4. What is the normal carotid anatomy?

The first branch off the aorta is the innominate artery, which then branches into the right common carotid artery (CCA) and right subclavian artery. The left CCA arises directly from the aortic arch as its second branch. The normal CCA diameter is 6–8 mm.

The common carotid artery runs deep to the sternocleidomastoid muscle and jugular vein. Near the middle of the neck, the common carotid dilates to form the carotid bulb before branching into the internal and external carotid arteries. The internal carotid artery (ICA) is positioned posteriorly and laterally, whereas the external carotid artery (ECA) is medial and anterior. The ICA does not have any branches in the neck (Fig. 1).

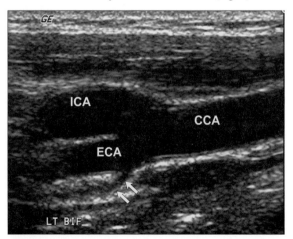

FIGURE 1. The carotid bifurcation. The common carotid artery divides into the internal carotid artery (ICA) and external carotid artery (ECA). The ECA is located more medially and anteriorly than the ICA. The ECA gives off branches (*arrows*) in the neck as can be seen in this image. *Note:* The normal thin (< 1 mm) echogenic mucosa lines the vessels.

5. What vessels are scanned for the carotid examination?

The carotid examination includes bilateral interrogation of the CCA, the ICA, the proximal ECA, and the vertebral artery (VA).

6. How should the patient be positioned?

The ideal patient position is supine with the chin extended and the head rotated away from the side being examined. It is also helpful to have the patient drop the shoulder of the side being examined by reaching down toward the knee.

7. What transducer frequency is used?

The operator should use the highest frequency that will provide adequate penetration, usually 7.5 MHz, (minimum 5 MHz) linear array transducer.

8. What are the scan planes?

Representative grayscale and color images are obtained in the transverse and sagittal or coronal planes. The transverse plane allows the sonographer to follow the course of the vessels, look for plaques, and plan the approach for the sagittal views. In the sagittal or coronal views, angle-corrected ($\leq 60°$) Doppler tracings are obtained of the CCA, the proximal ECA, the proximal, mid, and distal ICA, any areas of stenosis, and the VA.

9. What is the best approach to obtain the required views?

The vessels are scanned from the anterior, lateral, and posterolateral approaches to determine the best place for image acquisition. It is often necessary to change the approach from lateral to posterolateral to visualize as far into the ICA as possible.

10. When does the carotid examination become technically limited and what can be done?

The carotid examination becomes technically limited in the following settings:

- The patient has a neck brace limiting access to the vessels: The examination must wait until the collar can be removed.
- The patient has a large neck or high shoulders: In the case of a large neck, decrease the frequency to 5 MHz, and decrease the color Doppler frequency to 3.5–5 MHz to allow adequate penetration. In the case of high, broad shoulders, turn the head as far to the contralateral side as possible and scan posterolaterally; have the patient reach down toward the ipsilateral knee.
- The patient has a high bifurcation, limiting interrogation of the ICA: Follow the ICA as high as possible in the transverse axis with grayscale and color Doppler. Often only the proximal ICA is seen in the sagittal plane. It is also useful to turn the patient's head to the contralateral side and scan posterolaterally.
- The patient cannot turn his head: Often the patient can be turned to the side, allowing better access to a lateral or posterolateral approach to the vessels.
- The patient is unable to lie flat or cannot hold still: If the patient cannot lie flat, the examination can still be done with the patient upright and leaning back on a stretcher with the chin tilted up. If the patient cannot hold still, the examination will be technically limited at best.

11. What is the purpose of spectral Doppler tracings?

The purpose of Doppler tracings is to provide both direction of flow and flow velocity information.

12. What Doppler frequency is used?

The Doppler frequency used for spectral tracings is usually 5 MHz.

13. How are the most accurate velocity readings obtained?

It is important to keep the angle of the Doppler cursor to the vessel $< 60°$. The machine uses the insonating Doppler frequency and the angle of the vessel to that of the Doppler cursor to calculate velocity data. At angles $> 60°$, the velocity calculation becomes increasingly inaccurate and waveforms become damped. When possible, the CCA and ICA should be interrogated with a relatively constant angle.

14. When should Doppler frequency be changed?

The Doppler frequency should be decreased when more penetration is needed, for example, in patients with large necks. The Doppler frequency can be increased for shallow vessels to increase sensitivity.

15. What is the best technique to follow tortuous vessels?

Tortuous vessels should be first followed in the transverse axis using color flow Doppler. Once the vessel is located, turn the transducer to image the vessel in the sagittal plane and obtain the Doppler tracings. Power Doppler may also be useful to follow tortuous vessels.

16. What techniques are used for the evaluation of calcified vessels?

The presence of calcified plaque can obscure part of the distal CCA, bulb, or the ICA. In these cases, it is beneficial to turn the patient's head as far to the opposite side as possible and scan from as far posterior as possible in the sagittal plane. It is also helpful to scan the area in the transverse plane with color Doppler to ensure the vessel is patent.

17. How can artifacts in the lumen be eliminated?

Artifacts in the lumen can be resolved by decreasing the frequency of the transducer, decreasing the power, scanning from a different angle, or turning the head.

18. How does one distinguish the ICA from the ECA?

The ECA has branches, which are best seen with color Doppler. The ECA has a more pulsatile, higher resistance waveform, whereas the ICA has a low-resistance waveform. When using color Doppler, the color in the ECA flashes off and on and the color in the ICA tends to be persistent, indicating flow throughout diastole. The ICA courses more posteriorly, whereas the ECA courses toward the face. The ECA responds to a temporal tap.

19. What is a temporal tap and how is it performed?

The temporal tap is a means to distinguish the ECA from the ICA. When performing a temporal tap, the ipsilateral temporal artery is tapped while obtaining the ECA Doppler tracing. The Doppler tracing displays undulations representing the reflected tap from the temporal artery because it is a branch of the ECA (Fig. 2).

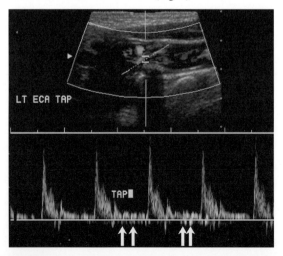

LT ECA TAP

TAP

FIGURE 2. Temporal tap. A temporal tap can be used to distinguish the external carotid artery (ECA) from the internal carotid artery. The ipsilateral temporal artery is tapped while obtaining the ECA Doppler tracing. The Doppler tracing displays undulations (*arrows*) representing the reflected tap from the temporal artery.

20. Are there pitfalls to using the temporal tap?

Yes. False-negative results occur when the tap is not properly performed. In some cases in the setting of normal vessels, the pulsations may be transmitted backward into the CCA and ICA.

21. What are the normal Doppler spectral waveforms for the CCA, ICA, and ECA?

The carotid arteries have forward flow throughout the cardiac cycle. The ICA has a smooth Doppler waveform with persistent flow throughout systole and diastole due to the low vascular resistance of the intracerebral vessels. The peak systolic velocities are normally 0.6–1.0 m/sec. The ECA has a sharp peak in systole and low velocity near the end of diastole due to the high resistance in its multiple branches. The CCA has mixed high and low resistance features with a sharp peak in systole as seen in the ECA and persistent diastolic flow as seen in the ICA (Fig. 3).

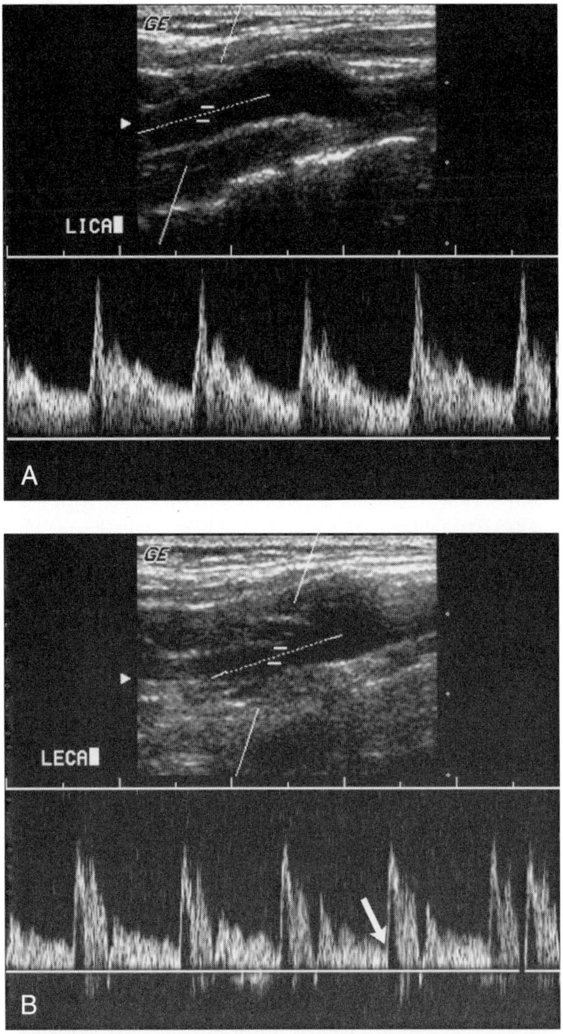

FIGURE 3. *A,* Normal internal carotid artery (ICA) waveform. The normal ICA has a smooth Doppler waveform with persistent flow throughout systole and diastole. *B,* Normal external carotid artery (ECA) waveform. The normal ECA waveform has a sharp peak in systole and low velocity near the end of diastole (*arrow*). (*continued*)

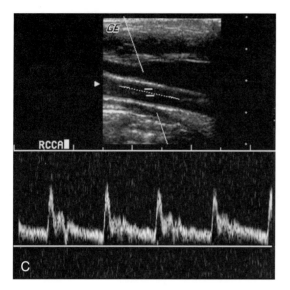

FIGURE 3. (*continued*) *C,* Normal common carotid artery (CCA). The normal CCA waveform demonstrates a sharp peak in systole and persistent diastolic flow.

22. What is the most common location for carotid stenosis to occur?
Most carotid stenoses occur at the origin of the ICA.

23. What is the basic principle upon which Doppler evaluation of stenosis is based?
Flow velocity in a stenotic lumen is elevated in proportion to the degree of narrowing. Therefore, by measuring the flow velocity by Doppler, the severity of narrowing can be indirectly determined. The velocity increase in a stenotic zone is small until the lumen diameter is reduced by 50%. Beyond 50% diameter reduction, the velocity rapidly increases as the degree of stenosis increases.

24. What three measurements are important in the stenotic zone?
- Peak systolic velocity (peak systole)
- End diastolic velocity (end diastole)
- Systolic velocity ratio (peak systole in stenotic zone divided by peak systole in ipsilateral CCA).

Tip: It is important to search the stenotic lumen for the highest velocity; otherwise, the severity of the stenosis may be underestimated.

25. What happens to the peak systolic velocity in a stenotic lumen?
As the lumen narrows, the velocity in the stenotic zone increases logarithmically up to a 90% diameter reduction. Beyond 95% diameter reduction, velocities rapidly decrease due to the effects of increased flow resistance. Therefore, in severe stenosis, the peak systolic velocity may actually be lower than expected. Careful correlation should be made with the size of the lumen seen on color flow images (Fig. 4).

26. How is the region of peak velocity identified?
The region with the highest velocity can be found by first using color Doppler to find the point at which the lumen is the most narrowed. The color Doppler scale (PRF) is maximized to determine whether there is aliasing in this segment. Spectral Doppler is then used to search for the highest velocity in the segment that narrowed or displays aliasing.

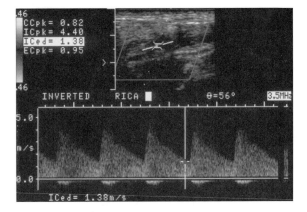

FIGURE 4. Severe internal carotid artery (ICA) stenosis with peak systolic velocity of 4.4 m/sec, elevated end-diastolic velocity of 1.38 m/sec, and ICA/common carotid artery ratio of 5.4

27. What is aliasing?

Aliasing is the inability to measure peak velocities because the Doppler sampling rate, or PRF, is too low. The Nyquist limit states that the maximum detectable frequency shift cannot exceed half the PRF.

28. How is aliasing manifested in the carotid examination?

Aliasing is seen in both the Doppler spectrum and the color Doppler image when high peak velocities are present. On the Doppler spectrum, the peak systolic velocities are cut off and displayed below the baseline. The color Doppler spectrum wraps around the four-color spectrum to include red, yellow, green, and blue (Fig. 5).

29. How is aliasing beneficial?

Aliasing can be used to locate the area of maximum velocity in a high-grade stenosis. This is done by using color Doppler and increasing the scale (PRF) to the maximum width, which still permits for areas of aliasing. The aliased image segment is then interrogated with spectral Doppler by scanning through the entire segment at an angle parallel to the segment, not the vessel wall, seeking the maximum systolic velocity. Triplex (live color and Doppler) is useful to find the maximum velocity and should be turned off before obtaining measurable Doppler tracings to improve the spectral signal. The spectral Doppler angle should be ≤ 60° (*see* Figure 5).

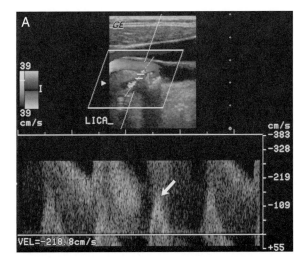

FIGURE 5. Severe internal carotid artery (ICA) stenosis at the level of the bifurcation. *A*, The Doppler waveform demonstrates markedly elevated peak systolic velocity (PSV) of greater than 380 cm/sec. *Note:* Aliasing of the Doppler spectrum where the systolic peak (*arrow*) wraps around and is written from below the baseline. The end-diastolic velocity is also elevated at 218 cm/sec (*cursor*). The common carotid artery velocity in this patient was 50 cm/sec resulting in an ICA/CCA PSV ratio of 7.6. This corresponds to a very high-grade stenosis of 80–99%. (*continued*)

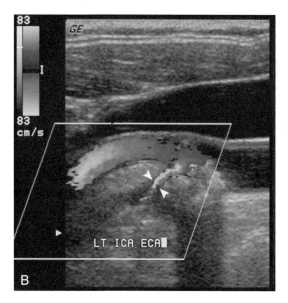

FIGURE 5. (*continued*) *B,* The color Doppler image in this same patient demonstrates severe narrowing of the internal carotid artery (*arrowheads*) by plaque.

30. How does flow reversal differ from aliasing?

Flow reversal is due to bidirectional flow in one plane of imaging. It is normally seen in the carotid bulb where the vessel widens, allowing the laminar stream to break up. The color spectrum only shows two colors with black in between (i.e., red and blue only indicating flow toward the probe and away from the probe.) The velocities in a region of flow reversal are normal. Aliasing is due to velocities exceeding the limit of the PRF. When the PRF is properly set, aliasing represents an area of extremely high velocity and therefore can be used to find the most stenotic zone of the vessel (Fig. 6).

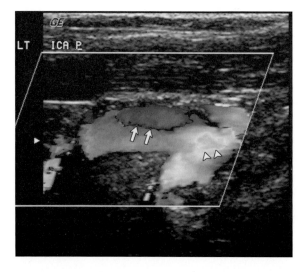

FIGURE 6. This normal internal carotid artery demonstrates flow reversal in the bulb (red to blue with a black line between) (*arrows*) and aliasing in the central high-velocity lumen of the bulb (red to yellow to blue to deep blue) (*arrowhead*). (See also Color Plates, Figure 15.)

31. What can be done to eliminate or decrease "artificial" aliasing?

To eliminate or decrease aliasing, several techniques are used:
- Increase the Doppler angles, thus decreasing the Doppler shift.
- Decrease the insonating frequency.
- Increase the PRF (scale), which increases the detectable frequency shift.
- Shift the zero baseline, being careful not to cut off flow signal below the baseline.

32. How can the degree of occlusion be measured when there is significant plaque shadowing the lumen of the vessel?

The degree of occlusion can be predicted by imaging the area in the transverse plane with color Doppler to locate the narrowest point of vessel lumen. The diameter of the lumen and the diameter of the vessel including the plaque are measured. The ratio of the lumen diameter to the entire vessel diameter is an indication of percent stenosis.

33. What other factors besides diameter reduction affect systolic velocity?

As the length of the stenosis increases, the velocity decreases. In patients with systemic hypertension, the velocity in the stenotic zone is higher than that of a normotensive patient with the same degree of diameter reduction. Decreased cardiac output can reduce the stenotic zone velocity. Therefore, a certain peak systolic velocity cannot precisely define a certain percent stenosis.

34. What are possible etiologies of decreased ICA systolic velocities?

Ipsilateral intracranial carotid stenosis, carotid dissection, stenosis at the carotid siphon, very high grade stenosis, stenosis at the origin of the CCA or innominate, and decreased cardiac output can all cause decreased ICA systolic velocities.

35. What happens to end diastole in the stenotic zone?

With less than a 50% diameter reduction, the diastolic velocity remains normal. Beyond 50% stenosis, diastolic velocities increase in proportion to the severity of the lumen narrowing due to the development of a pressure gradient in diastole. As the stenosis exceeds 70% diameter reduction, end-diastolic velocity increases rapidly (*see* Figures 4 and 5).

36. Why is the systolic velocity ratio valuable?

The systolic velocity ratio is the ratio of the peak systolic velocity in the stenotic zone divided by the peak systolic velocity in the ipsilateral CCA. Because systemic physiologic factors (e.g., blood pressure, cardiac output, peripheral resistance, and the development of collaterals) can affect the pulsatility and velocity in both normal and stenotic carotids, the ratio helps compensate for potential errors. The ratio is useful when there is decreased flow to the carotids, such as in decreased cardiac output and aortic stenosis. The ratio helps compensate for patient-to-patient physiologic variability. However, there is more room for error because two measurements are used. The ratio depends on accurate measurement of CCA and ICA velocities.

37. What happens to the systolic velocity ratio in stenosis?

The ratio increases as the stenosis severity increases. A ratio of 2 suggests a > 50% stenosis, whereas a ratio of 3 suggests > 75% stenosis (*see* Figures 4 and 5).

38. What happens to the CCA waveform and velocity in the setting of ipsilateral ICA stenosis (prestenotic waveforms)?

The CCA is the prestenotic vessel with corresponding changes in its waveform. It has more resistance, similar to an ECA waveform (i.e., more pulsatile with decreased diastolic flow). The peak systolic velocity of the Doppler signal may also be reduced because of overall decrease in flow on that side (Fig. 7).

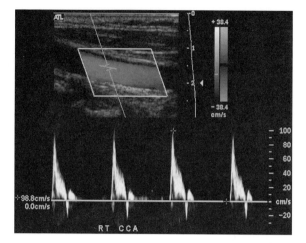

FIGURE 7. High resistive waveform in the common carotid artery proximal to an internal carotid artery stenosis. Note the lack of diastolic flow.

39. What happens to the ICA waveform with ipsilateral intracranial carotid stenosis?
The ICA becomes the prestenotic vessel and develops a low-velocity, high-resistance pattern.

40. What changes are seen in the post-stenotic region?
The spectral Doppler signal downstream from a stenosis shows spectral broadening and reversal of flow. This is caused by decrease in velocities and turbulence as the blood cells emerge from the point of stenosis.

41. What is turbulence?
Turbulence is a disruption in the laminar flow of blood through a vessel. It occurs in response to the change in diameter of the vessel. The most common sites for turbulence in the carotid artery are at the bifurcation and points distal to lumen narrowing due to plaque formation. Essentially, the laminar flow of blood is disturbed, creating a wider range of velocities.

42. How is turbulence useful?
In some cases, post-stenotic turbulence is the only indication of stenosis. This occurs when the stenotic area is obscured by shadowing from calcified plaque and only the post-stenotic region of the vessel can be seen.

43. What is spectral broadening?
Spectral broadening is the visual representation of the spectral Doppler tracing obtained from the turbulent part of a vessel. Spectral broadening is evident when the black space between the spectral tracing and the zero baseline fills in, indicating a large range of systolic velocities (Fig. 8).

44. What are the pitfalls associated with spectral broadening?
Spectral broadening can be artificially created by having the Doppler gain too high, the Doppler gate too wide, or sampling too close to the vessel wall.

45. Is spectral broadening useful for diagnosis?
Attempts have been made to correlate spectral broadening with the degree of stenosis; however, this currently has limited clinical utility for exact quantification of degree of stenosis. Spectral broadening usually increases in relationship to severity of stenosis. However, the criteria using spectral broadening to quantify stenosis are not well documented. With a stenosis > 70%, there are high-amplitude, low-frequency Doppler signals, flow reversal, and poor definition of the spectral border. Flow disturbance may be the only sign of carotid stenosis in some cases.

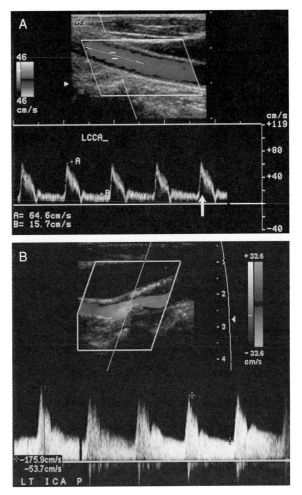

FIGURE 8. Spectral broadening. Compare the relatively clear "window" (*arrow*) of the internal carotid artery (ICA) (*A*) with that of an ICA with more turbulent flow (*B*) (spectral broadening). The greater number of velocities indicates less laminar flow.

46. What happens to ICA velocities in the setting of contralateral CCA or ICA obstruction?

Shunting of flow to the contralateral side may increase the stenotic zone velocity measurements, thereby causing an overestimation of the stenosis severity.

47. What happens to ICA velocities in the setting of ipsilateral proximal CCA stenosis?

Proximal CCA stenosis can reduce ipsilateral carotid flow and decrease the velocity in the ipsilateral ICA stenotic zone. Therefore, the degree of stenosis can be underestimated.

48. What are some reasons for false-positive (pseudostenosis) results?

With contralateral high-grade ICA stenosis, there is an increase in blood flow and velocity in the opposite carotid. High output states include hyperthyroidism, anemia, and exercise, which can increase carotid blood flow velocities. The peak systolic velocity ratio can be used to compensate for these physiologic variables.

49. What are some reasons for false-negative findings?

With very high-grade stenosis, the peak systolic velocity may be decreased and therefore the degree of stenosis is underestimated. Correlation should be made with color flow images for degree of diameter reduction. In addition, tandem stenosis proximal to the ICA (i.e., in the CCA, innominate artery, or aorta) can decrease flow and, therefore, decrease velocities, causing underestimation of the degree of stenosis.

50. Which parameter is best?

There is debate in the ultrasound literature regarding which parameter is most accurate in predicting the degree of carotid stenosis. Peak systolic velocity is the best documented parameter. However, at high degrees of stenosis, the velocity decreases, which may cause inaccuracy in measurements at the most critical degrees of stenosis. The peak systolic velocity ratio compensates for physiologic factors and the effects of collateralization; however, it uses two variables and therefore introduces more room for error. Because the end-diastolic velocity continues to increase as the degree of stenosis increases, this may be the most accurate parameter for stenosis > 75%, especially high-grade stenosis.

51. What are the difficulties in establishing universal parameters for evaluating carotid stenosis?

Physiologic differences, collaterals, arteriographic measurement variability, sonographer variability, and Doppler instrument variability combine to make establishing universal parameters difficult. For any degree of stenosis, a balance between sensitivity and specificity must be reached. As Doppler thresholds are raised, the sensitivity decreases and specificity increases. Based on NASCET outcome data, the relative cost of a false-negative finding is 17 times greater than that of a false-positive study, and parameters should reflect this.

In October 2002, the Society of Radiologists in Ultrasound issued a consensus statement with established parameters for defining degree of ICA stenosis.

Society of Radiologists in Ultrasound Consensus Conference on Carotid Ultrasound, October 22–23, 2002

DEGREE OF OCCLUSION	ICA PSV	PLAQUE	ICA/CCA PSV RATIO	ICA EDV
Normal	<125 cm/sec	None	<2.0	<40 cm/sec
<50%	<125 cm/sec	<50% diameter reduction	<2.0	<40 cm/sec
50–69%	125–230 cm/sec	≥50% diameter reduction	2.0–4.0	40–100 cm/sec
≥70% to near occlusion	230 cm/sec	≥50% diameter reduction	>4.0	>100 cm/sec
Near occlusion	May be low or undetectable	Visible	Variable	Variable
Total occlusion	Undetectable	Visible, no detectable lumen	Not applicable	Not applicable

52. Do the same parameters apply to CCA and ECA?

Peak systolic velocity values have only been defined for stenosis of the ICA, not the CCA or ECA.

53. What are the benefits of color Doppler?

Color Doppler improves the speed and accuracy of a carotid examination. Color Doppler is useful to assess the degree of stenosis visually to avoid errors and to cross check the Doppler spectrum. Using aliasing, the most stenotic zone is rapidly identified. Color Doppler may be useful in measuring carotid stenosis of less than 50% diameter reduction. Color Doppler is useful in distinguishing the ICA from the ECA.

54. Are plaque characteristics important in predicting the risk of stroke?

There are increasing data that plaque characterization may play a role in predicting stroke risk. Hypoechoic plaque is associated with lipid-rich material and intraplaque hemorrhage, and is associated with an increased risk of stroke. These data are based on surgical specimens and therefore on plaques associated with a 50% or greater stenosis. In patients presenting with acute neurologic symptoms, plaque surface characteristics may play an even more important role than plaque echogenicity. Ulcerated plaque on angiography has been reported to be an important prognostic indicator of cerebrovascular events. A plaque ulcer is an intraplaque defect or excavation measuring greater than 2×2 mm. However, both angiography and ultrasound have low sensitivity and specificity for plaque ulceration. Color Doppler may show areas of flow reversal within an ulcerated plaque (Fig. 9).

55. Does the thickness of the carotid wall matter?

Evaluation of wall thickness and changes may also play a role in predicting stroke risk because diffuse thickening of the intima and medial layers of the carotids is associated with atherosclerosis. Wall thickness may also serve as a subclinical marker of cardiovascular disease. The intimal-medial thickness is measured by determining the mean thickness or maximal thickness over the length of the vessel. Normal wall thickness is between 0.6 and 1.0 mm (Fig. 10).

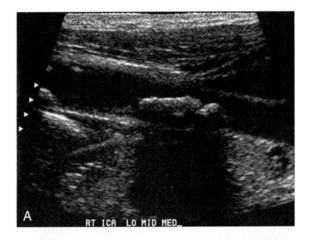

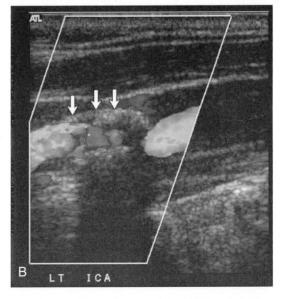

FIGURE 9. Carotid plaque. *A*, Calcified plaque with shadowing. *B*, Noncalcified (soft) plaque (*arrows*). (*continued*)

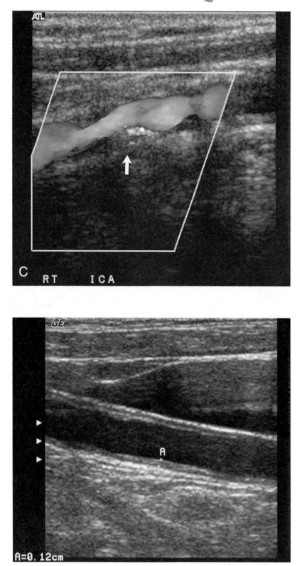

FIGURE 9. (*continued*) *C,* Ulcerated plaque demonstrating flow within it (*arrow*) (see also Color Plates, Figure 16).

FIGURE 10. Wall thickness. Note thickening of the intima and media in the common carotid artery (*cursors*).

56. How is ICA occlusion diagnosed by ultrasound?

ICA occlusion is suggested by the absence of arterial pulsations, the presence of echogenic material filling the lumen, the absence of flow on color or spectral Doppler, and small vessel size as seen in chronic occlusion. With ICA occlusion, the ECA and CCA have the same waveform. With internal carotid occlusion, a wall thump may be present in the distal CCA, which is a blunted low-velocity signal resulting from blood hitting the plaque (Fig. 11).

57. What are the causes of incorrect diagnosis of carotid occlusion?

A carotid occlusion can be missed if the artery is obscured by acoustic shadowing, image quality is poor, or Doppler signals are weak. Very high-grade stenosis with only a trickle of undetectable flow can cause a false-positive diagnosis of occlusion.

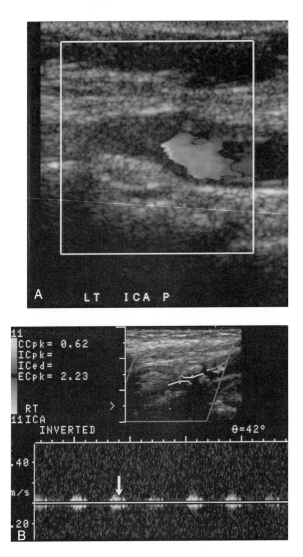

FIGURE 11. Internal carotid artery (ICA) occlusion. *A*, The absence of flow on color Doppler and the absent arterial pulsations suggest ICA occlusion (see also Color Plates, Figure 17). *B*, There is a wall thump present, which is a blunted low-velocity signal (*arrow*) resulting from blood hitting the plaque and thrombus in the occluded vessel.

58. What is the string sign?

Angiographically, the string sign is the pooling of contrast in the dependent portion of the vessel caused by slow-moving blood. The lumen is patent and the stenosis is located at the proximal end of the string. This is seen in very high-grade stenosis. Sonographically, the string sign is a low-velocity string of color with a damped waveform within the stenotic lumen and is an indicator of very high-grade stenosis (Fig. 12).

59. How can high-grade carotid stenosis be distinguished from occlusion on ultrasound?

If there is a flow signal present, there is a high-grade stenosis rather than occlusion. Color Doppler and power Doppler can be used to optimize a search for any flow signal. A low PRF and a low frequency filter should be used to detect minimal flow velocity. On the best possible view, the lumen should be carefully examined for any flow and then examined with spectral Doppler using high Doppler gain settings. False-positive results for occlusion can occur when flow is too slow to detect. In this situation, additional imaging should be considered.

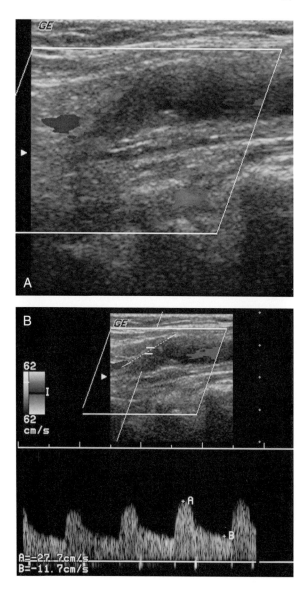

FIGURE 12. String sign. *A,* Low-velocity "string" of color indicating high-grade stenosis (see also Color Plates, Figure 18). *B,* Damped low-velocity spectral waveform within the stenotic lumen.

60. How does ultrasound compare with magnetic resonance imaging (MRA) and arteriography in the detection of carotid occlusion?

Many authors advocate operating on ultrasound results alone for stenosis > 70%. However, patients with total or near total occlusions still present a diagnostic dilemma in that focal near total occlusion is treated surgically and total occlusion is managed medically. The ability of ultrasound and MRA to differentiate between these two has not been definitively established. One recent study showed that ultrasound was able to accurately detect 100% of total occlusions but overestimated 14% of near total occlusions as completely occluded. MRA was able to detect 100% of near total occlusions but called 8% of total occlusions (all of which were distal to the bifurcation) as near total occlusions. Therefore, total or near total occlusions identified by one modality should be confirmed by a second modality. Currently, catheter angiography remains the gold standard.

61. What are the causes of carotid occlusion?

Carotid occlusion has multiple etiologies including atherosclerosis, arterial dissection, and fibromuscular dysplasia.

62. When should angiography, MRA, computed tomography (CT) angiography, or contrast-enhanced ultrasound be performed?

With severe pulsatility discrepancies in the CCAs and no apparent cause, MR imaging (MRI) or MRA should be considered to seek an obstructive lesion in the aortic arch. Preoperatively for carotid endarterectomy (CEA), MRA is performed to evaluate for intracranial stenosis (tandem stenosis). If ultrasound findings are equivocal, additional imaging should be considered. If the ICA appears occluded sonographically and the patient is a good surgical candidate, arteriography, CT angiography (CTA), or MRA may be indicated to differentiate between occlusion and high-grade stenosis.

63. What happens to the CCA and ICA waveforms with isolated ECA stenosis?

The CCA waveform is not significantly altered because the percentage of flow to the ECA is low and the ECA circulation is already a high-resistance circulation. However, with high-grade ECA stenosis, more blood is shunted to the ICA, causing increased ICA velocity.

64. What happens to the CCA waveform with CCA stenosis proximal to the clavicle or with innominate stenosis?

The CCA becomes the post-stenotic vessel and has damped waveforms. The waveform is low amplitude because flow is reduced.

65. What is the best way to quantify CCA waveform abnormalities?

The CCA waveform is best evaluated for abnormalities by visual comparison with the contralateral side. Symmetric CCA abnormalities can be seen in physiologic conditions. Symmetric increased pulsatility can be seen with hypertension, peripheral arterial disease, hyperthyroidism, and exercise. Symmetric damping of the CCA waveforms occurs with decreased cardiac output and severe aortic valve disease. With asymmetric abnormalities, a proximal stenosis, such as in the aortic arch, should be sought.

66. What are the ultrasound findings in carotid dissection?

When the intima is delaminated from the rest of the wall, a flap that moves with the cardiac cycle may be seen. A duplicated lumen may be visualized. The lumen may also appear narrowed or normal (Fig. 13).

67. What is the most common location for carotid dissection?

Dissection of the CCA can complicate dissection of the ascending aorta due to trauma or elastic tissue degeneration. Spontaneous or traumatic dissection originating in the carotids usually involves the ICA.

68. What are some possible vascular consequences of carotid dissection?

Stenosis, occlusion, and pseudoaneurysm formation can all complicate carotid dissection.

69. What are some etiologies of carotid dissection?

Carotid dissection has many possible etiologies including trauma, chiropractic manipulation, fibromuscular dysplasia, connective tissue disorders, Marfan's disease, exercise, and Ehlers-Danlos syndrome. Carotid dissection can also occur spontaneously.

70. What role does carotid ultrasound play in follow-up of CEA?

Interval carotid ultrasounds are performed following CEA. Following CEA, the ICA waveform can resemble the ECA waveform for unknown reasons. Early complications of CEA include

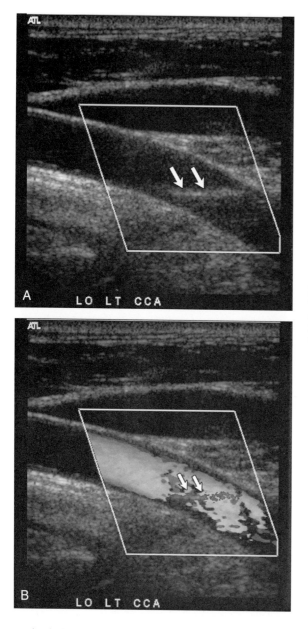

FIGURE 13. Carotid dissection. Grayscale (*A*) and color (*B*) images demonstrate an intimal flap (*arrows*) indicating carotid dissection (see also Color Plates, Figure 19).

retained plaque, arterial clamp injury, and intimal flap formation. Later complications include restenosis, 70% of which occur within 2 years of surgery. Restenosis is caused by intimal hyperplasia within the first 3 years; after 3 years, it resembles atherosclerotic plaque.

71. Can carotid ultrasound be used in the evaluation of carotid body tumors?

The normal carotid body is located in the carotid bifurcation and measures 1.0 × 1.5 mm. Paragangliomas can arise from the carotid body and present as neck pain with a palpable mass. These are highly vascular tumors with low malignant potential. Sonographically, they are highly vascular tumors within the carotid bifurcation. Ultrasound may be used to follow the growth of small tumors and to help define the relationship with surrounding vessels.

72. Can carotid ultrasound be used in the evaluation of connective tissue disorders, fibromuscular dysplasia (FMD), or arteritis?

FMD is a noninflammatory process with hypertrophy of muscular and fibrous walls of vessels and commonly involves the ICA. The ultrasound findings are nonspecific. Arteritis resulting from an autoimmune process such as temporal arteritis or Takayasu's arteritis can produce diffuse concentric thickening of the carotid walls, especially the CCA.

73. What are new ultrasound technologies for carotid imaging?

Three-dimensional reconstruction of acquired images may allow better definition of the extent of pathology and better depict tortuous carotid arteries and branches. Contrast-enhanced imaging following the injection of ultrasound contrast agents may increase the detection of blood flow signals, improve visualization and characterization of plaque, and define difficult anatomy.

74. What is the utility of vertebral ultrasound?

Vertebral ultrasound can be used in the workup of symptoms thought to be due to vertebral basilar insufficiency. It also plays a role in the evaluation of patients with subclavian steal. The vertebral arteries are evaluated as part of a routine carotid ultrasound evaluation to check for direction of flow. However, because of the nonspecific nature of posterior circulation symptoms and multiple technical considerations, overall ultrasound has a limited role in the evaluation of the vertebral arteries.

75. What are the neurologic symptoms classically attributed to the vertebral basilar system?

Dizziness, diplopia, dysarthria, and dysphagia are common symptoms of posterior circulation, or vertebral basilar, ischemia. Additional symptoms include hemiparesis, nystagmus, gaze palsy, Horner's syndrome, ataxia, hemisensory loss, and mental status change. These symptoms are manifestations of insufficient blood flow to the portions of the brain supplied by the vertebral and basilar arteries. These regions include the brainstem, cerebellum, and occipital lobes.

76. What are potential causes of vertebral basilar insufficiency (VBI)?
- Atherosclerosis of the vertebral or basilar arteries
- Embolization
- Atherosclerosis of small intracranial branches
- Hypotension in conjunction with vertebrobasilar and carotid occlusive disease
- Shedding of clot from vertebrobasilar ectasia
- Cardiac dysrhythmia
- Artery-to-artery steal syndromes
- Vertebral artery dissection
- Vertebral artery impingement due to large cervical osteophytes

77. What conditions other than VBI can cause similar neurologic signs and symptoms?

Migraine headache	Neoplasm
Cardiac dysfunction	Infection
Epilepsy	Carotid insufficiency

78. What is the normal anatomy of the vertebrobasilar system?

The vertebral arteries arise from the subclavian arteries distal to the thyrocervical trunk. The origin is often deep to the clavicle. They course through the neural foramina of C1 to C6. At the base of the skull, the two vertebrals join to form the basilar artery.

79. Are the vertebral arteries symmetric in size?

In approximately 75% of normal individuals, the vertebral arteries are asymmetric in size. In 80% of these cases, the left is the dominant vessel.

80. What are anatomic considerations of the vertebrobasilar system that make ultrasound evaluation of the vessels difficult?

The vertebral arteries cannot be directly evaluated by ultrasound because they pass through the foramina of the transverse processes. As they exit C1, they form a posteriorly oriented loop that is difficult to evaluate by ultrasound. Also, a short segment of each vertebral artery lies within the skull where it is inaccessible to routine ultrasound examination. In addition, the origin is deep to the clavicle, making it inaccessible to ultrasound evaluation. The origin is often tortuous in older individuals, causing confusing flow disturbances.

Because the two vertebrals join to form a single basilar artery, there is considerable opportunity for collateralization. Additional collateralization occurs through the circle of Willis. Therefore, unilateral vertebral occlusion is rarely clinically significant. Carotid occlusive disease can also increase the blood flow to the vertebrals. In addition, because the vertebral arteries are asymmetric in the majority of individuals, size discrepancies are of limited diagnostic value.

81. How is the vertebral artery located?

The patient is positioned the same way as for a carotid examination, supine with the head turned to the contralateral side. The transducer is placed longitudinal on the neck at the level of the mid CCA. The vertebral arteries are found slightly posterolateral to the CCA. The vertebral artery can be seen with color Doppler coursing through the foramen of the transverse process of the cervical spine. It is helpful to align the transducer in the plane of the shadows of the transverse processes. Only segments of the artery are seen at any one location (Fig. 14).

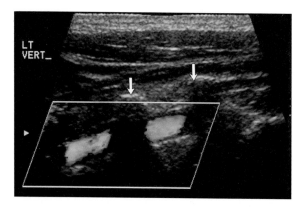

FIGURE 14. Normal vertebral artery. Normal flow is toward the head, in this case, away from the transducer. The transverse processes (*arrows*) prevent imaging the vessel within the foramina.

82. What frequency transducer is used?

For many patients, a 7.5-MHz linear transducer is adequate. For patients with larger necks, the increased penetration that a 5.0-MHz transducer offers is necessary to demonstrate color Doppler in the vertebral arteries.

83. What images are obtained?

For a routine carotid artery examination, it is sufficient to record one color Doppler and one spectral Doppler image of the vertebral artery on each side.

For indications specific to vertebrobasilar flow, the following protocol should be used:

- The flow direction is documented using both color and spectral Doppler.
- Measure the diameter of the artery in systole.
- If possible, angle-corrected spectral Doppler signals are obtained and peak systolic and end-diastolic velocities are recorded.
- The artery should be followed between each interspinous segment as far cephalad as possible noting the caliber of the vessel and flow characteristics.

- When possible, follow the artery to its origin and check the origin with color and spectral Doppler for stenosis.

84. What are technical limitations?
- Patients with a cervical collar cannot be examined.
- If the patient has a short neck, the examination is limited to only a partial look at the vertebral arteries.
- If the patient cannot turn his or her head, it is helpful to scan from a posterolateral approach.
- If the neck is thick, a lower frequency transducer is necessary (5.0 MHz).
- Because of the location of the origin (close to the clavicle), it may be helpful to use a sector transducer if stenosis is suspected.
- Often, musculoskeletal branches are mistaken for vertebral arteries. This can be prevented by first locating the plane of the transverse process shadows and the vertebral artery will be accompanied by the vertebral vein.

85. What is the normal vertebral waveform?
Vertebral artery waveforms have a low resistance pattern with persistent flow throughout diastole. They resemble ICA waveforms. Flow is cephalad throughout the cardiac cycle.

86. What is the significance of absent vertebral flow?
Absence of flow in a successfully imaged VA indicates occlusion of the vessel. False-positive diagnosis of occlusion can occur with high-grade stenosis with only a trickle of flow.

87. What is the significance of focal velocity elevation?
Increased peak systolic velocity > 40 cm/sec suggests a vertebral stenosis of 50% diameter reduction. However, velocity parameters have not been established for vertebral stenosis.

88. What is the significance of decreased velocity?
Distal to a severe VA stenosis, the velocity may be reduced and the waveform damped. With a severe stenosis distal to the site of examination (in the distal VA or basilar artery), the velocity may also be decreased. However, the waveform shows a high resistance pattern with sharp systolic peak and reduced diastolic flow.

89. What is the significance of abnormal pulsatility?
The waveform appears damped with both collateral flow and proximal occlusion. The VA waveform is large with elevated systolic and diastolic velocities when there is collateral flow such as seen with carotid occlusion. In proximal obstruction, such as in the subclavian, innominate artery, or proximal VA, the vertebral diameter is reduced, systolic and diastolic velocities are low, and flow is reduced.

90. When does flow reversal occur?
Flow reversal, or a to-and-fro pattern, occurs in vertebral to subclavian artery steal syndromes.

91. What is subclavian steal?
Vertebral-to-subclavian steal occurs when there is a stenosis of the subclavian artery proximal to the origin of the ipsilateral VA. In this setting, flow in the ipsilateral VA reverses. Then, blood flow can reverse to supply the subclavian artery distal to the occlusion through collateral circulation from the contralateral VA via the basilar artery. This involves the left subclavian artery 85% of the time. This rarely causes neurologic symptoms.

92. What are the ultrasound findings in vertebral-to-subclavian steal?
Flow may be reversed throughout the cardiac cycle, or it may be bidirectional (forward in systole and reverse in diastole). Flow may also be normal at rest, but can become abnormal with

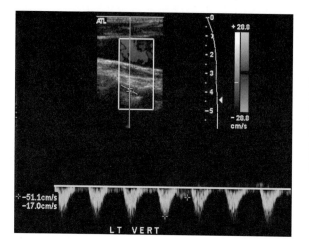

FIGURE 15. Subclavian steal. Flow in the vertebral artery is reversed (flowing toward the left arm) due to a stenosis of the ipsilateral subclavian artery proximal to the vertebral origin. Collateral flow occurs from the contralateral vertebral artery via the basilar artery.

exercise when the arm muscles require more blood flow. The steal may be more clearly demonstrated by inducing arm hyperemia with a blood pressure cuff inflated above systolic pressure for approximately 5 minutes. When the cuff is deflated, flow in the ipsilateral VA normally remains cephalad. If subclavian steal is present, the VA waveform reverses or becomes biphasic when the cuff is released (Fig. 15).

BIBLIOGRAPHY

1. Carroll BA: Carotid sonography. Radiology 178:303–313, 1991.
2. El-Saden S, Grant EG, Hathout GM, et al: Imaging of the internal carotid artery: The dilemma of total versus near total occlusion. Radiology 221:301–308, 2001.
3. Freed KS, Brown LK, Carroll BA: The extracranial cerebral vessels. In Rumack CM, Wilson SR, Charboneau JW (eds): Diagnostic Ultrasound, 2nd ed. St. Louis, Mosby, 1998, pp 885–919.
4. Grant EG, Duerinckx AJ, El Saden S, et al: Doppler sonographic parameters for detection of carotid stenosis: Is there an optimum method for their selection? Am J Roentgenol 172:1123–1129, 1999.
5. Polak JF: Carotid ultrasound. Radiol Clin North Am 39(3):569–589, 2001.
6. Polak JF: Neck arteries. In Polak JF (ed): Peripheral Vascular Sonography. Baltimore, Williams and Wilkins, 1992, pp 103–152.
7. Society of Radiologists in Ultrasound: Consensus Conference on Carotid Ultrasound. San Francisco, October 25–27, 2002.
8. Zwiebel WJ: Doppler evaluation of carotid stenosis. In Zwiebel WJ (ed): Introduction to Vascular Ultrasonography, 4th ed. Philadelphia, WB Saunders, 2000, pp 137–151.
9. Zwiebel WJ: Normal carotid arteries and carotid examination technique. In Zwiebel WJ (ed): Introduction to Vascular Ultrasonography, 4th ed. Philadelphia, WB Saunders, 2000, pp 113–124.
10. Zwiebel WJ: Ultrasound assessment of carotid plaque. In Zwiebel WJ (ed): Introduction to Vascular Ultrasonography, 4th ed. Philadelphia, WB Saunders, 2000, pp 125–135.
11. Zwiebel WJ: Ultrasound vertebral examination. In Zwiebel WJ (ed): Introduction to Vascular Ultrasonography, 4th ed. Philadelphia, WB Saunders, 2000, pp 167–176.

40. ULTRASOUND EVALUATION OF THE ABDOMINAL AORTA

William T. Kuo, M.D.

1. What are the indications for an aortic sonogram?

- Pulsatile abdominal mass
- Hemodynamic arterial compromise in the lower limb
- Abdominal pain
- Abdominal bruit

Ultrasound is also used to detect clinically silent abdominal aortic aneurysms and to follow known aneurysms for critical enlargement. Complications from aneurysm surgery may also be assessed.

2. What is the normal diameter of the abdominal aorta?

The abdominal aorta tapers from cranial to caudal, and 2 cm is the maximum normal diameter. The aorta is considered aneurysmal when the diameter exceeds 1.5 times an adjacent normal segment or when the distal aorta exceeds 3 cm. The upper limit of normal also varies with age, increasing by up to 25% in the seventh and eighth decades.

3. When is surgical or endoluminal intervention recommended for a nonruptured aneurysm?

Repair is recommended for aneurysms 5 cm or larger. Aneurysms less than 5 cm in diameter have only a 3–5% risk of rupture over a 10-year period. At 5 cm, the risk of rupture increases up to 5% per year. The average rate of aneurysm enlargement is 0.2–0.4 cm per year. Repair is also considered with significant aneurysm enlargement over time (> 0.5 cm over 6 months), associated pain, distal emboli, renal vascular compromise, and gastrointestinal bleeding.

4. What vessels should be assessed routinely with every ultrasound study of the abdominal aorta?

The common iliac arteries, normally 1 cm in diameter, should always be assessed for aneurysms. Although isolated iliac aneurysms are rare, they may be deadly because they are often difficult to palpate and symptoms of rupture are nonspecific (vague abdominal or pelvic pain). Iliac artery aneurysms 3 cm or larger should undergo surgical or endoluminal repair. Five percent of patients with distal aortic aneurysms have an associated iliac artery aneurysm.

5. Which acoustic windows are recommended for scanning the aorta?

- Midline upper abdomen
- Left flank with patient supine or right lateral decubitus
- Along the lateral aspects of the lower rectus abdominis muscles (evaluate iliacs)

6. What are the routine measurements and protocol?

Longitudinal:

- Examine the aorta from diaphragm to bifurcation.
- Document the length of the aneurysm and measure the anteroposterior (AP) diameter from outer wall to outer wall.
- Examine the iliac arteries to the iliac bifurcation and measure aneurysms from outer wall to outer wall.

Transverse:

- Document the maximum diameter of the aorta at the diaphragm, superior mesenteric artery (SMA), and distally.

- Measure AP and transverse diameters from outer wall to outer wall.
- Visualize the iliac arteries and measure aneurysms.

Coronal:

- Measure aortic aneurysm in transverse dimension from outer wall to outer wall.
n Examine iliac arteries and measure aneurysms.

7. What is the maximum interobserver variability for aortic measurements?

Maximum interobserver variability is 5 mm with mean variability of 2.5 mm. Thus, an increase in size less than 5 mm between examinations may not be significant.

8. How can aortic measurements change as much as 1 cm during the same examination and how should an aneurysm be measured?

A transducer held oblique to the true plane causes false measurements. This can be avoided by always measuring in the short axis. Aneurysms should be measured perpendicular to the main axis of the vessel (short axis) at the widest portion of the aneurysm (Figs. 1 and 2).

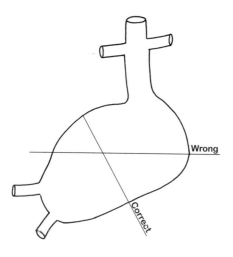

FIGURE 1. Aneurysm measurement technique. *A,* Correct measurement of diameter is from outer wall to outer wall, across the short axis of the lumen so as not to get a falsely elongated oblique measurement.

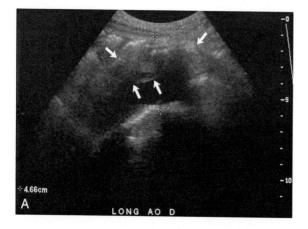

FIGURE 2. Abdominal aortic aneurysm. *A,* Longitudinal midline of the aorta shows typical hypoechoic mural atheroma (*arrows*) and anechoic lumen. The diameter (short axis, outer wall to outer wall) is 4.7 cm (*cursors*). (*continued*)

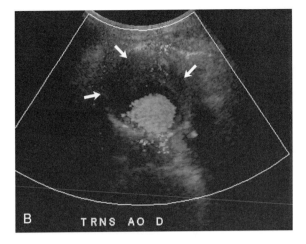

FIGURE 2. (*continued*) *B*, Color Doppler transverse image of the aorta shows the extent of the mural atheroma (*arrows*). The lumen fills with color.

9. If the renal arteries cannot be visualized, how can the position of an aneurysm be assessed relative to the renal vessels?

The distance from the SMA to the aneurysm should be measured. The renal arteries arise no more than 1.5 cm below the SMA.

10. What is the ultrasound appearance of aortic dissection?

The distinguishing finding is a visible intimal flap separating the true and false lumens. This membrane may flutter with arterial pulsation or become immobile in thrombosis. Color Doppler shows flow in both channels although flow rates may differ between the true and false lumens. Color Doppler is preferred because dissection is easily missed on grayscale (Fig. 3).

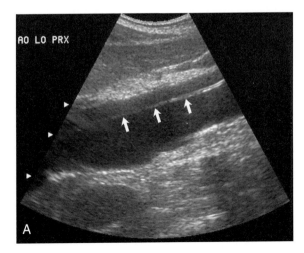

FIGURE 3. Aortic dissection. *A*, Longitudinal image in the mid-abdomen demonstrates the hyperechoic dissection flap (*arrows*) in the aorta. (*continued*)

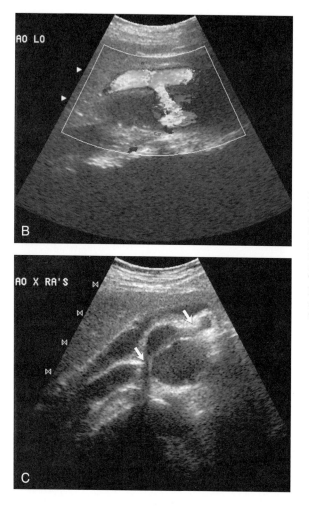

FIGURE 3. (*continued*) *B,* Color Doppler image at the same level shows flow toward the feet in the anterior true lumen, with filling of the posterior false lumen via a hole or fenestration in the dissection flap (see also Color Plates, Figure 20). *C,* Transverse image of the aorta at the level of the renal arteries (*arrows*) shows them originating from the anterior (true) lumen.

11. What is a pseudodissection on ultrasound?

A pseudodissection is a mirror image artifact seen in aneurysmal aortas during color Doppler examination. A heavily calcified aortic wall may act as a strong acoustic reflector, resulting in a mirror image artifact deep to the blood flow of the aortic lumen.

The artifact may be countered by using less color gain and decreasing the power output. Also, comparing the spectral analysis of Doppler signals from the aortic lumen and posterior artifactual echoes shows identical waveforms. The only difference is a lower signal amplitude from the artifactual echoes. Finally, grayscale images should be evaluated for movement of an intimal flap, which should be absent in pseudodissection.

12. What is the appearance of aortic rupture on ultrasound?

Acute rupture may be detected indirectly by searching for free fluid. Chronic rupture may be seen as retroperitoneal fluid collections. Overlying bowel gas renders ultrasound ineffective in detecting aortic rupture, and computed tomography (CT) remains the modality of choice.

13. How is ultrasound used to assess the aorta after aneurysm repair?

Although CT is widely used for postoperative evaluation, ultrasound is also useful in detecting the complications of graft surgery: hematoma, infection, stenosis, occlusion, aneurysms, and fluid collections. Color flow imaging is used to assess the entire length of the graft. Both the proximal and distal anastomoses are closely examined because most complications occur at the anastomoses.

14. What is the appearance and the most common site for graft stenosis?

The distal (iliac) anastomoses are the most common sites of stenosis, which may be seen as focal areas of increased velocity and flow disturbance.

15. What is the significance of perigraft fluid collections and how should they be evaluated?

A layer of perigraft fluid is normally present after graft placement and may persist for weeks or even months. The collection size should diminish over time. Interval fluid increase suggests graft infection.

16. What are the signs of graft infection?

Because hematomas and seromas cannot be sonographically differentiated from abscesses, other signs of infection should be recognized. These include inflammatory perigraft tissue, pseudoaneurysm formation, and fluid collections extending from the graft into surrounding tissues. If the collection is echogenic (containing gas) and increasing in size, fine needle aspiration may be indicated to exclude infection.

17. What is Takayasu's aortitis?

This typically affects young females. The abdominal aorta and its branches are involved in two thirds of patients. Sonographically there is diffuse wall thickening of the aorta, resulting in reduced caliber. Aneurysmal dilatation and, rarely, complete obstruction may result.

18. What is Leriche syndrome?

Leriche syndrome is infrarenal aortic occlusion. Patients present with thigh and buttock claudication, impotence, and absent femoral pulses.

BIBLIOGRAPHY

1. Cramer MM: Color flow duplex examination of the abdominal aorta: Atherosclerosis, aneurysm, and dissection. J Vasc Tech 19:249–260, 1995.
2. Crotty JM, Timken MJ: Pseudodissection of the abdominal aorta on color Doppler imaging. J Ultrasound Med 14:853–857, 1995.
3. Fillinger MF: Postoperative imaging after endovascular AAA repair. Semin Vasc Surg 12:327–338, 1999.
4. Hanely M, Ryley NG, Lewis P, Currie I: Can duplex accurately assess the relationship between the renal arteries and an abdominal aortic aneurysm using the superior mesenteric artery as a fixed point? J Vasc Tech 25:97–101, 2001.
5. Lederle FA, Wilson SE, Johnson JR, et al: Variability in measurement of abdominal aortic aneurysms. J Vasc Surg 21:945–952, 1995.
6. Orton DF, LeVeen RF, Saigh JA, et al: Aortic prosthetic graft infections: Radiologic manifestations and implications for management. RadioGraphics 20:977–993, 2000.
7. Ricci MA, Kleeman M, Case T, Pilcher DB: Normal aortic diameter by ultrasound. J Vasc Tech 19:17–19, 1995.
8. Rumack CM, Wilson SR, Charboneau JW: Diagnostic Ultrasound, vol 1, 2nd ed. St. Louis, Mosby-Year-Book, 1998, pp 464–478.
9. Takamyia M, Hirose Y: Growth curve of ruptured aortic aneurysm. J Cardiovasc Surg 39:9–13, 1998.
10. Yucel EK, Fillmore DJ, Knox TA, Waltman AC: Sonographic measurement of abdominal aortic diameter: Interobserver variability. J Ultrasound Med 10:681–683, 1991.

41. RENAL ARTERY DOPPLER ULTRASOUND

Mayumi Oka, M.D.

1. What are the clinical indications to assess renal arteries?

Evaluation of renal artery stenosis is indicated in patients with a clinical suspicion of renovascular hypertension. Renovascular hypertension is suspected when diastolic hypertension first develops in a patient younger than 30 years or older than 55 years, when previously stable hypertension abruptly accelerates, or when there is rapid progression to malignant hypertension within 6 months of onset.

2. What are the causes of renal artery stenosis (RAS)?

Atherosclerosis and fibromuscular dysplasia (FMD) account for approximately 95% of cases of significant RAS in the United States. Other disorders include neurofibromatosis, coarctation of the aorta, radiation injury, Takayasu's arteritis, and aortic dissection.

3. What is FMD?

FMD typically occurs in young women and affects both kidneys in about two thirds of patients. The most common histologic subtype of FMD is medial fibroplasia, which accounts for almost 85% of all cases of RAS. Most FMD lesions have a characteristic "string of beads" appearance on angiogram.

4. What part of the renal artery is involved in FMD?

FMD commonly involves the distal main renal artery, with extension into first-order branches in about 25% of patients.

5. What frequency transducer should be used for a renal artery study?

Use the highest frequency vector transducer possible.

6. How do you position a patient for a renal artery study?

Start the examination with the patient in the supine position. When bowel gas obscures the midline structures, including the aorta and origins of the renal arteries, the right lateral decubitus position or steep oblique position may be helpful. Owing to various factors such as gas interposition or the anatomy of the left renal artery, a complete examination of both renal arteries can be achieved in only 50–90% of cases.

7. Where are the renal arteries and how can they be found?

The superior mesenteric artery (SMA) can be used as a reference point because it is easier to find. The renal arteries are located slightly caudad to the SMA. The right renal artery usually arises from the anterolateral aspect of the aorta, whereas the left renal artery generally arises from the posterolateral aspect of the aorta. Use color Doppler to locate these vessels.

8. What is a normal renal arterial waveform?

It should have a rapidly rising upstroke with a gradual decline to a continuous lower velocity forward flow in diastole.

9. What percentage of hypertension is caused by renovascular disease?

Less than 2% is caused by renovascular disease. Although this seems a small number, hypertension affects more than 20% of people older than 20 years of age in the United States. Conversely, renovascular hypertension affects 15–30% of patients with clinical criteria suggestive of renovascular disease.

10. What percentage of patients are on hemodialysis because of renovascular disease?

Of patients on hemodialysis, approximately 15% are on therapy because of renovascular disease, and this number is increasing as the population grows older. These patients are older than other patients who are on dialysis and have the poorest survival estimates (25 months versus 52 months in total hemodialysis patient population).

11. What degree of stenosis is considered significant in the renal artery?

Doppler ultrasound criteria for significant renal artery stenosis corresponds to 60% diameter reduction. Angiogram and magnetic resonance angiography (MRA) currently use 50% diameter reduction as a cutoff for significant stenosis.

12. What are the limiting factors to using ultrasound as a screening tool for renal artery stenosis? What percentage of studies are adequate?

Doppler studies of the renal artery are technically demanding because of the difficulty visualizing the vessels in cases of large body habitus, deep location, and presence of bowel gas. These factors lead to difficulty obtaining accurate angle-corrected velocity. A complete examination of both renal arteries is achieved in the range of 50–90%.

13. What examination is considered the gold standard?

Conventional angiography is the gold standard. However, MRA has recently achieved the equivalent accuracy to be considered diagnostic for both a screening study and for presurgical assessment.

14. What Doppler criteria are used to make a diagnosis of RAS?

Most universally accepted Doppler criteria are:
- Peak systolic velocity (PSV) of $\geq$ 180–200 cm/sec
- Renal artery/aortic ratio (RAR) > 3.3–3.5. RAR is defined as the ratio of PSV in the renal artery divided by PSV in the aorta. However, accuracy of RAR is thought to be reduced when aortic PSV > 100 cm/sec.

15. What are other criteria for diagnosing RAS?

- Abnormal waveform of intrarenal arteries: Loss of early systolic peak with long acceleration time (AT) > 0.07 sec. This "tardus parvus" waveform was once considered a promising sign to detect RAS; however, later reports questioned the sensitivity and specificity of this finding.
- Acceleration index < 3.78 kHz/sec
- Size discrepancy > 3 cm between two kidneys
- Resistive index > 0.56

16. What is the sensitivity and specificity of Doppler ultrasound in the detection of RAS?

A wide range of sensitivity (0–98%) and specificity (37–99%) has been reported.

17. What are the potential causes of a false-negative examination in an adequate study?

- Nonvisualization of an accessory artery. An accessory renal artery is seen in up to 20% of the normal population, and it is a pitfall when evaluating a patient with suspected RAS. A search for accessory renal arteries is important especially when the main renal artery is normal.
- Stenosis in the intrarenal segmental artery seen in FMD or other vasculitides.

18. Can the same criteria be used for stenosis of a transplanted kidney?

No. PSV > 2.5 m/sec is considered the diagnostic threshold for a stenosis in a transplant kidney.

19. What is the cause of a false-negative for renal artery occlusion?

Collaterals (capsular or adrenal arteries) usually supply 10% of blood flow, but when there is an occluded main renal artery, they supply all blood flow and there are arterial Doppler signals within the renal parenchyma or even in the renal hilum.

BIBLIOGRAPHY

1. Baxter JM: Ultrasound imaging in renal transplantation. In Sidhu PS, Baxter GM (eds): Ultrasound of Abdominal Transplantation. New York, Thieme, 2002, pp 27–42.
2. Gottlieb RH, Snitzer EL, Hartley DF, Rubens DJ: Interobserver and intraobserver variation in determining the intrarenal parameters by Doppler sonography. Am J Roentgenol 168:217–221, 1997.
3. Kliewer MA, Tupler RH, Carroll BA, et al: Renal artery stenosis: Analysis of Doppler waveform parameters and tardus-parvus pattern. Radiology 189:779–787, 1993.
4. Kliewer MA, Tupler RH, Hertzberg BS, et al: Doppler evaluation of renal artery stenosis: Interobserver agreement in the interpretation of waveform morphology. AJR Am J Roentgenol 162:1371–1376, 1994.
5. Mailloux LU, Napolitano B, Belluci AG, et al: Renal vascular disease causing end-stage renal disease, incidence, clinical correlates, and outcomes: A 20-year clinical experience. Am J Kidney Dis 24:622–629, 1994.
6. Soulez G, Oliva VL, Turpin S, et al: Imaging of renovasucular hypertension: Respective values of renal scintigraphy, renal Doppler US, and MR angiography. Radiographics 20:1355–1368, 2000.
7. Stavros T, Harshfield D. Renal Doppler: Renal artery stenosis, and renovascular hypertension: Direct and indirect duplex sonographic abnormalities in patients with Renal Artery Stenosis. Ultrasound Q 12:217–263, 1994.
8. Zwiebel WJ: Duplex evaluation of native renal vessels and renal allografts. In Zwiebel WJ: Introduction to Vascular Ultrasonography, 4th ed. Philadelphia, W.B. Saunders, 2000, pp 455–475.

42. PSEUDOANEURYSMS AND ARTERIOVENOUS FISTULAS

Marat Bakman, M.D.

1. What is a pseudoaneurysm?

A pseudoaneurysm is a blood collection outside the vessel wall that communicates with an artery via a neck. This results in a swirling flow within the mass with a distinctive appearance on color Doppler. Waveform analysis demonstrates high-velocity inflow during systole and prolonged outflow throughout the entire diastole (Fig. 1).

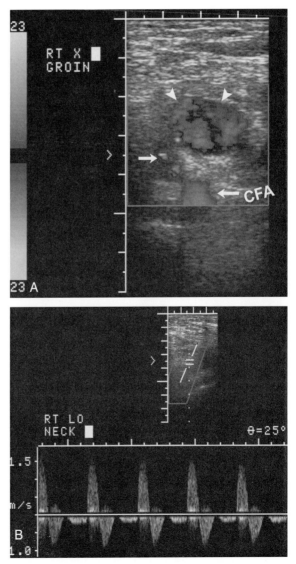

FIGURE 1. *A,* Transverse color Doppler image through the groin shows the common femoral artery (CFA), the aneurysm neck (*arrow*), and the pseudoaneurysm anteriorly (*arrowheads*) with typical "yin-yang" red and blue colors caused by blood swirling in and out (see also Color Plates, Figure 21). *B,* Spectral Doppler tracing through the pseudoaneurysm neck documents the diagnostic to-and-fro flow pattern.

2. What causes a pseudoaneurysm?

Pseudoaneurysms can be caused iatrogenically, following either peripheral or cardiac endovascular catheterization procedures, which use a percutaneous femoral approach. Any other trauma, surgery, or infection to an artery may also cause a pseudoaneurysm.

3. What are the common locations?

The most common locations include the common femoral artery, superficial femoral artery, popliteal artery, radial artery, renal artery, and splenic artery. Pseudoaneurysms may also arise from artificial arteries, such as grafts (Fig. 2).

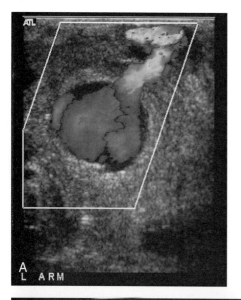

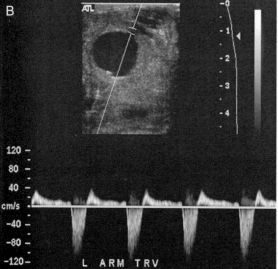

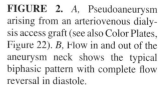

FIGURE 2. *A,* Pseudoaneurysm arising from an arteriovenous dialysis access graft (see also Color Plates, Figure 22). *B,* Flow in and out of the aneurysm neck shows the typical biphasic pattern with complete flow reversal in diastole.

4. What is an anastomotic aneurysm?

Anastomotic pseudoaneurysms occur at the site of anastomosis when synthetic vascular bypass grafts are used. They usually occur late, on average 5–10 years after graft placement, and preferentially develop at the femoral anastomosis of aortofemoral grafts.

5. How is grayscale ultrasound helpful?

Grayscale ultrasound identifies a blind-ending pouch arising from an artery. The largest single pseudoaneurysm dimension, number of lobes, neck length, and width should be measured. Images should be obtained in a transverse and longitudinal relationship to the artery in question.

6. What are the Doppler waveform findings in pseudoaneurysm?

The Doppler waveform finding of a "to-and-fro" flow in the neck of the pseudoaneurysm confirms the diagnosis. The "to" component is due to the expansion of the cavity of the pseudoaneurysm as blood enters during systole. The "fro" component is seen during diastole as the blood stored in the pseudoaneurysm is ejected back into the artery (Fig. 1).

7. What are the color Doppler findings in a pseudoaneurysm?

Color Doppler exhibits classic bidirectional color flow, with flow into and out of the pseudoaneurysm in each cardiac cycle. This appearance is called a "yin-yang" sign.

8. When might a typical yin-yang sign be absent?

- When the pseudoaneurysm is multilobed and has more than one entry from the artery, the blood flow in one lobe may be unidirectional.
- When the pseudoaneurysm is thrombosed, no flow is appreciated.

9. What transducer should be used?

A high-frequency 5–7 MHz linear probe, or, if edema is present, a 3-MHz curvilinear probe should be used. Search the soft tissues surrounding the pseudoaneurysm for evidence of arteriovenous fistula or multiple interconnecting pseudoaneurysm lobes. Look above and below the connection with the artery for additional connections.

10. What are the common treatments for pseudoaneurysms?

Surgery, ultrasound-guided compression, and percutaneous ultrasound-guided thrombin injection are the common treatments for pseudoaneurysms.

11. How is ultrasound-guided compression performed?

A vascular surgery consult is required before beginning compression. Document dorsalis pedis and posterior tibialis arterial pulses before, during, and after treatment. Manual compression with a transducer is applied to the pseudoaneurysm neck for 10 minutes in patients who are not anticoagulated and 20 minutes in those who are. Compression should be sufficient to completely stop flow into the pseudoaneurysm and continued until thrombosis results. Compression is released briefly between cycles to assess thrombosis, reposition the transducer, or switch operators. After compression, patients are instructed to lie in bed with the affected leg straight for 4–6 hours. The success rate for ultrasound-guided compression is 70–74%.

12. What are the indications for ultrasound-guided compression?

A pseudoaneurysm of < 4 cm, a pseudoaneurysm neck of > 5 mm, and duration of less than 1 week are suitable indications for ultrasound-guided compression.

13. What are the contraindications to ultrasound-guided compression?

A pseudoaneurysm present for more than a month (due to epithelialization of the tract) is a contraindication that diminishes success. Skin ischemia or infection are also relative contraindications. Clinical signs of rapid expansion, such as a compartment syndrome or neuropathy, should triage the patient to vascular surgery.

14. What are the disadvantages?

This is a lengthy procedure that is tiresome for both patients and operators. The success rate is reduced in anticoagulated patients. In some cases, even with best effort, flow through the pseudoaneurysm neck cannot be arrested. Recurrence is most common within 72 hours of ultrasound-guided compression.

15. What is ultrasound-guided thrombin therapy?

An intravenous line and vascular surgery consult are required. Document dorsalis pedis and posterior tibialis arterial pulses before, during, and after treatment.

Characterize the pseudoaneurysm as described above. The area of needle insertion is anesthetized with lidocaine. A 22-gauge spinal needle is used, preloaded with bovine thrombin (1000 μ/ml), and attached to a 1-ml syringe, also preloaded with thrombin. Under ultrasound guidance, the needle is advanced into the pseudoaneurysm lumen. The needle should be placed where the direction of flow is away from the pseudoaneurysm neck, which decreases the possibility of escape of free thrombin from the flow lumen into the artery with resultant distal embolization. It is also important to avoid puncture of or injection into the pseudoaneurysm neck, the feeding artery, or its branches. An injection of 0.1–0.3 ml (100–300 units) of thrombin is given over 3–5 seconds. Flow in the lumen is monitored with color Doppler ultrasound for development of thrombus. If partial thrombosis occurs, a second injection is done. After the pseudoaneurysm is thrombosed, the needle is removed. Patients are instructed to lie in bed for 6 hours with the affected leg straight; frequent groin and pulse checks are made.

16. What are the advantages compared to compression?

Thrombosis occurs quickly within 3–20 seconds. There is no need for conscious sedation. The success rate is > 96%. Thrombin injections can be performed in the pseudoaneurysm above the inguinal ligament, which is contraindicated for compression because of the risk of intraperitoneal or extraperitoneal rupture. Thrombosis is also effective in cases of systemic anticoagulation with heparin because heparin acts earlier in the coagulation cycle by inhibiting conversion of prothrombin to thrombin.

17. What are the contraindications to thrombin therapy?

- Arteriovenous fistula
- Known allergy to bovine thrombin
- Previous exposure to bovine thrombin, resulting in a possible development of antibody to bovine factor V and coagulopathy
- Wide pseudoaneurysm neck (relative)
- Superimposed infection

18. What is an arteriovenous fistula (AVF)?

AVF is described as an abnormal area of communication between the arterial and venous circulation with resultant shunting of blood from the high-pressure arterial side to the low-resistance venous side.

19. What causes an AVF?

These are mostly iatrogenic and include percutaneous vascular interventions such as cardiac catheterizations, trauma, and surgery. The risk of developing an AVF is increased when, in addition to a femoral artery puncture, the femoral vein is accessed for catheterization of the right heart. Additionally, when the arterial puncture is below the bifurcation of the common femoral artery, a needle can easily pass through the artery and vein simultaneously.

20. What are common sites for AVFs?

Common sites include the common femoral artery, superficial femoral artery, and profunda femoris artery. The kidney and liver also commonly develop AVFs subsequent to biopsy. Congenital AVFs may exist anywhere, but are most common in the brain.

21. What transducer should be used?

A 5–7 MHz high-frequency linear array transducer is suitable to detect AVFs.

Tip: If looking in a solid organ, lower the velocity scale and look for high-velocity venous flow.

22. What are the diagnostic criteria for an AVF?

- In a peripheral artery, this is an area of persistent intra-arterial flow throughout the cardiac cycle. This can be best seen in diastole when normal arterial flow should stop. In addition, the normal triphasic waveform is lost.
- In arteries of solid organs, continuous, high-velocity flow is present in the vein. This flow often lacks respiratory variation and shows a pulsatile arterialized waveform (Fig. 3). With large AVFs, the vein can dilate and venous blood flow signal persists during Valsalva's maneuver (normally it disappears.)

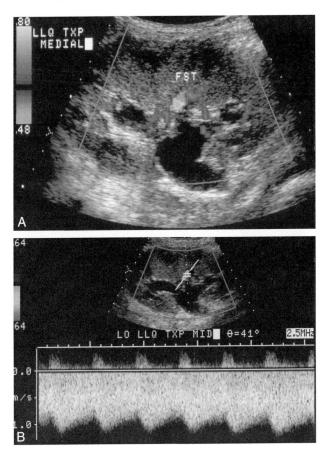

FIGURE 3. *A,* Longitudinal ultrasound of a renal transplant shows high-velocity venous flow (blue) appearing when all other vessels are arterial (red) and directed into the kidney (see also Color Plates, Figure 23). *B,* Spectral tracing shows an angle-corrected venous velocity of 1 m/sec. Note the arterialized waveform in the vein, which is slightly delayed compared with the renal artery tracing about the baseline. (*continued*)

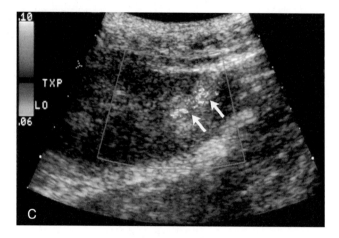

FIGURE 3. (*continued*) *C,* An arteriovenous fistula at the lower pole of a renal transplant after biopsy demonstrates a typical color Doppler "bruit" with mixed color pixels indicating turbulent flow and vibration in the surrounding parenchyma (see also Color Plates, Figure 24). The actual size of the fistula is much smaller and is invisible on grayscale. This fistula was asymptomatic and closed spontaneously.

- For all AVFs, look for turbulent high-velocity area of communication between artery and vein.
- Diameter of supplying artery may be increased proximal to the fistula.
- There may be focal venous dilatation at the site of the fistula.
- A focal perivascular vibration artifact (bruit) may occur due to high-velocity turbulent flow, which causes vibration in the surrounding tissue. This creates color Doppler noise around the AVF at normal scale settings.

23. What are symptoms and potential complications of AVF?
Patients may present with congestive heart failure secondary to shunting of blood.

24. What is the treatment of AVF?
Many small AVFs resolve spontaneously, especially in solid organs. Complete cessation of blood flow signals during the Vasalva maneuver indicates a high likelihood that the fistula will spontaneously occlude during the next few weeks. Ultrasound-guided compression over the fistula has been used for a period of 20–60 minutes with a success rate of < 30%. Surgical ligation can be performed if ultrasound-guided compression is unsuccessful. Arterial stent to bypass the anomalous connection can also be used.

BIBLIOGRAPHY

1. Brophy DP, Sheiman RG, Amatulle P, Akbari CM: Iatrogenic femoral pseudoaneurysms: Thrombin injection after failed US-guided compression. Radiology 214:278–282, 2000.
2. Igibashian VN, Mitchell DG, Middleton WD, et al: Iatrogenic femoral arteriovenous fistula: Diagnosis with color Doppler imaging. Radiology 170:749–752, 1989.
3. Li JC, Cai S, Jiang YX, et al: Diagnostic criteria for locating acquired arteriovenous fistulas with color Doppler sonography. J Clin Ultrasound 30:336–342, 2002.
4. Paulson EK, Sheafor DH, Kliewer MA, et al: Treatment of iatrogenic femoral arterial pseudoaneurysms: Comparison of US-guided thrombin injection with compression repair. Radiology 215:403–408, 2000.
5. Roubidoux MA, Hertzberg BS, Carroll BA, Hedgepeth CA. Color flow and image-directed Doppler ultrasound evaluation of iatrogenic arteriovenous fistulas in the groin. J Clin Ultrasound 18:463–469, 1990.
6. Thalhammer C, Kirchher AS, Uhlich F, et al: Postcatheterization pseudoaneurysms and arteriovenous fistulas: Repair with percutaneous implantation of endovascular covered stents. Radiology 214:127–131, 2000.

43. MESENTERIC CIRCULATION EVALUATION

Mayumi Oka, M.D.

1. What are the clinical indications for mesenteric artery Doppler?

One indication is clinical suspicion of chronic mesenteric ischemia. Patients with acute mesenteric ischemia are usually in critical condition, and Doppler ultrasound adds little or no data to their management. Patients should be evaluated by computed tomography (CT), which often has suggestive findings such as bowel wall edema, pneumatosis, presence of air in the portal or mesenteric vein, or thrombi in mesenteric vessels when intravenous contrast is given.

2. What is the clinical presentation of acute mesenteric ischemia?

In acute mesenteric ischemia, the patient presents with acute onset of severe abdominal pain often associated with bleeding and progression to a life-threatening condition. Unless there is a bowel perforation, abdominal examination is benign.

3. What is the hallmark of chronic mesenteric ischemia?

In chronic mesenteric ischemia, patients classically have symptoms of intestinal angina; in the long term, postprandial abdominal pain causes weight loss secondary to decreased food intake.

4. What causes acute mesenteric ischemia?

Acute mesenteric ischemia can be occlusive or nonocclusive. Occlusive ischemia may be secondary to thromboembolism, aortic dissection, or venous thrombosis. Nonocclusive ischemia is secondary to systemic hypotension of various causes, such as cardiac or septic shock.

5. What is the etiology of chronic mesenteric ischemia?

Chronic mesenteric ischemia is most often associated with atherosclerotic stenosis of two of the three major splanchnic arteries, although patients with occlusion of those arteries can be asymptomatic because of collateralization.

6. What is a splanchnic artery? Which vessels should be evaluated to diagnose mesenteric ischemia?

Splanchnic arteries are the vessels that supply the bowel with blood: the celiac artery, the superior mesenteric artery (SMA), and the inferior mesenteric artery (IMA). The celiac artery should be evaluated from its origin to its bifurcation at the splenic and common hepatic arteries. The SMA should be followed as far distally as possible. The IMA is rarely seen in normal subjects; however, it can be quite large and meandering when it serves as a collateral with stenosis of the celiac artery and SMA.

7. What is median arcuate ligament syndrome?

This controversial disease is thought to cause mesenteric ischemia secondary to compression of the proximal celiac artery just beyond its origin by the median arcuate ligament of the diaphragm. Clinical features include postprandial epigastric pain, weight loss, and abdominal bruit, which grows louder with expiration. The typical angiographic finding is a characteristic smooth concave extrinsic compression on the ventral border of the celiac artery. Stenosis is usually greater with expiration. This syndrome is controversial because isolated stenosis or even occlusion of the celiac artery is always compensated by collateral circulation from the SMA. Also, the angiographic finding of compression of the celiac axis is frequently demonstrated in asymptomatic patients. Neural origin of the clinical symptoms has also been postulated. When one needs to evaluate this syndrome, it is essential to demonstrate a stenosis in the proximal celiac artery that reduces or resolves with inspiration.

8. Do patients need any preparation?

A clear liquid diet on the day before the examination and overnight fasting are recommended to evaluate chronic mesenteric ischemia. (Sonographic evaluation is rarely indicated in case of acute mesenteric ischemia.) This is done to reduce interference from bowel gas. Also, velocity criteria for mesenteric stenosis are based on data obtained in the fasting state.

9. What are the main collaterals for celiac and SMA stenosis and occlusion?
- Marginal artery of Drummond (SMA to IMA)
- Arc of Riolan (SMA to IMA)
- Pancreaticoduodenal arcade (celiac to SMA)

10. What is a normal spectral waveform of the mesenteric arteries?

High-resistance flow with early diastolic flow reversal and late diastolic forward flow (triphasic) characterize the SMA and IMA in the fasting state. This changes to a low-resistance pattern after a meal. Persistent low-resistance flow is seen in the celiac artery pre- or postprandial because it supplies blood to the liver and spleen.

11. What are the ultrasound findings in the patient with chronic mesenteric ischemia?
- Low-resistance flow is seen in the SMA or IMA in the fasting state.
- In the case of celiac artery occlusion, reversed direction of flow in the common hepatic artery or gastroduodenal artery secondary to collaterals through the pancreaticoduodenal arcade is seen.

12. What degree of stenosis is considered significant in the mesenteric arteries?

Greater than 70% diameter reduction by angiogram is considered significant.

13. What are the velocity criteria for significant stenosis of the mesenteric arteries?
- For the SMA, a PSV > 275 cm/sec indicates a > 70% stenosis.
- For the celiac artery, a PSV > 200 cm/sec indicates a > 70% stenosis.

BIBLIOGRAPHY

1. Cognet F, Salcm DB, Dranssart M, et al: Chronic mesenteric ischemia: Imaging and percutaneous treatment. Radiographics 22:863–880, 2002.
2. Foley WD: Mesenteric ischemia. Ultrasound Q 17:103–111, 2001.
3. Moneta GL: Diagnosis of chronic intestinal ischemia. Semin Vasc Surg 3:176–185, 1990.
4. Moneta GL, Yeager RA, Dalman R, et al: Duplex ultrasound criteria for diagnosis of splanchnic artery stenosis or occlusion. J Vasc Surg 14:511–520, 1991.
5. Ralls PW: Doppler sonography: Clinical usefulness in abdominal vascular disease. In RSNA Categorical Course in Vascular Imaging. Oak Brook, IL, Radiological Society of North America, 1998, pp 201–209.
6. Zwiebel WJ: Ultrasound assessment of the splanchnic arteries. In Zwiebel WJ (ed): Introduction to Vascular Ultrasound, 4th ed. Philadelphia, WB Saunders, 2000, pp 421–429.
7. Zwiebel WJ: Anatomy and normal Doppler signature of abdominal vessels. In Zwiebel WJ (ed): Introduction to Vascular Ultrasound, 4th ed. Philadelphia, WB Saunders, 2000, pp 379–395.

44. HEMODIALYSIS ACCESS: GRAFTS AND FISTULAS

Nancy L. Carson, M.B.A., RDMS, R.V.T., and Susan L. Voci, M.D.

1. What are the types of hemodialysis access?
There are two major types of hemodialysis access: synthetic arteriovenous grafts and native arteriovenous fistulas (AVFs).

2. What are the indications for ultrasound evaluation of hemodialysis access?
Indications include but are not limited to:
- Difficult needle placement during dialysis
- Elevated venous pressure
- Abnormal laboratory values
- Underdeveloped fistula
- Loss of graft thrill
- Swelling
- Perigraft mass

3. What is the role of ultrasound in evaluating hemodialysis grafts and fistulas?
Ultrasound is used to evaluate both grafts and fistulas internally for stenosis, intimal flaps, and occlusion. Extraluminal findings include pseudoaneurysm, hematoma, and abscess. Ultrasound is also used to evaluate the anastomotic sites as well as the draining veins for stenosis or occlusion.

GRAFTS

4. Where are grafts typically placed?
Grafts can be placed in either the forearm or the upper arm. If possible, it is helpful to get a drawing from the referring physician indicating the course of the graft. If not, the graft can be followed quickly with grayscale to determine placement.

5. What are the most common graft placements found in the arm?
Three placements are the forearm loop graft, the upper arm straight graft, and the forearm straight graft. There are several other possible attachments and it is helpful to obtain a diagram from the surgeon (Fig. 1).

6. What type of transducer is used to analyze a graft?
A linear transducer should be used with the highest frequency possible, usually 7.5 MHz.

7. What is the best way to start a graft analysis with ultrasound?
It is best to scan the graft first in the transverse plane with grayscale to determine its orientation and follow its course. While in the transverse plane, the graft can also be evaluated for intraluminal pathology and extraluminal masses.

8. What is the normal sonographic appearance of a graft?
A graft consists of two parallel echogenic lines just under the surface of the skin. The center of a patent graft is anechoic (Fig. 2).

9. What is the purpose of color Doppler in graft analysis?
Color Doppler is used to look for areas of stenosis, occlusion, and pseudoaneurysms. Color Doppler should be performed both transverse and longitudinal to the graft. Color Doppler should also be used to assess any perigraft masses to evaluate for pseudoaneurysm or hematoma.

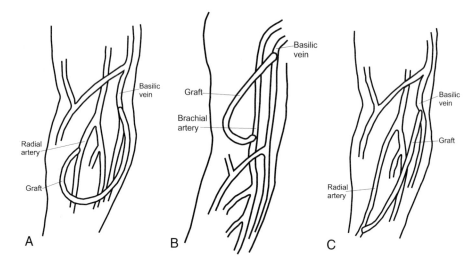

FIGURE 1. *A,* The forearm loop graft is attached to the radial artery and one of the antecubital veins (in this case, the basilic vein), and the loop is tunneled through the forearm. *B,* The upper arm straight graft is attached to the brachial artery just proximal to the antecubital fossa and the basilic vein. The venous end may also be attached to the brachial or axillary vein. *C,* The forearm straight graft is attached to the radial artery and an antecubital vein such as the basilic vein.

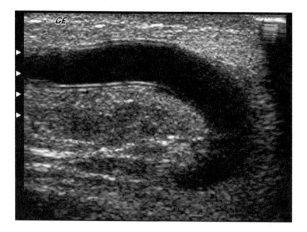

FIGURE 2. Normal graft appearance. Note echogenic walls.

10. What does a hematoma look like?

A hematoma appears as an area of mixed echogenicity around the lumen of the graft or adjacent to the graft. Often there is a palpable bump on the extremity (Fig. 3).

11. What does a pseudoaneurysm look like?

A pseudoaneurysm presents as a hypoechoic mass outside the lumen of the graft. Color Doppler shows bidirectional flow, and spectral Doppler in the neck should show alternating flow above and below the baseline. Every effort should be made to find the neck of the pseudoaneurysm where it arises from the graft (Fig. 4).

12. How does color Doppler differentiate between pseudoaneurysms and fluid collections?

A pseudoaneurysm demonstrates the typical mosaic swirling of blood in the mass. Fluid collections are hypoechoic and will not display any color Doppler signal.

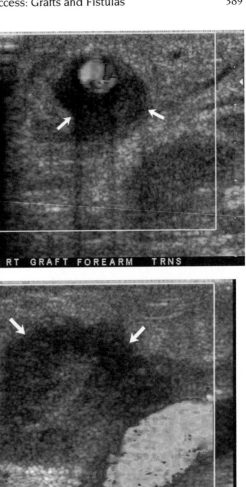

Figure 3. *A,* Hematoma *(arrows)* surrounding the graft lumen. *B,* Hematoma *(arrows)* adjacent to the graft.

13. Where should spectral Doppler tracings be taken?

Spectral Doppler tracings (all angle corrected to ≤ 60° to the graft) are taken at the venous and arterial anastomotic sites, at several representative sites within the graft, and specifically at any areas of stenosis. Angle-corrected Doppler tracings are also taken 2 cm caudal to the venous anastomosis in the draining vein and 2 cm cranial to the arterial anastomosis in the feeding artery.

14. What does a normal graft spectral waveform look like?

The waveform is generally monophasic with low-resistance arterial characteristics (high diastolic flow, slightly pulsatile) (Fig. 5).

15. What does the Doppler waveform taken at the draining vein typically look like?

Draining veins demonstrate arterial pulsations with velocities ranging from 30 to 100 cm/sec.

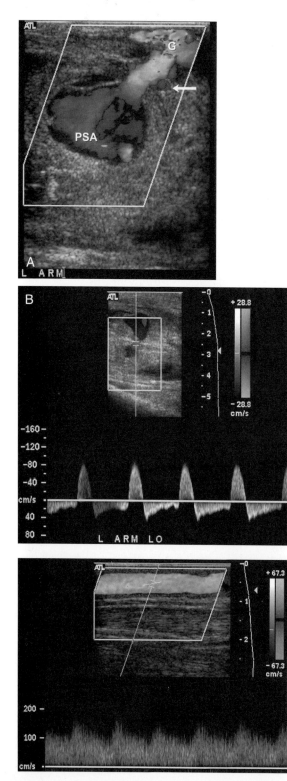

FIGURE 4. *A*, Color Doppler showing the graft (*G*) with a neck (*arrow*) connecting to a pseudoaneurysm (*PSA*). *B*, Spectral Doppler waveform from pseudoaneurysm neck. Note to-and-fro characteristics with flow above and below the baseline as the blood enters and exits the pseudoaneurysm.

FIGURE 5. Normal graft spectral Doppler waveform.

16. What velocities are measured from the Doppler tracings?

Each institution may have different required measurements and criteria that are used to report stenoses. Common measurements are peak systolic and end-diastolic velocities. Peak systolic velocities (PSVs) within the graft typically range from 100 to 400 cm/sec and end-diastolic velocities range from 60 to 200 cm/sec.

17. What velocity ratios are calculated and how are they obtained?

PSV ratios can be calculated for the venous and arterial anastomoses using the PSVs recorded at the anastomoses and the PSVs of the feeding artery and draining veins, respectively.
- PSV ratio arterial anastomosis = peak velocity anastomosis/peak velocity 2 cm cranial to arterial anastomosis
- PSV ratio venous anastomosis = peak velocity venous anastomosis/peak velocity 2 cm caudal to venous anastomosis.

18. What causes stenosis and where does it occur?

Graft stenoses most commonly occur secondary to intimal hyperplasia and are seen most frequently at the venous anastomosis and the draining vein (Fig. 6).

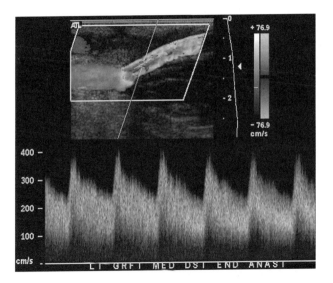

FIGURE 6. Graft end stenosis at the venous anastomosis. Peak systolic velocity is approaching 4.0 m/sec.

19. What other vessels should be interrogated and why?

The subclavian vein and the jugular vein of the ipsilateral side should be interrogated with color Doppler and spectral Doppler to provide information on vein patency central to the graft.

20. Describe pitfalls of performing ultrasound on patients with grafts.

Central stenosis: Doppler interrogation of the jugular vein and subclavian veins in patients with grafts may not show the typical pulsations and respiratory phasicity that is seen in patients without grafts. This is due to the high volume of blood flowing through the graft. In these patients, a change in the waveform pattern from previous studies or the presence of small-caliber tortuous veins may indicate stenosis or occlusion centrally.

Graft patency: Slow flow may be mistaken for graft thrombosis; it is helpful to use power Doppler when color Doppler does not show graft patency. Spectral Doppler with slow flow settings and a wide gate can be used to search for patency.

Graft stenosis: Most of the stenoses can be seen visually with either grayscale or color Doppler. When grafts form a loop, however, this area may alias and demonstrate increased velocities with spectral Doppler, even though the graft is patent in the loop. This should be considered technical unless there is a visible narrowing of the graft.

FISTULAS

21. **What are the common types of AVF anastomoses?**
    - Forearm radiocephalic fistula: This is an anastomosis between the radial artery and cephalic vein at the wrist.
    - Upper arm cephalic vein: This is an anastomosis of the brachial artery and cephalic vein near the antecubital fossa.
    - Basilic vein transposition: The basilic vein is transposed to a more central position and there the anastomosis is between the basilic vein and the brachial artery at the antecubital fossa.

22. **What are the common anastomotic connections between artery and vein?**
    - Side-to-side anastomosis: The side of the artery is anastomosed to the side of the vein (Fig. 7A).
    - End-to-side anastomosis: The end of the vein is anastomosed to the side of the artery (*see* Fig. 7B). The end of the artery is anastomosed to the side of the vein (*see* Fig. 7C).
    - End-to-end anastomosis: The ends of the artery and vein are anastomosed together (*see* Fig. 7D).

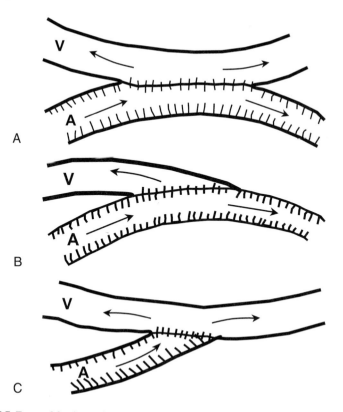

FIGURE 7. Types of fistula arterio-venous anastomoses. *A,* Side-to-side anastomosis. Note the side of the artery (*A*) is anastomosed to the side of the vein (*V*). *B,* End-to-side anastomosis. Note the end of the vein (*V*) is anastomosed to the side of the artery (*A*) *C,* The end of the artery (*A*) is anastomosed to the side of the vein (*V*) (*continued*)

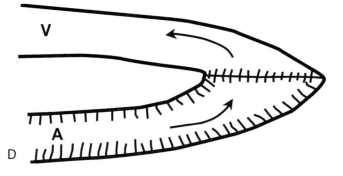

FIGURE 7. (*continued*) *D,* End-to-end anastomosis. Note the ends of the artery (*A*) and vein (*V*) are anastomosed together.

23. What are the advantages of using ultrasound for evaluation of hemodialysis access grafts and fistulas?

Ultrasound is noninvasive, inexpensive, portable, and does not require iodinated contrast.

24. What are the advantages of native AVFs over grafts?

Fistulas have increased longevity. The complications of stenosis, thrombosis, and infections occur less frequently in fistulas.

25. What are the disadvantages of native AVFs over grafts?

Fistulas require more time to mature before being able to use them, that is, 3 months versus 3 weeks for grafts. Temporary catheters are required for dialysis access during this time. Fistulas have a higher rate of early thrombosis.

26. What are the complications that occur in fistulas?

- Stenosis
- Thrombosis
- Pseudoaneurysm formation
- Fluid collections

27. What are the ultrasound findings of AVF stenosis?

On grayscale there is a visual narrowing. There is an increased PSV at the site of stenosis, as well as an increased PSV ratio. This ratio is the PSV measured at the suspected stenosis divided by the PSV measured 2 cm proximally.

28. What is considered an abnormal PSV ratio?

A ratio of 2–3 is thought to be abnormal. This corresponds to a 50–75% narrowing, and a ratio > 3 corresponds to a > 75% stenosis.

29. Where do the majority of stenoses occur?

The majority of stenoses in AVFs occur at the anastomosis.

BIBLIOGRAPHY

1. Finlay D, Longley D, Foshagen M, Letourneu J: Duplex and color Doppler sonography of hemodialysis arteriovenous fistula and grafts. Radiographics 13:983–989, 1993.
2. Lockhart M, Robbin M: Hemodialysis access ultrasound. Ultrasound Q 17:157–167, 2001.
3. Rumack CM, Wilson SR, Charboneau JW (eds): Diagnostic Ultrasound, 2nd ed. St. Louis, Mosby, 933–939, 1998.

45. TRANSCRANIAL DOPPLER ULTRASOUND

Nancy L. Carson, M.B.A., RDMS, R.V.T., and Susan L. Voci, M.D.

1. What is a transcranial Doppler examination?

A complete transcranial Doppler (TCD) examination is the evaluation of several intracranial arteries (Fig. 1). Included in the examination are the middle cerebral artery (MCA), the anterior cerebral artery (ACA), the posterior cerebral artery (PCA), the distal internal carotid artery (dICA), the basilar artery (BA), the ophthalmic artery (OA), the vertebral arteries (VA), and in some cases the extracranial internal carotid artery (eICA).

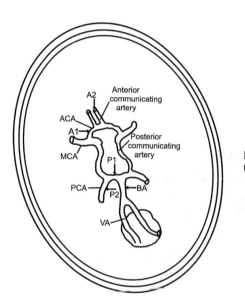

FIGURE 1. Intracranial arteries. Axial diagram at the level of the circle of Willis.

2. What are the indications for performing a TCD?

Indications for the TCD examination vary between institutions. Some of the most common indications follow:

- Detect intracranial stenosis
- Follow the course of vasospasm in the setting of subarachnoid hemorrhage
- Confirm the diagnosis of brain death
- Assess collateral pathways
- Monitor intraoperatively
- Detect cerebral microembolism
- Predict stroke associated with sickle cell disease
- Evaluate of the vertebrobasilar system
- Evaluate migraine headaches
- Evaluate possible emboli from a patent foramen ovale

3. What kind of equipment is used for a TCD examination?

TCD examination is done with a 2-MHz, focused, bidirectional, pulsed Doppler transducer, which displays only a spectral waveform. Transcranial imaging (TCI) can also be done using duplex ultrasound with a 2-MHz transducer, which provides direct color visualization of the vessels in addition to the spectral waveforms.

4. What information is recorded on a TCD examination?

When using spectral Doppler only, several tracings are recorded as the vessels are followed. Key information includes the velocity and direction of the blood flow. The velocity measurements obtained from the spectral tracings include the peak systolic velocity, the end-diastolic velocity, and the mean velocity. Because the velocities are obtained assuming the Doppler angle is zero, the mean velocity is the most important measurement and is calculated by the machine. In some laboratories, the pulsatility index is recorded, which provides information regarding distal resistance. In the setting of vasospasm, the ratio of the MCA to the extracranial ICA is also reported. When performing transcranial imaging, color images of the vessels are recorded as are the Doppler tracings.

5. With transcranial imaging, what windows are used to evaluate the vessels?

A complete TCD examination involves four windows: the transtemporal, the transorbital, the suboccipital, and the submandibular (Fig. 2).

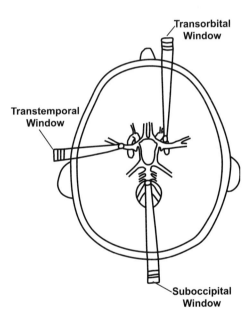

FIGURE 2. Diagram of the acoustic windows.

6. How does one find the transtemporal window?

The transtemporal window varies with each patient and the ability to penetrate the temporal bone varies with age, sex, and ethnicity. The thinnest part of the bone tends to be just above the zygomatic arch. It is helpful to rotate the transducer in a circular manner just above the arch to find the best window. Once the window is located, small angling adjustments are necessary to optimize the signal as the vessels are followed.

7. Which vessels are interrogated through the transtemporal window?

The vessels interrogated through this window include the MCA, the ACA, the PCA, and the dICA.

8. What is the best depth to start the initial search for the transtemporal window?

It is often easier to pick up a signal at the level of the bifurcation, 56–66 mm, and then follow the MCA to the shallowest depth possible before beginning to record Doppler tracings.

MCA: The MCA is the first vessel to be interrogated after the best transtemporal window is located. The MCA can be found at a depth as shallow as 45–52 mm and can be followed to a depth of about 56–60 mm until it joins the ACA at the level of the distal ICA bifurcation. Flow in the MCA should be toward the transducer and thus displayed above the baseline. At the level of the bifurcation of the distal ICA, MCA flow is above the baseline and ACA flow is depicted below the baseline, signifying flow away from the transducer (Fig. 3).

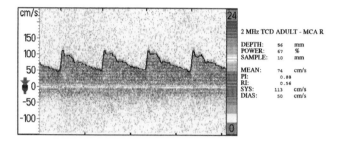

FIGURE 3. Normal middle cerebral artery. Waveform obtained at a depth of 56 mm. Mean velocity is equal to 74 cm/sec.

ACA: From the bifurcation, 56–60 mm, the ACA can be followed. Flow continues to be away from the transducer and it is often necessary to angle the transducer slightly superiorly or anteriorly to follow the ACA. It may be traced to depths of about 68–72 mm. As the ACA is followed, the MCA signal disappears from above the baseline (Fig. 4).

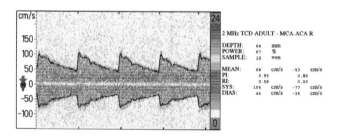

FIGURE 4. Normal bifurcation. Spectral Doppler waveform obtained at 64 mm. Middle cerebral artery is above the baseline. Anterior cerebral artery (ACA) is below the baseline. The ACA mean velocity is 68 cm/sec.

Distal ICA: Doppler signals can be obtained from the distal ICA at the level of the bifurcation, or 58–62 mm. At this level, the transducer should be angled slightly inferiorly and the signal from the dICA is toward the transducer and damped (lower amplitude) compared with that of the MCA and ACA.

PCA: The PCA is found by returning the sample volume to the level of the bifurcation then angling posteriorly. Flow is above the baseline, and the PCA can be followed to about 68–72 mm where the flow is bidirectional. At this point, the PCA has been traced to the top of the basilar artery (TOB), at its point of bifurcation. The signal below the baseline represents the contralateral PCA. Note that only the P-1 segment of the PCA is interrogated because of the sharp angle of the P-2 segment as it wraps around the midbrain (Fig. 5).

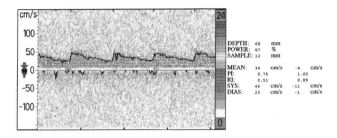

FIGURE 5. Normal posterior cerebral artery (PCA). Spectral Doppler angled slightly posterior at a depth of 68 mm. This shows a normal PCA waveform above the baseline with a mean of 34 cm/sec.

9. How can the PCA signal be distinguished from the MCA signal if they are both above the baseline?

The PCA has a lower velocity than the MCA and it can be followed posteriorly to 68–70 mm. The MCA can only be followed to about 62–64 mm at best, at which point the signal also displays the ACA below the baseline.

10. If no signal is obtained, what factors can be changed to ensure maximum penetration?

The power should be set at maximum and the Doppler frequency chosen should be the lowest available. Other factors include increasing the scale (or pulse repetition frequency), opening the Doppler gate, increasing the gain, and, if available, increasing the amplitude.

11. If no signal is obtained using the transtemporal window on one side, should the examination be terminated?

No. Often the patient has an adequate window on at least one side. If that is the case, the contralateral MCA and ACA can be interrogated by crossing the midline.

12. How do the Doppler signals appear when insonating the contralateral vessels?

The Doppler signals are reversed. The MCA appears below the baseline, indicating flow away from the transducer, and the ACA is above the baseline, indicating flow toward the transducer.

13. Are the anterior communicating and posterior communicating arteries interrogated?

No. Usually the only time a signal is detected in the anterior and posterior communicating arteries is when they are functioning as collaterals. If detected, flow in the anterior communicating artery is at a depth of 70–80 mm and the direction is away from the side supplying the blood. Flow in a posterior communicating artery is turbulent with a higher velocity than a normal PCA.

14. Which vessels are interrogated from the suboccipital window?

The intracranial vertebral arteries and the basilar artery can be evaluated with the suboccipital approach.

15. How is the patient positioned?

The patient is seated with the head tipped slightly forward. The transducer is placed at the nape of the neck and the foramen magnum is used as the window. If the patient cannot sit up, the patient can lie on his or her side as long as the spine is kept in a horizontal plane. The chin is again tipped forward.

16. At what depth is the signal from the vertebral arteries seen?

The vertebral artery signals are obtained at a depth of about 60–85 mm. The transducer must be angled slightly to the right or left of midline to follow the vessels. The net direction of flow is away from the transducer, but occasionally the signal may be bidirectional as the arteries course through the foramina of the transverse spinous processes.

17. At what level do the vertebral arteries join to become the BA?

From the suboccipital window, the BA begins at about 85 mm and can be followed distally to a depth of 100–108 mm. The Doppler signal is below the baseline with a higher mean velocity than the vertebrals (Fig. 6).

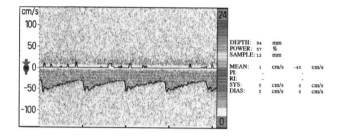

FIGURE 6. Normal basilar artery. Doppler tracing obtained from the suboccipital window at a depth of 94 mm. The basilar artery is below the baseline within a mean velocity of 40 cm/sec.

18. What if, after several attempts, no signal is obtained from the suboccipital window?

Possibly the chin is tipped too far forward. The head should be tipped back and angle the transducer angled in the same plane as the orbits.

19. Which vessels are interrogated from the transorbital window?

Doppler signals from the OA and the siphon of the internal carotid artery can be obtained using the transorbital approach.

20. What are the technical considerations when using the transorbital window?

When using this window, the ultrasound beam travels through the eye. To minimize exposure to the eye, the acoustic power must be reduced to a low setting, 10–25% of maximum, and the examination time should be as short as possible.

21. How is the transorbital window used?

The transducer is placed directly on the closed eyelid. The depth of the sample volume should be at about 40–50 mm with a slight medial angle.

22. In which direction does the OA flow?

Flow in the OA is toward the transducer. The waveform is highly pulsatile because it supplies blood to the globe of the eye.

23. How deep is the carotid siphon?

The carotid siphon is about 56–70 mm deep. The angle of the transducer must be adjusted slightly as the depth is increased.

24. How does the signal from the carotid siphon differ from that of the OA?

The signal from the carotid siphon changes from highly pulsatile in the OA to low resistance in the carotid siphon. The direction of the signal in the siphon depends on which part of the siphon the Doppler gate is in.

25. What are the different areas of the siphon?

The carotid siphon is "S" shaped and is divided into three parts, the parasellar, the genu, and the supraclinoid. The signal from the parasellar region is toward the transducer, the signal is bidirectional in the genu, and the signal is away from the transducer in the supraclinoid section. All three sections may not be represented in each transorbital examination.

26. When is the submandibular window used in the TCD examination?

The submandibular window is used to obtain a signal from the extracranial portion of the internal carotid artery. With the patient's head tilted slightly to the contralateral side, the transducer is placed at the angle of the mandible aiming toward the head with a slight medial angle. The depth of the sample volume is 56–70 mm and the direction of flow is away from the transducer.

27. What are the normal values for the arteries interrogated?

There are several references for normal values published. Our laboratory uses the following criteria for adults:

TCD Adult Normal Values

ARTERY	TRANSDUCER POSITION	DEPTH OF SAMPLE VOLUME (MM)	DIRECTION OF FLOW	MEAN VELOCITY (CM/SEC)
MCA	Transtemporal	30–60	Toward	62 ± 12
ACA/MCA	Transtemporal	55–65	Bidirectional	—
ACA	Transtemporal	60–80	Away	51 ± 13
PCA (P1)	Transtemporal	60–70	Toward	38 ± 10
diCA	Transtemporal	55–65	Toward	37 ± 8
Extracranial ICA	Submandibular	45–55	Away	36 ± 8
OA	Transorbital	40–60	Toward	22 ± 4
Vertebral Artery	Suboccipital	60–90	Away	37 ± 10
BA	Suboccipital	80–120	Away	39 ± 9

28. How does the TCI examination differ from the TCD examination?

The same vessels can be interrogated from the same windows for both examinations. The TCI examination uses a 2.0–2.5-MHz phased-array transducer. In addition to the Doppler spectrum, TCI provides both grayscale and color Doppler images.

29. What value does the color image add?

The color image makes it easier to locate the intracranial arteries for spectral Doppler analysis.

30. What are the grayscale landmarks seen before turning on the color when using the transtemporal window?

Once the transtemporal window is located, if the transducer is tipped inferiorly, several reflective bony landmarks can be seen. The petrous ridges of the temporal bone extend posteriorly and the lesser wings of the sphenoid bone extend anteriorly.

31. From these landmarks, where will the vessels be located?

The terminal ICA can be seen with color Doppler at the level of the bony landmarks mentioned previously. To visualize the MCA and ACA, the transducer must be angled anteriorly and superiorly. The PCA can be detected with color Doppler by angling the transducer slightly posterior and inferior using the cerebral peduncles as a landmark.

32. If the vessels are visible with color Doppler, should the spectral Doppler angle be corrected to that of the vessel?

No. The angle should not be corrected. Angle-corrected velocities tend to be elevated compared to the criteria that has been set up assuming a 0° angle.

33. Is there a grayscale landmark for the suboccipital window?

With the transducer placed at the nape of the neck, the chin tilted toward the chest, and the beam directed toward the bridge of the nose, there would be a circular anechoic or hypoechoic region on the grayscale image, which represents the foramen magnum. The vertebral arteries can be seen by angling slightly from side to side, and the BA is more distal in the midline.

34. How does the normal velocity of the MCA compare with the velocities of the ACA, PCA, and ICA?

The normal velocity of the MCA is greater than the velocity of the ACA and PCA. The velocity of the PCA is greater than the velocity of the ICA.

35. In the evaluation of vasospasm secondary to subarachnoid hemorrhage, what is the mean MCA velocity that corresponds to a mild degree of narrowing (> 25%), moderate narrowing (25–50%), and severe vessel narrowing (< 50%)?

- Mean MCA velocities up to 120 cm/sec correlate with a mild degree of narrowing.
- Mean MCA velocities of 120–200 cm/sec correlate with moderate narrowing (Fig. 7).
- Mean MCA velocities greater than 200 cm/sec correlate with severe vessel narrowing.

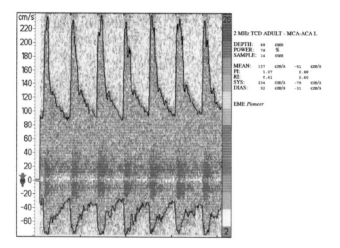

FIGURE 7. Vasospasm. Spectral Doppler obtained at a depth of 68 mm in an adult who is postaneurysm clipping. The mean velocity of the middle cerebral artery is 137 cm/sec.

36. In the evaluation of vasospasm secondary to subarachnoid hemorrhage, how do side-to-side differences in velocities assist the interpretation?

A discrepancy of > 14% of the VMCA or VICA is abnormal. A discrepancy of > 24% of the VACA is abnormal, and a discrepancy of > 34% of the VPCA is abnormal (V = velocity).

37. Why is the hemispheric ratio of the VMCA/VICA useful in making the diagnosis of vasospasm in the setting of subarachnoid hemorrhage?

The ratio is independent of flow. The velocities in both vessels increase with volume. Therefore, if the velocities of the ICA and MCA are increased, the ratio remains normal, and a false-positive diagnosis of vasospasm is avoided.

38. What is a normal hemispheric ratio?

A hemispheric ratio < 3.0 is normal.

39. What is an abnormal hemispheric ratio?

A ratio $> 3.0–6.0$ is seen in vasospasm. A ratio > 6.0 is seen in severe vasospasm.

40. What is a subarachnoid hemorrhage (SAH)?

A subarachnoid hemorrhage is due to blood leaking into the subarachnoid space from a ruptured artery, vein, or intracranial hemorrhage that dissects through the parenchyma to the surface of the brain or ventricles.

41. What is the incidence of a subarachnoid hemorrhage secondary to an aneurysm?

The incidence of subarachnoid hemorrhage secondary to an aneurysm is 10 in 100,000 in the United States.

42. What is cerebral vasospasm?

Cerebral vasospasm is the abnormal constriction of the basal intracranial arteries that can lead to cerebral ischemia or infarction.

43. If vasospasm occurs as a complication of subarachnoid hemorrhage, when would it typically occur?

Vasospasm occurs between days 2 and 7 after a subarachnoid hemorrhage with maximum severity between days 7 and 12.

44. In the management of vasospasm, when and how often are TCD examinations performed?

Typically, a baseline study is performed, then follow-up studies are performed every other day. Mean flow velocities of the MCA, PCA, ACA, dICA, and extracranial ICA are recorded.

45. Why is TCD examination performed on children with sickle cell disease (SCD)?

Cerebral infarction in children with SCD is associated with occlusive vasculopathy. The vessels most commonly involved are the distal ICA, proximal MCA, and the ACA. TCD examination can detect intracranial lesions by demonstrating elevated velocities in the aforementioned vessels. TCD is safe and noninvasive, and can be tolerated by most children.

46. What is the incidence of stroke in SCD?

Stroke is one of the most serious complications of SCD. It occurs in 11% of patients with homozygous SCD by the age of 20 years.

47. What is the most common type of stroke in SCD and what is its etiology?

Cerebral infarction is the most common type of stroke in children with SCD. It results from occlusion stenosis of the large arteries of the brain. The distal intracranial portions of the ICA and the proximal MCA are especially susceptible to stenosis.

48. What is the STOP protocol?

The STOP protocol is a standardized protocol used in performing TCD in clinical SCD.

49. According to the STOP protocol, what are the velocities used to classify a study as normal or abnormal?

Mean velocities less then 170 cm/sec are classified as normal, those greater than 170 but less than 200 cm/sec are considered conditional, and those greater than 200 cm/sec are considered abnormal (Fig. 8).

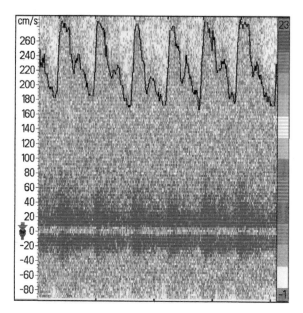

FIGURE 8. Vasospasm. Spectral Doppler tracing from a child with sickle cell. The mean velocity of the middle cerebral artery at a depth of 54 mm is 224 cm/sec.

50. What factors influence cerebral blood flow velocity?

Age	Blood pressure
Hematocrit	Cardiac output
Carbon dioxide	Proximal arterial obstruction
Oxygen	Distal arterial stenosis
Hypoglycemia	Rhythmic oscillations
Fever	Arteriovenous malformations

BIBLIOGRAPHY

1. Babikian VL, Wechsler LR: Transcranial Doppler Ultrasonography, 2nd ed. Woburn, MA: Butterworth-Heinemann, 1999, pp 9–27.
2. Becker G, Bogdahn U: Transcranial color-coded real-time ultrasonography in adults. In Babikian VL, Wechsler LR (eds): Transcranial Doppler Sonography. St Louis, Mosby-Year Book, 1993, pp 11–28.
3. Lindegaard K-F, Bakke SJ, Sorteberg W, et al: A noninvasive Doppler ultrasound method for the evaluation of patients with subarachnoid hemorrhage. Acta Radiol Suppl 369:96–98, 1986.
4. Lindegaad K-F, Nornes H, Bakke SJ, et al: Cerebral vasospasm diagnosis by means of angiography and blood velocity measurements. Acta Neurochir (Wien) 100(1–2):24, 1989.
5. Lindegaard K-F, Nornes H, Bakke SJ, et al: Cerebral vasospasm after subarachnoid hemorrhage investigated by means of transcranial Doppler ultrasound. Acta Neurochir Suppl (Wien) 42:81–84, 1988.
6. Otis SM, Ringelstein EB: Transcranial Doppler sonography. In Zwiebel WJ (ed): Introduction to Vascular Ultrasonography, 4th ed. Philadelphia, WB Saunders, 2000, pp 177–199.
7. Saver JL, Feldman E: Basic transcranial Doppler examination: Technique and anatomy. In Babikian VL, Wechsler LR (eds): Transcranial Doppler Sonography. St. Louis, Mosby-Year Book, 1993, pp 11–28.
8. TCD in Children with Sickle Cell Disease: An Intensive Training Course. Presented by School of Medicine, Medical College of Georgia, the Alumni Center, Augusta, GA, January 27–30, 1998.
9. Vollrath K: Whaaz up in TCD! Atlanta, Society of Diagnostic Medical Sonography Conference Proceedings, 2002, pp 553–559.

46. DOPPLER EVALUATION OF LIVER AND TRANSJUGULAR INTRAHEPATIC PORTOSYSTEMIC SHUNTS

Deborah J. Rubens, M.D., and Nancy L. Carson, M.B.A., RDMS, R.V.T.

1. Why is Doppler used to scan the liver?

Doppler is used to distinguish vascular from nonvascular structures, to find vessels that are invisible on grayscale, and to make diagnoses based on arterial or venous spectral flow patterns.

2. What scanning parameters should be used?

A 3-MHz transducer small footprint is often preferred for intercostal approaches. The Doppler gain should be as high as possible without image or spectral noise and the wall filter as low as possible to avoid false diagnosis of thrombosis.

Scale (pulse repetition frequency) should be as low as possible to localize vessels quickly with color, then to sample and angle-correct for spectral Doppler.

3. Which type of Doppler should be used?

Spectral Doppler is most sensitive to flow, but is inefficient for quick overview of flow direction. It requires precise gate placement and is best with suspended respiration. It can sometimes detect small hepatic arteries that cannot be seen with color or power Doppler. For this application, the Doppler sample gate should be opened wide in the anatomic vicinity of the vessel (hepatic artery) without color.

Color Doppler is most useful for flow direction of portal and hepatic veins due to less flash artifact than that of power Doppler. With a low wall filter, it can usually localize hepatic arteries quickly for spectral sampling. Aliasing is useful to identify areas of stenosis for spectral sampling in hepatic arteries and transjugular intrahepatic portosystemic shunts (TIPS).

Power Doppler is best used in TIPS (which often have poor Doppler angles) and in portal vessels with slow flow, but it is limited by motion artifact.

4. What can be done to improve Doppler sensitivity when no flow is detected in a vessel?

- Change the acoustic window to decrease the angle to the vessel to as close to zero as possible.
- Increase penetration by lowering the frequency of the transducer.
- Use the highest power setting for both color and spectral Doppler.
- Lower the pulse repetition frequency (PRF) and the scale.
- Decrease the wall filter settings for both color Doppler and spectral Doppler.
- Increase color and spectral gain to just below the point where noise is detected.
- Use power Doppler.

5. What is the normal vasculature of the hepatic arteries, portal veins, and hepatic veins?

Hepatic arteries: The hepatic arteries have a low resistance arterial waveform. Their normal resistive index is ≥ 0.5, but it is usually in the 0.6–0.7 range. Higher numbers (0.7–1.0) are normal postprandial because the blood is diverted to the mesenteric circulation and away from the liver. High resistance may also be seen immediately after transplantation, and does not correlate with rejection. Low resistance (<0.5) is indicative of shunt flow, hepatic artery thrombosis, or stenosis. Hepatic arterial flow increases in cirrhosis and in some tumors (Fig. 1).

Portal vein: A monotonous continuous waveform is normally directed into the liver (hepatopedal). Color Doppler should fill out the entire vessel to exclude portal vein thrombosis, which may be anechoic. Spectral Doppler velocities are typically low (15–40 cm/sec) and may

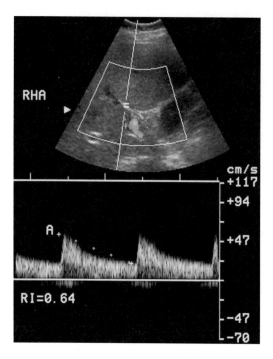

FIGURE 1. Normal hepatic artery. Normal hepatic artery spectral Doppler tracing; note: resistive index (RI) is 0.64.

even be bidirectional as a result of swirling flow in a large slow-flowing vein. Portal vein flow reverses (out of the liver, hepatofugal) in portal hypertension and in, well-functioning portosystemic shunts (Fig. 2).

Hepatic veins: There are right, middle, and left hepatic veins with a variable accessory right. The middle and left hepatic veins frequently share a short common trunk at the inferior vena cava (IVC) confluence. These provide anatomic landmarks for segmental resection for live liver donation. Normal flow is triphasic, reflecting cardiac activity, with forward flow in systole and diastole and a small reversal during atrial emptying. Monotonous (damped) flow is seen in cirrhosis, and veins may be difficult to locate because of parenchymal compression. Color Doppler should be used to localize veins that are invisible on grayscale (Fig.3).

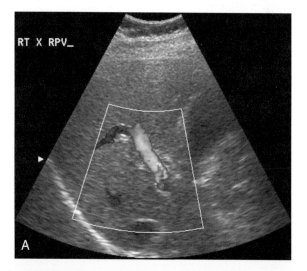

FIGURE 2. Normal portal vein. *A,* Color Doppler of normal right portal vein, flow direction is hepatopedal (into the liver). (*continued*)

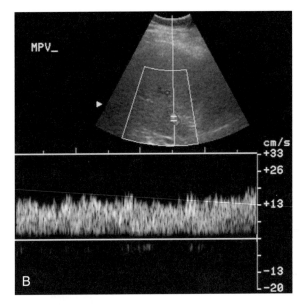

FIGURE 2. (*continued*) *B,* Normal portal venous Doppler waveform.

PORTAL HYPERTENSION

6. What is portal hypertension?

Portal hypertension is a condition that results from impedance of blood flow through the liver causing elevated pressure in the portal venous system. In this setting, blood normally directed toward the liver through the portal system is redirected through collateral channels to lower pressure systemic vessels.

7. What are the causes of portal hypertension?

The causes of portal hypertension are broken down into three levels: (1) prehepatic (inflow), (2) intrahepatic (liver, sinusoids, and hepatocytes), and (3) posthepatic (outflow).

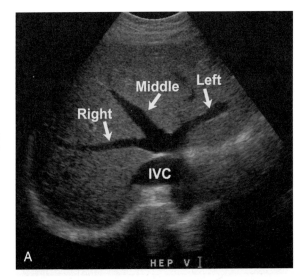

FIGURE 3. Normal hepatic veins. *A,* Grayscale image demonstrating the normal relationship of the hepatic veins. (*continued*)

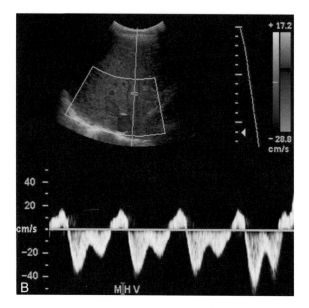

FIGURE 3. (*continued*) *B*, Spectral Doppler tracing demonstrating normal hepatic venous flow.

Some of the most common prehepatic causes are portal vein and splenic vein thrombosis and portal vein compression. The most common intrahepatic cause is cirrhosis, but hepatic fibrosis, malignancies, veno-occlusive disease, lymphoma, and sarcoidosis can also cause portal hypertension. Posthepatic causes include but are not limited to chronic heart failure (CHF), IVC obstruction, and Budd-Chiari syndrome.

8. What is the role of ultrasound in portal hypertension?

Color and spectral Doppler can be used to detect portal vein thrombosis, the presence of collaterals, and direction of portal vein flow, and to evaluate bypass shunts (portocaval, splenorenal, mesocaval, and TIPS) for patency.

9. How does the portal vein appear in the setting of acute and subacute portal hypertension?

The portal vein increases in diameter as a result of elevated portal pressure, resulting in decreased average velocities and a continuous waveform (i.e., no respiratory variation). As pressures continue to increase, flow may become to-and-fro (biphasic) and eventually reverse to become hepatofugal (Fig. 4).

10. What is the best way to measure the diameter of the portal vein?

The portal vein should be measured with the patient supine in quiet respiration. Making sure the portal vein is in its long axis, measurement should be taken at or close to the point where it crosses the IVC.

11. What are the normal and abnormal measurements of the portal vein?

The portal vein is considered normal with a measurement of ≤ 13 mm in quiet respiration and an increase up to 50% during deep inspiration. A dilated portal vein measures > 15 mm during quiet respiration.

12. Does a dilated portal vein always signify portal hypertension?

No. Because of backpressure from the heart through the hepatic veins, the portal vein can be dilated in cases of long-standing CHF. In this setting, the portal flow demonstrates increased pulsatility on spectral Doppler and the IVC is dilated (Fig. 5).

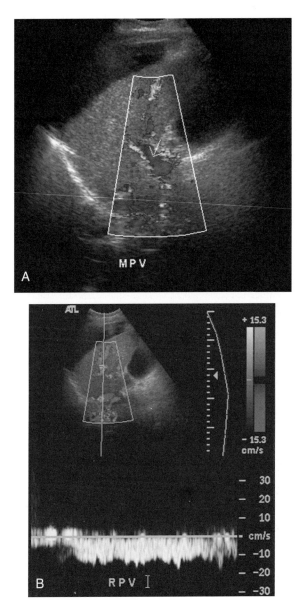

FIGURE 4. Portal hypertension. *A,* Color Doppler showing portal venous flow directed away from the liver (hepatofugal) (*arrow*). *B,* Spectral Doppler obtained from the right portal vein confirming flow direction is hepatofugal.

13. What are some of the complications resulting from portal hypertension?

Portal vein thrombosis

Slow or reversed portal vein flow

Portosystemic collaterals

Splenomegaly

Variceal hemorrhage

PORTAL VEIN THROMBOSIS

14. What are the sonographic findings in the setting of acute portal vein thrombosis?

Early thrombosis tends to be hypoechoic and may be partial or complete. The portal vein as well as the distal branches can be dilated. Color Doppler demonstrates partial or complete

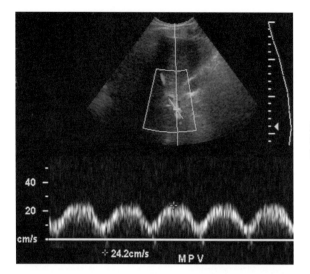

FIGURE 5. Pulsitile portal venous flow. Doppler signal from the main portal vein demonstrating pulsatility.

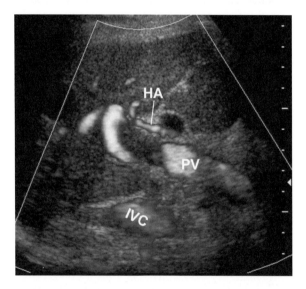

FIGURE 6. Portal vein clot. Power Doppler demonstrates a non-occlusive clot in the main portal vein (see also Color Plates, Figure 25).

occlusion. Spectral Doppler demonstrates increased velocities if there is partial occlusion as the blood courses around the clot (Fig. 6).

15. What are the sonographic findings of chronic portal vein thrombosis?

In chronic portal vein thrombosis, the thrombus appears hyperechoic as it becomes fibrotic. Ultrasound may be unable to detect the fibrotic, occluded portal vein. The vein may eventually recanalize or form collaterals in which color Doppler and spectral Doppler can detect venous flow from small, tortuous veins.

16. What is cavernous transformation and how can it be detected?

Cavernous transformation is a result of portal vein thrombosis in which a mass of tortuous vessels forms in the porta hepatis, usually 6–20 days after the portal vein is thrombosed. Color flow Doppler demonstrates flow in the vessels and spectral Doppler indicates portal venous flow; otherwise, they may be mistaken for biliary dilatation.

17. What is the best way to detect portal vein thrombosis?

The best way to detect portal vein thrombosis is with the use of color flow Doppler, making sure the settings are optimized for slow flow. It is useful to scan transverse to the portal vein with color Doppler to look for non-occlusive thrombosis. In cases of absence of flow, power Doppler and spectral Doppler should be used to search for slow flow. It is also helpful to reposition the patient and scan from different angles to minimize the Doppler angle to the portal vein ($< 60°$) and decrease the depth to the vessel.

18. How can tumor invasion of the portal vein be distinguished from portal vein thrombosis?

Spectral Doppler can be used to detect an arterial waveform from within a soft tissue mass in the portal vein. The settings should be maximized for increased sensitivity. The arterial signals are not present in portal vein thrombosis. A partially recanalized portal vein gives portal venous signals from the vascular channels in the clot.

19. When portal vein pressure increases resulting in decreased portal vein flow or portal vein thrombosis, what happens to hepatic arterial flow?

Hepatic artery flow increases in response to decreased portal vein flow to maintain hepatic perfusion. This is referred to as *arterialization*. Color Doppler demonstrates an enlarged hepatic artery, often with turbulent flow (Fig. 7).

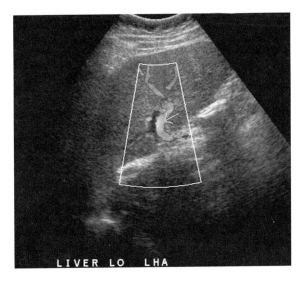

FIGURE 7. Arterialization. Patient with cirrhosis. Color Doppler shows increased arterial flow (*arrow*) in relationship to the scant flow in the adjacent portal vein.

PORTOSYSTEMIC COLLATERALS

20. Why do portosystemic collaterals form and how sensitive is ultrasound for detection of portosystemic collaterals?

Portosystemic collaterals form so that blood from the gut has an alternative route to bypass a congested liver on its way to the heart. Ultrasound is extremely sensitive in detecting collaterals when color Doppler is used.

21. What are the most common collaterals that can be seen with ultrasound?

The most common collateral noted with ultrasound is the umbilical vein, which can be followed anteriorly and medially from the falciform ligament toward the umbilicus, carrying blood

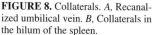

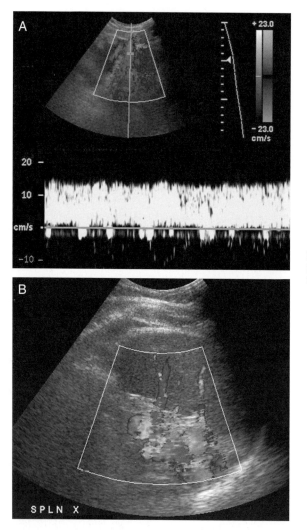

FIGURE 8. Collaterals. *A*, Recanalized umbilical vein. *B*, Collaterals in the hilum of the spleen.

away from the liver. Other common sites where portosystemic collaterals are detected include the gastroesophageal junction in the midepigastrium, and splenorenal and gastrorenal collaterals in the left upper quadrant (Fig. 8).

PORTOSYSTEMIC SHUNTS

22. What is the role of ultrasound in evaluating portosystemic shunts?

The primary role of ultrasound is to evaluate shunt patency using color Doppler, spectral Doppler, and possibly power Doppler. TIPS can be consistently evaluated with ultrasound; however, mesocaval, portocaval, and splenorenal shunts are often obscured by overlying bowel gas (Fig. 9).

23. What is TIPS?

Transjugular intrahepatic portosystemic shunt, which is an intrahepatic portacaval shunt placed to decompress the portal venous system. The shunt is created percutaneously and is the most common portosystemic shunt used.

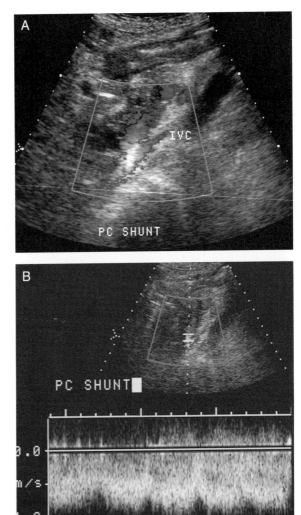

FIGURE 9. Portocaval (PC) shunt. *A,* Color Doppler demonstrating a patent PC shunt between the distal portal vein and the inferior vena cava (IVC). *B,* Spectral Doppler indicating shunt flow is directed away from the liver into the IVC.

24. What is the purpose of a TIPS?

Primarily, a TIPS is placed in patients with end-stage liver disease to avoid some of the complications while awaiting a liver transplant. A working shunt reduces ascites, decreases portal hypertension, and prevents esophageal variceal hemorrhage, but the shunts are susceptible to stenosis and occlusion.

25. Where are the proximal and distal ends of the TIPS located?

The proximal end is usually found in the main or right portal vein and the distal end is located in the right hepatic vein near its junction with the IVC (Fig. 10).

26. When obtaining a Doppler signal from the proximal end of the shunt, where should the cursor be placed to avoid abnormally low velocities?

The cursor is placed far enough into the shunt from its portal vein end so that the cursor is in the intrahepatic portion of the shunt. At this point, the spectral Doppler signal has characteristic "shunt flow" and is not characteristic of portal vein flow (Fig. 11).

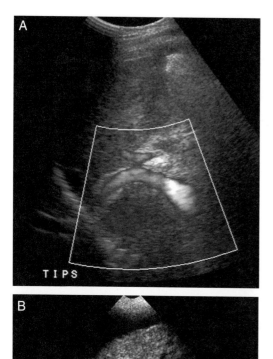

FIGURE 10. Normal transjugular intrahepatic portosystemic shunt (TIPS). *A*, Power Doppler demonstrating a patent TIPS. *B*, Typical appearance of a TIPS with grayscale imaging.

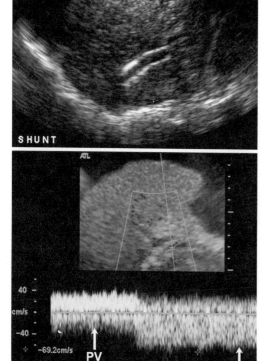

FIGURE 11. Proximal transjugular intrahepatic portosystemic shunt (TIPS) velocity. Doppler signal from the proximal end of the TIPS. Note the increase in flow velocity as the cursor is moved from the main portal vein into the shunt.

27. What type of transducer is best for shunt imaging and what images of the shunt are required?

The best transducer for shunt imaging is a 3.5-MHz curved array that has the capability to be powered down to 2–2.5 MHz. The shunt must be imaged in grayscale and both spectral and color Doppler. The Doppler signals must be taken from the lumen of the shunt with a Doppler angle of less than 60°.

28. What other vessels should be interrogated with a TIPS examination?

The vessels that should be imaged in addition to the shunt are the main, right, and left portal veins; the main, right, and left hepatic veins; the main, right and left hepatic arteries; the IVC; any collaterals. Both color Doppler and spectral Doppler images should be recorded. The spectral Doppler of the main portal vein should be angle corrected at an angle of ≤ 60°.

29. If the shunt cannot be interrogated at a Doppler angle of ≤ 60° from the subcostal or intercostal approach, what are other options?

It is helpful to turn the patient on his or her left side and image from the front, or intercostal window from a posterior approach.

30. What are the normal ultrasound findings in the shunt after placement?

- Color Doppler flow should fill the entire lumen of the shunt (*see* Fig. 10A).
- There should be a monophasic, slightly pulsatile spectral flow pattern through the length of the shunt with peak shunt velocities > 60 cm/sec, typically ranging from 90–120 cm/sec (Fig. 12).
- Velocities at the proximal midline distal ends of the shunt should be similar as long as the proximal end is not sampled too close to the portal vein.

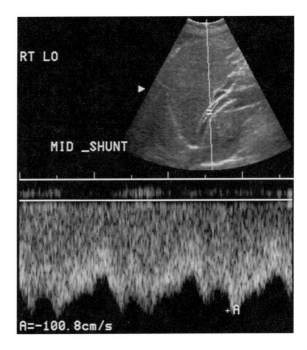

FIGURE 12. Normal transjugular intrahepatic portosystemic shunt (TIPS). Angle-corrected spectral Doppler tracing from the mid portion of a TIPS.

31. What direction should flow be in the portal system after shunt placement?

The direction of flow should be hepatofugal in the right and left branches, indicating diversion of portal venous flow from the liver into the shunt. Flow in the main portal vein remains hepatopedal, or toward the liver (Fig. 13).

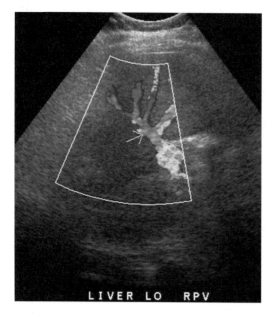

FIGURE 13. Portal venous flow in a patient with a transjugular intrahepatic portosystemic shunt (TIPS). Color Doppler shows the portal venous flow is directed away from the liver (hepatofugal).

32. If the shunt appears to be thrombosed using color Doppler, what can be done to optimize for slower flow?
- Decrease the color filter
- Decrease the Doppler frequency
- Scan from a different window to decrease the depth
- Decrease the Doppler angle
- Use power Doppler
- Use spectral Doppler with a wide gate to pick up slow flow.

33. What are the direct indications for shunt stenosis or thrombosis?
Lack of color Doppler signal in the shunt indicates thrombosis (Fig. 14). Stenosis is indicated by the following:

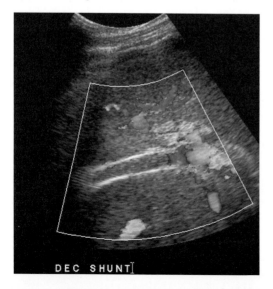

FIGURE 14. Occluded transjugular intrahepatic portosystemic shunt (TIPS). Color Doppler demonstrating an occluded TIPS (see also Color Plates, Figure 26). This was confirmed with angiography.

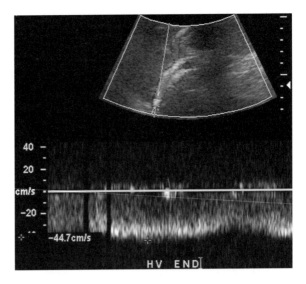

FIGURE 15. Abnormal transjugular intrahepatic portosystemic shunt (TIPS) flow. Spectral Doppler signal obtained from the distal end of a TIPS indicating an abnormally low shunt velocity of 44.7 cm/sec.

- Change of velocity within the shunt of a factor ≥ 2.
- Maximum velocity within the shunt of < 60 cm/sec or > 2 m/sec (Fig. 15).
- Greater than 50% change in velocity within the shunt compared to the baseline examination.

34. What are the indirect indicators of shunt stenosis?
- Change in direction of flow in the MPV, LPV, or RPV from baseline post-shunt examination. (Normal flow should be toward the shunt in all vessels. Flow away from the shunt indicates shunt malfunction.)
- Worsening ascites or splenomegaly.
- Reappearance of collaterals or a recanalized umbilical vein.
- Reversed flow in the draining hepatic vein. This indicates shunt outflow obstruction either in the vein or in the IVC.

35. What is the accuracy of ultrasound as compared with angiography for detecting TIPS stenosis or thrombosis?
Reports range from 25% sensitivity and 90% specificity to numbers as high as sensitivity of 94% in a long-term clinical outcome study. The angiographic gold standard of degree of shunt narrowing or portal pressure gradients varies within studies, as do the Doppler criteria. Typical middle end values are 92% sensitivity and 92% specificity using the angiographic diagnostic criteria of 50% shunt narrowing, without portal pressure gradients. Ultrasound contrast enhanced Doppler has been found to be 82% sensitive and specific as compared with angiographic portosystemic gradients of greater than 15 mmHg.

36. What is the most common site of stenosis?
The most common site for stenosis is at the hepatic vein (distal) end of the shunt, usually within the shunt (Fig. 16).

37. What is the most common reason for TIPS stenosis?
Pseudointimal hyperplasia is the most common cause of stenosis or occlusion. This can be seen as early as a few weeks after insertion.

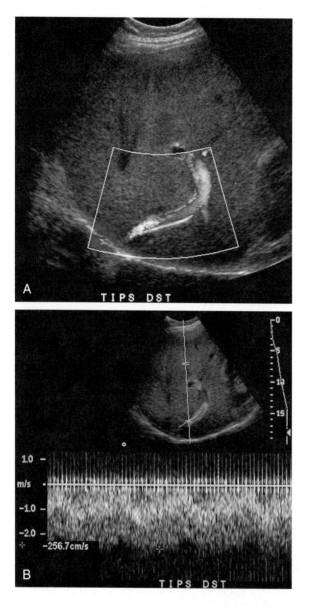

FIGURE 16. Transjugular intrahepatic portosystemic shunt stenosis. *A,* Increased shunt velocity at the distal end of the shunt indicated by color Doppler aliasing. *B,* Spectral Doppler signal demonstrates the focal distal shunt stenosis; velocity is 256.7 cm/sec.

38. What is a patency rate of a TIPS at 1 year?

It has been reported that the patency rate at 1 year without revision ranges from 23–66%. With intervention for occlusion or stenosis by balloon angioplasty and thrombolysis, the patency rate at 1 year is about 85%.

39. What are the pitfalls of shunt imaging?

Shunts that are curved or sharply angled may result in high Doppler shifts, which could result in a false-positive examination. This may be resolved by scanning from different angles to get a more accurate Doppler tracing. Shunts can be easily located, but often the lumen appears to be thrombosed because of the lack of color Doppler signal. In these cases, the shunt may be parallel to the beam or too deep. The patient should be scanned in different positions and from different angles to decrease the angle of the shunt to the beam and place it closer to the beam. The color Doppler scale should be set low enough to detect slow flow and the lowest Doppler frequency available should be used to ensure maximum penetration.

HEPATIC ARTERIES

40. How can color flow be optimized to locate the hepatic arteries?

The hepatic arteries can be located with color flow Doppler by maximizing sensitivity for slow flow. This varies on different equipment, but the main factors to adjust are (1) decrease the scale (PRF), (2) decrease the filter, (3) adjust the color gain until there is just a small amount of noise, (4) open the color gate, and (5) change the Doppler frequency depending on the depth of the vessel. For longer depths, decreasing the sensitivity allows for more penetration; for shallower depths, increasing the frequency increases the color sensitivity (*see* Fig. 1).

41. If color Doppler is unsuccessful in demonstrating the hepatic arteries, how can spectral Doppler be used?

Spectral Doppler can be used by searching adjacent to the portal vein until arterial flow is detected. Often the hepatic artery can be seen as a tiny hypoechoic structure running adjacent to the portal vein. It is helpful to scan in planes both transverse to and longitudinal to the vessel axis.

HEPATIC VEINS

42. How can hepatic veins be located in a cirrhotic liver?

Hepatic veins can be found by scanning with color Doppler (optimized for slow flow) or power Doppler. If the veins are not visible with color Doppler, use spectral Doppler to search where they are normally located.

43. What positioning techniques can be used to search for hepatic veins?

It often helps to turn the patient, left side down or left posterior oblique, and scan from a lateral intercostal approach or from the front from a subcostal approach. It may also be helpful to sit the patient up and scan from the bare area of the liver.

44. How does the hepatic vein spectral Doppler tracing appear in a cirrhotic liver?

The spectral tracing tends to be more monophasic (Fig. 17).

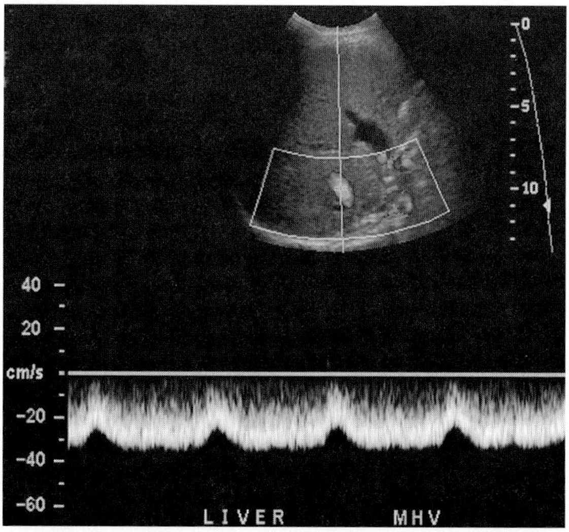

FIGURE 17. Abnormal hepatic vein. Spectral Doppler from a patient with cirrhosis. The signal is damped compared to that of a normal hepatic vein (*see* Figure 3B).

45. How does the Doppler signal differ in patients with hepatomegaly and nodular regeneration?

The hepatic veins may be compressed and have a more monophasic waveform.

46. What is Budd-Chiari syndrome?

Budd-Chiari syndrome refers to both clinical and histologic responses to acute obstruction of hepatic vein flow. Several causes of obstruction determine the level of obstruction in the hepatic venous system (sinusoids, hepatic veins, or IVC) (Fig. 18).

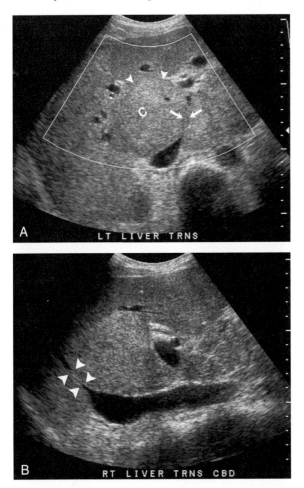

FIGURE 18. Budd Chiari syndrome. *A,* Transverse image at the level of the inferior vena cava (IVC) shows a narrowed hepatic vein with color Doppler (*arrows*) and enlarged caudate lobe (*C*) (*arrowheads*) (see also Color Plates, Figure 27). *B,* Longitudinal ultrasound through the right lobe shows marked narrowing of the IVC (*arrowheads*).

47. What are the sonographic signs of Budd-Chiari syndrome?

The hepatic vein waveform may be absent, reversed, turbulent, or monophasic. Sonographic signs show the following:

- Hepatic vein wall thickening
- Abnormal hepatic vein course
- Intrahepatic collaterals
- Dilatation of the IVC or hepatic veins with intraluminal echoes
- Enlarged caudate lobe
- Slow or reversed flow in the portal vein

- Ascites
- Splenomegaly
- Portosystemic collaterals

48. Is ultrasound specific for Budd-Chiari syndrome?

No. Nonvisualization of flow in the hepatic veins can often be related to a technical factor in larger patients or in patients with diseased livers. Budd-Chiari can be excluded only when the patency of the major hepatic vein branches can be confirmed without question.

BIBLIOGRAPHY

1. Brown BP, Abu-Yousef M, Farner R, et al: Doppler sonography: A noninvasive method for evaluation of hepatic venocclusive disease. Am J Roentgenol 154:721–724, 1990.
2. Dodd GD, Memel DS, Baron RL, et al: Portal vein thrombosis in patients with cirrhosis: Does sonographic detection of intrathrombus flow allow differentiation of benign and malignant thrombus? Am J Roentgenol 165:573–577, 1995.
3. Dodd GD, Memel DS, Zajko AB, et al: Hepatic artery stenosis and thrombosis in transplant recipients: Doppler diagnosis with resistive index and systolic acceleration time. Radiology 192:657–661, 1994.
4. Dodd GD, Zajko AB, Orons PD, et al: Detection of transjugular intrahepatic portosystemic shunt dysfunction: Value of duplex doppler sonography. Am J Roentgenol 164:1119–1124, 1995.
5. Duerinckx A, Grant E, Perrella R, et al: The pulsatile portal vein: Correlation of duplex Doppler with right atrial pressures. Radiology 176:655–658, 1990.
6. Feldstein VA, LaBerge JM. Hepatic vein flow reversal at duplex sonography: A sign of transjugular intrahepatic portosystemic shunt dysfunction. Am J Roentgenol 162:839–841, 1994.
7. Foshager MC, Ferral H, Nazarian GK, et al: Duplex sonography after transjugular intrahepatic portosystemic shunts (TIPS): Normal hemodynamic findings and efficacy in predicting shunt patency and stenosis. Am J Roentgenol 165:1–7, 1995.
8. Furst G, Malms J, Heyer T, et al: Transjugular intrahepatic portosystematic shunts: Improved evaluation with echo-enhanced color Doppler sonography, power Doppler sonography, and spectral duplex sonography. Am J Roentgenol. 170(4):1047–1054, 1998.
9. Joynt LK, Platt JF, Rubin JM, et al: Hepatic artery resistance before and after standard meal in subjects with diseased and healthy livers. Radiology 196:489–492, 1995.
10. Kanterman RY, Darcy MD, Middleton WD, et al: Doppler sonography findings associated with transjugular intrahepatic portosystemic shunt malfunction. Am J Roentgenol 168:467–472, 1997.
11. Murphy TP, Beecham RP, Kim HM, et al: Long-term follow-up after TIPS: Use of Doppler velocity criteria for detecting elevation of the portosystematic gradient. J Vasc Intervent Radiology 9(2):275–281, 1998.
12. Ralls PW: Color Doppler sonography of the hepatic artery and portal venous sytem. Am J Roentgenol 155:517–525, 1990.
13. Ralls PW, Johnson MB, Radin DR, et al: Budd-Chiari syndrome: Detection with color Doppler sonography. Am J Roentgenol 159:113–116, 1992.
14. Tessler FN, Gehring BJ, Gomes AS, et al: Diagnosis of portal vein thrombosis: Value of color Doppler imaging. Am J Roentgenol 157:293–296, 1991.
15. Uggowitzer MM, Kugler C, Machan L, et al: Value of echo-enhanced Doppler sonography in evaluation of transjugular intrahepatic portosystematic shunts. Am J Roentgenol 70(4):1041–1046, 1998.
16. Wachsberg RH, Obolevich AT: Blood flow characteristics of vessels in the ligamentum teres fissure at color Doppler sonography: Findings in healthy volunteers and in patients with portal hypertension. Am J Roentgenol 164:1403, 1995.
17. Zizka J, Elias P, Krajina A, et al: Value of Doppler sonography in revealing transjugular intrahepatic portosystematic shunt malfunction: A 5-year experience in 216 patients. Am J Roentgenol 75(1):141–148, 2000.
18. Zwiebel WJ: Vascular disorders of the liver. In Zwiebel WJ (ed): Introduction to Vascular Ultrasonography, 4th ed. Philadelphia, W.B. Saunders, 2000, pp 431–451.

47. ERECTILE DYSFUNCTION AND PRIAPISM

Vikram Dogra, M.D., and Shweta Bhatt, DMRD, DMRE

1. What is erectile dysfunction (ED)?

ED is defined as the consistent or recurrent inability to attain or maintain penile erection sufficient for sexual performance.

2. What are the indications of penile Doppler evaluation?

Doppler evaluation is indicated when arterial or venous insufficiency is suspected as a cause of ED. The other indications include priapism, Peyronie's disease, and penile trauma.

3. Describe the sonographic anatomy of the penis.

The penis is composed of two dorsal corpora cavernosa (CC) and one ventral corpus spongiosum (CS), which surround the urethra. The two CC are enclosed in a fibrous sheath called tunica albuginea. Buck's fascia envelops the two CC and CS, forming the penis. A cavernosal artery travels through each CC. The venous drainage is via the deep dorsal vein and cutaneous dorsal vein. The cavernosal arteries are interrogated in the evaluation of ED (Fig. 1).

4. Describe the vascular supply to the penis.

The penile blood vessels arise from the internal pudendal artery. The penile artery divides into the dorsal penile artery and the cavernosal artery (CA). The CA enters the corpus cavernosum on the superomedial surface of the penis. The branches of this artery are called the *helicine arteries,* which subsequently divide in smaller vessels that communicate with the lacunae of the corpus cavernosum. The venous blood flow is drained into the venous plexus beneath the tunica albuginea. The emissary veins perforate the tunica albuginea and the blood is drained by the venae circumflexae into the deep dorsal vein.

5. What transducer is used to perform the Doppler evaluation for ED?

Using a 7-MHz linear transducer, evaluation of the cavernosal arteries is performed before and after intracavernosal injection of a vasoactive drug such as prostaglandin E.

6. Name the stages of penile erection.

- Flaccid state
- Filling phase
- Tumescent phase
- Rigid phase

7. Describe the normal spectral Doppler findings in various stages of penile erection.

In the **flaccid state,** the spectral Doppler waveform is of high resistance with no antegrade flow during diastole. The velocities are 5–15 cm/sec.

In the **filling phase,** there is marked increase in both the systolic and diastolic flow components, with evidence of very low resistance to flow.

During the **tumescent phase,** the systolic velocities increase, and diastolic flow ceases and becomes reversed. During the late phase of tumescence, the systolic velocity decreases and the **rigid phase** is obtained (Fig. 2).

8. How is a penile Doppler examination performed?

Grayscale examination of the penis is performed to exclude Peyronie's disease. On the ventral side, the CC and CA within the CC are identified. The diameter of the CA is measured on both sides and the spectral Doppler waveform is recorded. The vasoactive substance (prostaglandin E

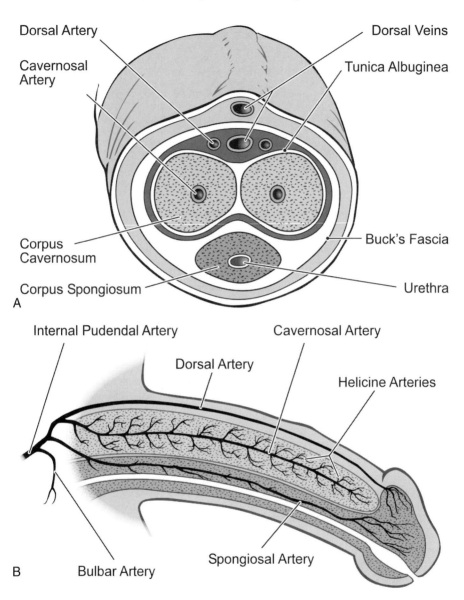

FIGURE 1. Diagrammatic representation of penile anatomy in cross-section (*A*) and longitudinal (*B*) views. (From Fitzgerald SW, Erickson SJ, Foley WD, et al: Color Doppler sonography in the evaluation of erectile dysfunction. Radiographics 12:3–17, 1992, with permission.)

or papaverine) is then injected in one CC and the spectral waveform in each CA is recorded. Penile response in terms of full erection, partial erection, and no erection after the injection of vasoactive substance is also observed. Spectral waveform in dorsal penile vein is recorded.

9. Describe the method of injecting vasoactive substance in the CC.

Prostaglandin E_1, also called *caverject,* an important vasodilating agent, is injected in the distal two thirds of the shaft in one CC using a small needle of 27–30 gauge. The total quantity of prostaglandin injected is 10–20 µg.

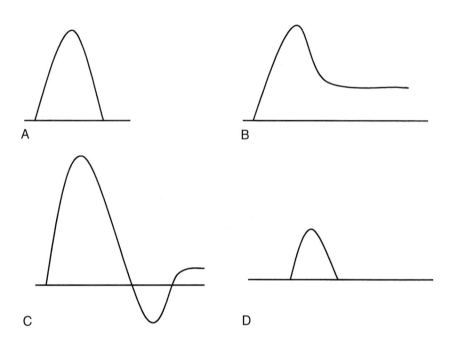

FIGURE 2. *A,* Flaccid state. Spectral waveform demonstrates high-resistance waveform. *B,* Filling phase. Spectral waveform demonstrates increased systolic velocity and increased diastolic flow. *C,* Tumescent phase. Spectral waveform demonstrates decrease in the diastolic flow as seen by the reversal of diastolic notch. *D,* Rigid phase. Spectral waveform demonstrates high-resistance waveform with no diastolic flow and minimal systolic flow.

10. Are there any side effects of injecting intracavernosal prostaglandin E or papaverine?

Yes. Priapism is a known side effect of these drugs after intracavernosal injection. This can be relieved by intracavernosal injection of phenylephrine.

11. What is the best place for recording the CA peak systolic velocity?

The peak systolic velocity of the CA should be recorded near the proximal one third of the shaft because the velocities are greatest at this level. If velocities are recorded in the distal shaft, the velocities are lower.

12. How long after prostaglandin injection should the spectral Doppler of the CA be scanned and recorded?

Spectral Doppler waveforms should be recorded in both CAs starting 5 minutes after injection and should continue every 5 minutes until 25 minutes elapse.

13. What is the normal peak systolic velocity recorded after injection of vasoactive substance?

Velocities greater than 25 cm/sec probably are adequate when papaverine is injected; however, velocities in the 35–40 cm/sec range probably are normal when substances containing prostaglandin are injected.

14. What are the standard diagnostic criteria for arterial insufficiency?

A peak systolic velocity < 25 cm/sec in the CA and waveform dampening are the standard diagnostic criteria.

Secondary diagnostic criteria include failure of CA dilatation and asymmetry of cavernosal flow velocities $> 10\%$.

15. When should venous leak be suspected?

A venous leak is suspected when there is adequate arterial inflow and an erection is obtained, but the duration is short and there is persistent antegrade diastolic flow throughout the examination.

16. What is an indeterminate result?

A venous leak is the suspected but uncertain diagnosis when arterial inflow is normal but the erectile response is poor and there is antegrade diastolic flow throughout the examination; this is called an indeterminate result.

17. What constitutes persistent antegrade diastolic flow?

An arterial diastolic velocity > 5 cm/sec throughout all phases of erection constitutes persistent arterial diastolic flow and suggests of venous leak. This is angle-corrected velocity.

18. If a diagnosis of venous leak is made by ultrasound, are there any other options for further evaluation?

A venous leak can be evaluated by cavernosonography and cavernosometry.

19. Describe the significance of flow in the dorsal vein of the penis.

Persistence of flow in the dorsal vein reflects veno-occlusive insufficiency. This has an 80% sensitivity and 100% specificity for venous leakage at cavernosography.

20. Describe nocturnal penile tumescence test (NPT).

A normal healthy man develops NPT during rapid eye movement stage of sleep. Various tests have been designed to evaluate NPT to diagnose ED, but all the tests have limitations and there is no universal agreement on which test to perform for NPT; hence, these tests are not favored.

21. Describe the penile brachial pressure index (PBI).

The PBI represents the penile systolic blood pressure divided by the brachial arterial systolic blood pressure. A PBI of 0.7 or less has been used to indicate arteriogenic impotence.

22. Is there a role of resistive index (RI) in the diagnosis of ED?

An RI measured at 20 minutes after the injection of vasoactive substance is a reliable noninvasive method to diagnose cavernosal venous leakage. An $RI < 0.75$ is associated with venous leakage in 95% of patients. An $RI > 0.9$ is associated with normal results in 90% of patients.

23. What is Peyronie's disease?

This disease commonly presents with a fibrous plaque lining the upper or lower regions of the penis. This fibrous plaque usually involves the tunica albuginea. During erection, the area affected by the plaque restricts the affected side of the penis, causing curvature toward that side. This bending or indentation caused by the plaque creates a painful sensation or even a loss of erection, which is why Peyronie's disease is classified as a form of ED.

24. Describe the sonographic findings of Peyronie's disease.

Sonographic findings typical of Peyronie's disease include plaque appearing hyperechoic near the peripheral margin of the cavernosa, usually along the dorsal aspect. There may be foci of calcification.

25. What is priapism?

Priapism is characterized by persistent tumescence of the penis that is not associated with sexual desire or stimulation.

26. What are types of priapism?

There are two types: low-flow and high-flow types. Low flow is most common.

27. Describe low-flow priapism.

Low-flow priapism is secondary to inadequate venous outflow. This is a urologic emergency, because prolonged hypoxia and ischemia secondary to poor venous outflow leads to corporeal fibrosis and ED.

28. How does low-flow priapism present?

In patients with low-flow priapism, the penis is erect and painful.

29. What is high-flow priapism?

This is characterized by a fistula formation between the cavernosal artery and lacunae in the CC called *arterial-lacunar fistula*. This is usually secondary to penile or perineal trauma.

30. Describe the clinical presentation patients with high-flow priapism.

Patients present with painless partial erection and are able to increase the rigidity of the penis with sexual stimulation. This is not a urologic emergency.

31. Name a test other than ultrasound examination for high-flow priapism.

Corporeal aspiration of oxygenated blood is confirmatory for high-flow priapism.

BIBLIOGRAPHY

1. Benson CB, Aruny JE, Vickers MA Jr: Correlation of duplex sonography with arteriography in patients with erectile dysfunction. Am J Roentgenol 160:71–73, 1993.
2. Chung WS, Shim BS, Park YY: Hemodynamic insult by vascular risk factors and pharmacologic erection in men with erectile dysfunction: Doppler sonography study. World J Urol 18:427–430, 2000.
3. Erdogru T, Kaplancan T, Aker O, Aras N: Cavernosal arterial anatomic variations and its effect on penile hemodynamic status. Eur J Ultrasound 14:141–148, 2001.
4. Fitzgerald SW, Erickson SJ, Foley WD, et al: Color Doppler sonography in the evaluation of erectile dysfunction. Radiographics 12:3–17, 1992.

INDEX

Page numbers in **boldface type** indicate complete chapters.